HYDROSOLS
The Next Aromatherapy

HYDROSOLS
The Next Aromatherapy

SUZANNE CATTY

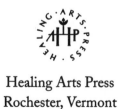

Healing Arts Press
Rochester, Vermont

Healing Arts Press
One Park Street
Rochester, Vermont 05767
www.InnerTraditions.com

Healing Arts Press is a division of Inner Traditions International

Note to the reader: This book is intended as an informational guide. The remedies, approaches, and techniques described herein are meant to supplement, and not to be a substitute for, professional medical care or treatment. They should not be used to treat a serious ailment without prior consultation with a qualified health care professional.

Library of Congress Cataloging-in-Publication Data

Catty, Suzanne.
    Hydrosols : the next aromatherapy / Suzanne Catty.
        p. ; cm.
    Includes bibliographical references and index.
    ISBN 0-89281-946-4 (alk. paper)
    1. Aromatherapy. 2. Colloids. I. Title.
    [DNLM: 1. Plant Extracts. 2. Aromatherapy. 3. Oils, Volatile—isolation & purification.
    QV 766 C355h 2001]
    RM666.A68 C38 2001
    615'.321—dc21

                                        00-054180

Printed and bound in Canada

10 9 8 7 6 5 4 3 2 1

Text design and layout by Priscilla Baker
This book was typeset in Caslon and Agenda, with Bernhard Tango as a display face

To Gaia: with love and hopes for the future

To Pierre Mainguy: pure heart, pure light, adieu

Contents

Foreword

Hydrosols, the subject of this book, do something rather unique. They bring the aromatic compounds of aromatherapy to the healing process in a precisely defined concentration, namely in the maximum amount possible to be dissolved homogenously in water. Upon superficial examination, essential oils and their components seem to be insoluble in water. But that is not 100 percent true. On more precise examination, it becomes obvious that a small fraction of the aromatic compounds recovered from a plant in the distillation process actually end up in the distillation water. Every aromatic substance has a maximum solubility in water, and only after this point is reached will these aromatic compounds, the essential oils, start to separate into a distinct layer on top of the distillation water.

Much has been written about the use of essential oils in aromatherapy. A recurring concern in all of aromatherapy is the potential of essential oils to irritate the various tissues with which they come in contact, and the discussion about the proper dilution of essential oils to avoid such irritation is still raging. The appropriate application of aromatic substances in their dissolved state most elegantly avoids these problems. Because hydrosols are dissolved there is no oily or lipophilic phase to irritate tissue. On the contrary, it is not too much of a simplification to state that hydrosols not only do not irritate, but for the most part they are anti-inflammatory: they relieve irritation. It has been known in aromatherapy for quite some time that hydrosols, for this reason, often are better suited for treatments of sensitive patients. This theoretical knowledge, however, was only occasionally translated into fruitful reality, because detailed experiences in the use of hydrosols had never been published, nor had the all-important questions about shelf life and viability ever been addressed in any concise form. All of this is now changing. *Hydrosols: The Next Aromatherapy* puts aromatherapy in its safest form at the disposal of every interested enthusiast. The sheer wealth of carefully assembled empirical data will answer many hitherto unanswered questions about how to use hydrosols for many different conditions. While this contribution of *Hydrosols* is of obvious benefit to the reader, there is an equally important—and for those in the field maybe even more exhilarating—aspect to *Hydrosols*: it alters the evolution of aromatherapy itself.

Consider the following. At the beginning of this new century, the fate of aromatherapy hangs in the balance. The initial supply of enthusiasm that spawned the French "medical" approach as well as the popular British "massage" approach has become depleted. Yes, the indisputably fantastic fundamentals of aromatherapy—namely putting low-cost healing of many diseases at the fingertips of everyone, not just experts—are still in place. But the idealistic small business operators who made it their mission to bring this spectacular modality to a broader public are gradually running out of cash to finance their good will. Lavender and tea tree oils work as well as ever for rashes and toe fungus, but their potential to generate sizable capital gains has been vastly overestimated. To make things worse, the adoption of aromatherapy concepts by larger commercial interests has led to the seemingly unpreventable loss of quality and substance. The initial wave of aromatherapy entrepreneurialism has become a victim of its narrow and exclusive focus on sales.

Focused on building the business, aromatherapy activists accepted whatever popular books appeared on the market as authoritative representations of "aromatherapy" not realizing that these books were mostly written by other entrepreneurs concerned with maximizing business. An apparently endless stream of encyclopedias on how to use this and that oil paraded as a representation of the discipline of aromatherapy but really served as glorified sales literature. This did indeed serve to bring essential oils to more interested individuals, but it did predictably little to advance aromatherapy as an independent faculty of learning. Recipes in most books were often based on the decree of the author. Rationales for given uses or reasons in terms

of cause and effect are often glaringly absent: the pressures of marketing mandated-simplicity without a theory. Initially, this did not appear to be much of a drawback because short of turning murky randomness into pop intuition, essential oils will work without precision in percent and accuracy in language. But a maturing field deserves more.

Aromatherapy will undergo the developments that many of its supporters so feverishly hope for only if it grows up to be a "real" discipline, a true faculty of learning. This is where *Hydrosols* breaks most important and exciting new ground. To appreciate its contribution I would like to invoke a statement from eminent biologist E. O. Wilson's latest work, *Consilience*. In the context of this work, Wilson opines that for a faculty of learning to be successful and to be able to arrive at meaningful predictions it should have its units and processes clearly defined and solidly in place. Checking aroma-therapy for units and processes, we find a bleak picture. Even in the relatively simple case of agreeing on a unit of volume the only common denominator aromatherapy has to offer is the marketing-mandated "drop." Rather obviously, a drop is not a very precise unit of volume. As far as processes go, a rather unexciting and mostly trivial process, the mixing together of various essential oils, was awarded near cult status by renaming it "blending." From Goddess blends to weight-loss blends, clear definition was again sacrificed in favor of marketing-mandated simplicity.

Hydrosols takes aromatherapy to a new degree of self-understanding. It moves aromatherapy literature away from the limitations of sales literature by introducing units and processes adequate to the phenomena they describe. *Hydrosols* transcends these limits by speaking to the competency of the reader. It makes aromatherapy more real by naming the names of the contributors to the field and by describing the processes by which the concepts they contributed came about. The air of an anonymous superauthority that simply has to be believed is banished. Instead, *Hydrosols* describes in an unpretentious and matter-of-fact way what real people did and how their experiments shaped their conclusions. In many cases this is not complex science but simply accurate observation, which makes it even more real and usable.

If we understand aromatherapy as a low-risk healing modality with the potential to empower the lay person, these descriptions of the processes in which empirical observation are made are essential stages in the maturing of aromatherapy. These narratives are necessary for aromatherapy to come into its own and will ultimately contribute to a much needed theoretical framework. Not, as one would expect, one oil or one specific compound is universally effective for any given disease or condition. Realizing that many chemically diverse essential oil components are effective provides the necessary stimulus for considerations that go past a simple pharmacological approach. If nothing else it proves that essential oils can work by physiological mechanisms vastly different from those understood by conventional knowledge.

Hydrosols: The Next Aromatherapy is unique in that for the first time in a popular work the author establishes processes special to aromatherapy with a rigor that would be adequate—even exemplary—for many older and more established faculties of learning.

Kurt Schnaubelt
Author of Advanced Aromatherapy *and*
Medical Aromatherapy

Preface

Far below the plane, the blackness of the north Atlantic stretches below me in all directions and I can't help feeling that there is no small serendipity in the ways that water has dominated my life this year. The wet slushy winter of 1999 to 2000 was spent in front of the computer writing this book—living, breathing, and consuming hydrosols day after day. Torrential rains and thunderstorms started in early spring in Toronto and continued throughout our normally hot and dry summer, repeatedly flooding my stockrooms and wreaking havoc in the garden. Then the autumn arrived and the rains, perversely, stopped at home, but conferences took me to both Seattle (the rainy city) and England (the rainy country), which experienced some of its worst flooding on record throughout my stay. And so it goes.

Of course, my relationship with water has gone on for a very long time, and hydrosols, the aromatic waters that are the subject of this book, have dominated my life for several years, but the downpours of this year are something else again. From a metaphysical point of view, water is the element related to emotions. Water images, themes, and dreams always stem from emotional issues bubbling to the surface, whether unresolved, unexpressed, or needing attention in

some way. We also get emotional support from water, whether it's luxuriating in a hot bath or walking on a seashore. The feeling of floating, the colors, smells, movements, and sounds of water create a positive resonance that can soothe the soul. It is also about movement: stepping into the current, going with the flow, and charting a new course are all positive steps we can take for our development. With the movement comes sustenance and growth. Without water most living things will quickly die—plants, animals, and people alike. Water is our succor, our nourishment, and a large part of our physical makeup. In 2000 the world's water problems came to the forefront of our consciousness. Perhaps this is not just my year of water but every one's.

There has also been a lot of movement and flow in the world of aromatherapy during the past twelve months. Two years ago, when I went out into the aromatherapy world with my hydrosol information, interest in these substances was almost nonexistent. Today, many different people are talking about hydrosols and their amazing uses. With this increased public interest, product demand has grown, and more and more distillers are preserving hydrolates as a coproduct of essential oil manufacture. The perception of aromatherapy has also changed, and today people understand that this is not just bubble-bath, but a viable therapy option for treating a huge range of health concerns. At international aromatherapy conferences, clinical scientists stand beside professional aromatherapists and shamanic healers discussing everything from receptor-site research to the mind-body-spirit connection, from essential oils and hormone modulation to preserving the integrity of the immune system. Guidelines for eliminating the guesswork in preserving hydrosols are my contribution to this information explosion. We've come a long way from pretty smells.

Someone recently asked me if I still use essential oils or whether my practice only includes hydrosols. The answer is that I use both—and

more. Aromatherapy is a form of phytotherapy, and there is compelling evidence that we experience synergistic effects when we combine oils and waters along with herbs, tinctures, homeopathic remedies, vibrational healing methods, and good nutrition. Just like the endless depths of the ocean below, these modalities offer vast opportunities for healing and growth. We will not be able to control every aspect of the adventure to come, but it will be exhilarating, mind expanding, and life enhancing at the very least. I hope this book inspires you to join in shaping what is yet to be. My year of water is almost over, but the journey has just begun.

Acknowledgments

~

There are many who contributed to this book: from the earth to the plants, the spring waters, the distillers, the teachers, the practitioners, the researchers, and, of course, the users of all things aromatic. However, a few deserve my very special thanks. First, my staff: Jan Scanlon-Coles, who believed from first meeting; I'm still honored. Jessica Cullingham— thrown in at the deep end, she swam; go girl. And Kelly Teigrob, who wasn't satisfied with half the story so sought out the other half. They are the best, and I hope I tell them often enough. Yea team!

Ariane France Smith, whose generosity and friendship are beyond words and who has provided continuous inspiration by her fine example; merci, Madame. Lucie and Pierre Mainguy and their very extended family, who adopted another witch into their truly magic circle; I love you all. Kerry Doyle, a truly dedicated aromatherapist who helped show me a road neither of us knew was there. Chris Chanter for her clinical work and humor; love you, babe. Kurt Schnaubelt, for his peer review and inspiration. Delwyn Higgens, artist and aromatherapist, who plowed through the first draft and gave honest opinions and a great edit. Shauna Rae and Adrienne Leong, two more goddess gals whose art helped shape my own vision and who can't get enough of the waters. Simone Zrihen and Miriam Erlichman, great practitioners who understood from the start; thanks for the recipes, ladies. C. J. Puotinen, for her early support and outstanding work with animals. Pam Parsons, for the surprise of my millennium. Erwin Pearlman, who helped me with myself, and thus with everything. Rosemary, Kate, Maryanne, Kathleen, M.A., Gilberte, Annette, David, Frank, Kirsten, Anna, John, Doug, Wendy, and Phoebe—my first willing guinea pigs, who took what I thought and showed me the real truth underneath. And everyone at Healing Arts Press for making my reality concrete. Thank you, one and all.

ONE

In the Beginning Was Smell

Our sense of smell, like so many of our other body functions,
is a throwback to the time, early in evolution, when we thrived in the oceans.
Diane Ackerman, *A Natural History of the Senses*

This is an aromatherapy book. And because aromatherapy is a holistic health-care practice, concerning itself with the whole being, I consider it an inclusive practice. Everyone has the ability to use or benefit from aromatherapy. This book is also inclusive; it is written for anyone with an interest in, or curiosity about, the aromatic world and what it has to offer: for the serious practitioner seeking more knowledge and a broader scope of practice, for the nonprofessional adept wanting to dive headlong into the aromatic waters that are my theme, and for those simply interested in taking care of their health and needing clarification concerning what "aromatherapy" is all about.

Aromatherapy is perhaps the hottest word in marketing as we enter the twenty-first century. Every kind of scented product, from air freshener to hand soap to perfumes, is being sold with the tag "aromatherapy," "aromatology," or even "aromachology." At the same time, the environmental sensitivities experienced by many people who come into contact with synthetic fragrance is causing the creation of scent-free zones and, in some cases, laws restricting the use of scents by individuals in their workplace, on public transportation, and in restaurants, stores, and schools. It is time to define what we are talking about when we say "aromatherapy" and, hopefully, clear up a few misconceptions about things that smell.

WHAT IS AROMATHERAPY?

Aromatherapy is a branch of phytotherapy, or plant therapy, just as herbalism, homeopathy, flower remedies, traditional Chinese medicine, and many other treatments are also phytotherapy. Aromatherapy is holistic, concerning itself with the whole of the person and attempting to create balance for the whole of the body.

Aromatherapy practice has been documented in some form or another for more than four thousand years but went through a major reassessment and earned its modern name during the First World War. This renaissance has taken aromatherapy into many worlds: the chemical explorations of hard science, the hallowed halls of modern medicine, and the metaphysical realms of spirituality. Now, as we enter the twenty-first century, I believe it is changing again. The aromatherapy of the future will no longer segregate the different avenues of aromatic practice but will allow them to coalesce into one broad modality. Even now aromatherapy exhibits its own synergy, a blend of thoughts and methods in which the total is greater than the sum of the parts, magic cohabits with chemistry, botany lives with bodywork, and layperson practitioners have as much chance of healing themselves as professionals. It lives and breathes and grows just as the plants from which it comes.

Aromatherapy, in the truest sense of the word, is the use of 100 percent natural, whole, unadulterated, aromatic essences obtained from specific botanical sources by steam distillation or expression for the benefits of mind, body, and spiritual health. These essences may be pure essential oils, the non–water-soluble, volatile, aromatic compounds found in flowers, leaves, branches, seeds, roots, barks, resins, and fruits and obtained by gentle steam distillation. They may also be the expressed oils found in the rinds of citrus fruits like lemon, orange, bergamot, and grapefruit, which are gathered by squeezing the oil from the peel. Aromatherapy also involves the use of the nonvolatile fatty oils (carrier oils) found in avocados, sesame seeds, and exotics such as rose hips and hazelnuts. Last but not least, aromatherapy uses hydrosols, the aromatic waters coproduced during the steam distillation of essential oils. What is most important is that the substances used in the creation and maintenance of health be totally pure and from very specific plants. In this book I will spend a great deal of time giving you all the different parameters that must be met for true aromatherapy products. Here you will find information enabling you to ask intelligent questions about the quality of any hydrosols, oils, or other preparations you may encounter.

What aromatherapy is not is the use of synthetic substances such as perfumes and fragrance oils, nor is it simply the use of "anything that smells." Aromatherapy products are not made in a plant (factory) but in a plant (living, growing, green thing). They are not merely perfumes. The bulk of items marketed as aromatherapy on the shelves of pharmacies, department stores, cosmetics suppliers, spas, and even health-food stores are *not* true aromatherapy. They may be "smelly," but they are not exclusively natural. Many have never seen a plant (living, growing, green thing), and some may contain ingredients linked to, or suspected of causing, serious health problems and allergic reactions, yet the labels call them aromatherapy all the same. Given all that's out there, what's a person to do?

The bottom line is that we are in uncharted territory. We are working in a world where no clear differentiation exists between things that are natural and aromatic and things that are synthetic and aromatic, a zone where there is no perceived difference between smells that heal and smells that harm and where no laws exist. At present there are few controls on the creative license used by those who write the labels and market the products, unless they are medicines. A bottle may say that it contains "100 percent pure essential oil" but contain only a small percentage; it doesn't say it contains *"only* 100 percent essential oil." There are no requirements that other ingredients, such as carrier oils, perfume-industry chemicals, or even common alcohol, be listed on the label. You may buy this bottle thinking that what you are getting is the real thing, but that real thing contributes only a fraction to the price you are paying.

THE EDUCATED CONSUMER

When a well-known natural-body-care company opened its first store in Toronto, I visited this beautiful boutique with a colleague. We explored the store, sniffing merrily away until we came to the essential oils. There were testers, so, of course, a drop instantly went on the hand, and . . . lo and behold, it contained carrier oil, a vegetable oil used to dilute the pure essential oil. When we asked the salesperson about this, we were told that these were the purest oils available, and no, they were not diluted in any way. Even when we

pointed out that although they were certainly good quality, they were actually "oily," or greasy to the touch, and not completely volatile, as true essential oils should be, the salesperson referred to the label copy, which said they were pure and did not mention any dilution. Obviously we were mistaken, for these were clearly undiluted. Unconvinced, we asked the salesperson to make a call, just to check. Four phone calls later she finally found someone who could tell her that, indeed, these oils were diluted, in fractionated coconut oil, to be precise, and that they were at 30 percent concentration. That was in 1996. Since then the labeling has been changed, and all this company's essential oils now state very clearly that they are diluted in coconut oil.

If a reputable "natural-health" company can do this, what is being done by companies that have no interest in the bigger picture but just want to make a profit using the most effective marketing tag? The truth is that no one is going to protect you and your health except you. The more information you have, the better able you will be to make good choices, thus controlling your exposure to synthetics, carcinogens, preservatives, and toxins of all kinds. This level of awareness is the minimum necessary if your intention is to preserve and maintain health.

The inclination of a growing proportion of the world's population is to return to more-natural, less-processed products, whether they be food, drinks, body-care items, or supplements. True aromatherapy is one of these natural-product families; synthetic fragrances are not. It is up to you, the consumer, to know what it is you are looking for, to do your own homework and not just rely on the information provided on labels and by store staff. Although some store employees are extremely knowledgeable, in other cases a little knowledge is a dangerous thing. Sometimes you will be given wrong information; other times you may be deliberately misled. In fact, there is probably more misinformation than good information out there, or maybe the good information is just harder to get.

CHEMICALS: FRIENDS OR FOES?

In this book you will find talk of chemicals and chemistry. After what I have just said, this may seem incongruous, but there is no contradiction here. Knowledge of the chemical composition of aromatherapy products is actually of vital importance, since this is a major factor in how they work on our health. It is also one of the keys to empowerment in consumer decision making.

Every plant contains a wide variety of chemical compounds. Some of these chemicals exist in the form of aromatic essential-oil molecules, some are alkaloids, others are water-soluble or complex polysaccharides, and there are many more besides. We know that therapeutic chemicals from plant material can be extracted by soaking the material in cold water (cold infusion), heating the material in water (decoction or tea), infusing the material in oil (maceration), extract-

ing components in alcohol (tinctures), or distillation (essential oils and hydrosols). It is important to remember that there are many ways to extract the therapeutic benefits from plant material because each method will release different qualities and chemicals of the plant and therefore have different properties and applications in health and healing.

The primary issue here is not only that these are naturally occurring chemicals manufactured by the plants as part of their desire to grow, flourish, and propagate themselves, but also that they appear in complex combinations, not as single or isolated compounds. Rose contains over 400 different chemicals, clary sage around 250, and lavender more than 100. Herein lies the rub! Mother Nature is incredibly intelligent, and plants have spent millions of years evolving and using their chemicals to communicate with each other and with the world at large. Some of their chemicals protect them from predators, others alert them to weather changes and soil conditions, still others send messages about potential pollinators and seed carriers. These chemicals exist in combinations because that's how they work best, together in synergy, like an orchestra. A solo violin is nice, but Beethoven sounds better with a full complement of instruments.

When we talk about chemical sensitivities or even, specifically, about fragrance sensitivities, we often forget to note whether these chemicals and fragrances are natural or synthetic, isolated or in combination. And that makes all the difference! The smell of chamomile is added to many shampoos that contain chamomile "extracts." The smell has to be added because the extracts are usually isolated chemicals chosen for a specific action, and they may have no odor or a nonchamomile odor. The smell component may or may not be natural; if it is natural, it may again be an isolated chemical chosen for scent only. What we have is not what nature created. While 100 percent natural chamomile may not cause an allergic reaction in people, some of its chemicals taken in isolation—out of context, if you will—*can* cause an allergic response. And synthetic versions of chamomile will almost certainly cause a reaction in sensitive people.

The prescription drug Valium illustrates this point most clearly. There is an herb called valerian that has been used for thousands of years for its relaxing, antianxiety, and sedative properties, and valerian products can be found in most health-food stores. Recognizing its therapeutic value, scientists studied valerian in order to isolate the one chemical they felt was responsible for its desirable effects. They then worked on this chemical in the lab and finally came up with a drug they called Valium. It was a huge success, and millions of people, mostly women, were prescribed Valium for many years. We now know that this drug, for all its benefits, has some pretty serious side effects and, for many, is highly addictive. Worldwide, there are thousands of people still suffering its ill effects. In Britain there were so many lawsuits that the government withdrew legal aid for Valium cases in the early 1990s. What went wrong? Is it possible that science, in its desire to find absolute answers, ignored the possibility that more than one chemical may contribute to an herb's beneficial effects? Is it that some of the natural chemical combinations in a plant can prevent side effects, one chemical acting as a buffer for another? The scientists were doing their best, but even science is imperfect and is growing, changing, and learning all the time.

It is the same with aromas. If you make a synthetic smell, or isolate just one aromatic chemical from a natural source, you may well end up with a smell that harms. The chemical creating the odor may have a negative effect on health, causing headache, allergies, skin reactions, nausea, and so on. It is not the odor per se that harms but the chemical creating the odor when it is taken out of context. People want scent-free zones because isolated and synthetic chemicals are making them sick. It is not nature, but what we have done to nature, that causes harm!

CHEMICAL-FREE, NOT SCENT-FREE

I adore smells; it is a consuming passion with me. Odors, aromas, and scents, at least the natural kind, affect every aspect of my life every day. However, I have difficulty going near perfume counters and can barely bring myself to approach most commercial body-care products and stores. When I do, there is an instantaneous tightness across my forehead, my temporal lobes start to throb, the muscles in my neck and shoulders tense up, and I want to run from the onslaught of the so-called fragrance that threatens my being. My body displays all the autonomic nervous system fight-or-flight responses that are triggered by danger. And . . . I don't have allergies and . . . it's getting worse!

Because the health risks are real and the ability to control the marketing of smells impossible, the pendulum of caution is swinging to the very far right. Scent-free zones seem to offer people the only way to avoid the life-threatening responses that chemical scents trigger in their bodies. It has gotten so bad, and people are becoming so afraid of smell, that they can't see the forest for the trees. If we used only unpolluted, totally natural, unadulterated smells, the chances of negative health reactions would be dramatically reduced, if not completely removed. I tried to explain this to a woman sitting beside me on an airplane when she panicked as I sprayed organic rose hydrosol on my face. She told me rose fragrance was one of the most irritating to her. I explained that, because of its high cost, real rose was rare and that it was likely that synthetic rose was the cause of her irritations. She was unwilling to listen. As far as she was concerned, all rose smells and, indeed, roses were horrible poisons. My heart ached at the thought that she would live the rest of her life not understanding the real cause of her problem, never allowing herself to "smell the roses."

Aromatherapy is a complex subject. It deals with smell, chemistry, plants, humans, and the beautiful web that links us all together. Hydrosols, the aromatic waters used in aromatherapy, are just one part of the whole and must be taken in context if they are to be understood. All life is about balance, and we still have much to learn from and about the natural balance of our world.

Until recently, hydrosols and their therapeutic actions have been largely overlooked. Although in the early development of distillation products like rosewater (a hydrosol) were the primary goal, somewhere along the line it became clear that the essential oils had a value far greater than that of the waters. So hydrosols slowly fell out of use and only the distillers and their friends and neighbors continued to benefit from their properties. In recent years, however, hydrosols have been rapidly gaining in popularity, and there has been a resurgence of interest in these plant waters, principally owing to the broad nature of their therapeutic applications. Like the villagers in Bulgaria who fill pools with rose hydrolate, we will want to surround ourselves with these healing substances.

INFLUENCES

In 1995 I received a pamphlet from the Aromatic Plant Project titled *101 Ways to Use Hydrosols*. Most of the brochure concerned itself with spraying the waters on your face and body or drinking them because they taste good, but my curiosity was piqued by a world I felt was waiting to be discovered. Up to that point I had experienced only a few of the so-called floral waters: lavender, rose, orange blossom, rosemary, cornflower, and Roman chamomile. But I had learned enough about distillation to know that, theoretically, every plant that produces an essential oil will, when distilled, produce a hydrosol, and I began to wonder where all this water went and why it wasn't available.

I also instinctively felt that just spraying hydrosols on your face was ignoring the real possibility that these waters were as therapeutic as the oils, or at least as healing as herbs, tisanes, and other plant-based remedies. I began a search for hydrosols from every source I could find. One organic Italian neroli was particularly surprising, with an intensity of flavor and scent much closer to that of the oil than anything I had encountered previously. In retrospect I realized that the "hydrosols" I had been buying up to that point probably contained preservatives and/or alcohol, were far from fresh, and could easily have been synthetic. After trying the *real* neroli water, I was gone . . . totally, utterly in love.

Then came the discovery of a company that offered no fewer than *twenty* different true aromatic waters. This was a revelation! An Aladdin's cave of hydrosols! I now had waters for oils that I barely knew: winter savory, *Satureja montana;* chemotype-specific hydrosols of rosemary and four different thymes; the expensive and elusive *Inula graveolens* and rock rose, *Cistus ladaniferus.* But what to do with them all? I had already begun my studies of French aromatherapy, in which essential oils are seen as plant medicines and are used internally, topically, and aerially, not just for massage, as I had learned in England and Canada. So it was to the French that I turned to learn more about the hydrosols in my fridge.

Nelly Grosjean

Nelly Grosjean was my first teacher on the possibilities of using aromatic waters therapeutically. Her book *Aromatherapy: Essential Oils for Your Health* discusses their use and methods of application as well as treatment protocols for specific health concerns. In her work Grosjean combines oils, hydrosols, diet, and lifestyle, as well as massage. Unfortunately the English edition of the book eliminated most of the discussion of internal use; as drinking hydrosols is one of the best ways to use them therapeutically, it is a great shame that the original text is not more widely available. Under Nelly's tutelage I undertook a period of experimentation during which I consumed most of my stock in three-week sequences, two tablespoons of hydrosol dissolved in one liter of distilled water daily for twenty-one days, with a week off in between. I drank liters of hydrosol, took copious notes, and experienced a gamut of effects.

A course with Nelly followed, during which her autodidactic approach became clearer. She works with a series of twelve essential-oil synergies, one for each month of the year, one for each of the body systems, one for each sign of the zodiac. She calls the blends frictions, and in most cases they are used both internally and topically for a three-week treatment period. Each friction works with one or several possible hydrosols that provide supporting therapy, and as part of the protocol these hydrosols are to be consumed daily diluted in water (thirty milliliters of hydrosol per 1.5 liters of water). Depending on the health concern being treated, Grosjean includes suggestions for raw-food diets and juicing. Anyone who has heard her speak or has read her books will know her list of Ten Golden Rules by heart.

The approach made sense to me, and what coalesced in my mind is that for all we talk of using whole, authentic, unadulterated, organic, complete essential oils, if we are not using the distillation water as well, there is a portion of the plant therapeutics that is missing. It has also become abundantly clear to me, as a lifelong adherent of homeopathic remedies, that the hydrosols are more akin to homeopathics, on a number of levels, than to the essential oils. Nelly credits a dream with providing the recipes for her frictions and the combinations in which they are used, and she speaks frequently about the vibrational aspects of aromatherapy. It is gratifying to hear someone discuss the energetic aspect of the waters as part of his or her rationale. There are those who have discounted her work because of this seemingly unscientific approach, but we are in a new millennium now, so perhaps we've learned better.

Franchomme and Penoel

From Grosjean I went to Pierre Franchomme and Daniel Penoel or, rather, to their book *L'Aromathérapie exactemente*. I had attended a workshop with Franchomme in 1996 and been overwhelmed by the intensely medical nature of the presentation. If this was what the French called aromatherapy, what on earth was I doing? Undaunted, I plowed through the heavily scientific tome, devouring every shred of information, particularly where it concerned hydrosols. This is where I got my first information on hydrosol pH readings, the significance of which I came to appreciate only much later (see chapter 3). But at this time my brother gave me a pH meter, and Franchomme and Penoel listed some data, so I started taking readings too. It just seemed like the thing to do. Now, years later, I know that even these two academic gentlemen recognize the vibrational aspects of aromatherapy and the link with the plant and human worlds. Dr. Penoel, in particular, has pursued this area of study, as evidenced in his later work.

After *L'Aromathérapie exactemente* I had no choice but to pursue my own experiments. My family, my friends, my dogs, and virtually every single client began to receive hydrosols as part of their aromatherapy treatments. My fridge was filled with bottles from top to bottom. Hydrosols went into every glass of water, on every pore of skin, in most body orifices, and in all my recipes, and they were combined and blended in the same way that I worked with oils. By early 1997 I had a fairly clear understanding of the properties of my original twenty, plus another handful, and was beginning to feel that I needed a new approach and some additional science to back up my experiments.

Kurt Schnaubelt

Enter Kurt Schnaubelt. Schnaubelt's approach to life, the universe, and aromatherapy appeals to me. His excellent conferences bring together presenters from many fields and modalities, creating a bigger picture for aromatherapy within the context of holistic health. During his intensive course he explained the science of aromatherapy in an accessible way, never getting stuck in rigid paradigms. Schnaubelt lets nature and the intention of the products play their part, promoting the view that flexibility is key when dealing with aromatics. As a chemist he knows better than most the importance of working from an informed position, and as a humanist he honors all of life and what it means to be alive. As he says in his 1999 book *Medical Aromatherapy,* "It is the most blatant admission of hubris, that scientific proof amounts to the act of creation."

With more science under my belt I finally understood why bay leaf hydrosol clears swollen lymph nodes in breast tissue and why green myrtle hydrosol can be put in the eyes. The connection between homeopathy and hydrosols also became clearer. Hydrosols can be seen as microdoses of oil, and if used in the manner prescribed by Grosjean and others, this microdose is further diluted in water. In homeopathy, the more you dilute, the stronger the remedy. When you drink a liter of water containing hydrosols over the course of a day, you are taking multiple microdoses of your "remedy." In homeopathy, multiple doses at frequent intervals are the most powerful and potent way to take remedies. And as Schnaubelt

points out, a microdose can achieve the same thing as a megadose in the appropriate situation.

There are many people and hundreds of events that have influenced my learning path and direction in the world of aromatherapy, but in the context of hydrosols, my encounters with Grosjean, Penoel, Franchomme, and Schnaubelt have most dramatically altered my thinking.

WHAT IS A HYDROSOL?

The word *hydrosol* is a chemistry term meaning "water solution." It is derived from the Latin *hydro,* meaning "water," and *sol,* for "solution." The chemistry term does not refer specifically to a distillate and can be applied to any aqueous solution.

In the world of aromatherapy, hydrosols are also known as hydrolates, hydrolats, floral waters, and plant waters. *Hydrolate* uses *hydro,* "water," and *late,* from the French *lait,* for "milk." When a hydrolate first comes off the still, and often for some time afterward, it will be slightly milky, owing to the quantity and nature of the various plant substances and essential oils dissolved in the water. All of these terms are basically interchangeable, and to avoid boredom they will all be used throughout the book. However, I should say that I am less fond of the term *flower* or *floral water* for a number of reasons. First, hydrosols do not come just from flowers any more than essential oils come only from flowers. Roots, bark, branches, wood, needles and leaves, even fruit and seeds can produce both oils and hydrosols. Thus hydrosols are not strictly "flower" or "floral" waters.

I would propose the following definition for aromatherapy purposes: "Hydrosols are the condensate water coproduced during the steam- or hydro-distillation of plant material for aromatherapeutic purposes." A longer definition would add, "Usually the distillation is undertaken to obtain the essential oils contained in the plant material, but occasionally the distillation is undertaken specifically to produce the plant water that results. Hydrosol production should use certified organic or pesticide- and chemical-free plant material harvested in a sustainable manner and composed of one distinct identifiable botanical species only. The distillation should be slow and under low or atmospheric pressure over sustained periods and use pure, uncontaminated water to preserve all the therapeutic components of the plant material, with an intention that the products produced be for therapeutic use without further processing."

Although hydrosols have been around for as long as distillation has and may even have been the intended product for which distillation was invented, their use in aromatherapy is still quite new. But bearing in mind that all essential-oil production has hydrosols as a coproduct, it is safe to assume that as interest continues to grow the variety and availability of these products will also grow. I have received samples of no fewer than twenty "new" hydrosols in the past six months alone.

I also think of hydrosols as holograms of the plant. The concept of the interconnectedness of the entire universe is not new, and it shows up everywhere, from quantum physics to Amazonian shamanic practice. Viewing this interconnectedness as one big hologram, where every tiny part actually contains all the information of the whole, seems perfectly reasonable. In holistic health we view the body as a whole, all parts affected by each other and all parts equally affected by the world in which we live. Now go one step further and consider that the world in which we live is, in turn, affected by the universe in which it exists, and the universe is affected by whatever may be next up the ladder. These are the basic concepts found throughout the religious and philosophical history of humankind, even throughout our evolutionary history, some might say. The term *holistic* is derived from the word *hologram*. And the hologram is so clear that acupuncture has, for nearly five thousand years, seen the whole of the body in the ear; reflexology sees it in the feet and hands; iridology in the eye; and researchers in Germany have developed a database that can scan the fingerprints of parents to look for any of nearly fifty distinctive patterns known to be linked to hereditary health problems.[1]

Hydrosols contain all of the plant in every drop, just like a hologram. Here we have the water-soluble components, the essential-oil molecules, the very fluid that was flowing through the plant cells when the plant was collected. It's all there in a matrix of water that is so much more than water, one of the most recognized holographic substances in healing.

Another way of looking at this is to think of

hydrosols as fractals. Several years ago I presented a paper at the Third Aromatherapy Conference on Therapeutic Uses of Essential Oils in San Francisco. Another speaker, Dorothy L. Severns, talked about fractals and chaos theory in relation to health and healing. As she spoke I was transfixed by the implications of her subject. "Nature is full of locally unpredictable, but wholistically stable, non-linear systems. These dynamic processes produce non-Euclidean geometric shapes which are called fractal."[2] Nature is inherently fractal: "Trees with their branching and sub-branching forms are classically fractal."[3] What may appear to be a chaotic form can be seen, when viewed as a fractal, to have an order that is so complex and advanced that it is not necessarily visible through normal observations. The human heartbeat is an irregular rhythm, but analyzed over a long period it will show the inherent patterns deep within this chaos. The energy field over the chakras, when measured, will also display this chaos pattern. Nonlocal similarities are also evident in the body, where each system is doing its own thing, say cell metabolism, which will be locally different from the liver to the skin to the lungs but holistically similar because together these organs make up the functioning of the whole body. In fact, there is significant new research indicating that disease is often heralded by a move toward regularity, or periodicity. Severns states, "Indeed this decomplexification of systems with disease may be a defining feature of pathology." Since synthetic compounds exhibit little or no fractal

nature, it can be assumed that the complexity of essential oils is what allows them to work when these substances fall short. "It appears that some molecules, or more exactly, some systems of molecules, are capable of fine-tuning human subtle and energetic health, as well as the health of the physical body. It seems reasonable to suppose that consciousness itself is a fractal process which may be enhanced by the use of fractal agents."[4] Fractals and chaos theory have only become understandable through the incredible analytic capabilities of computers and the genius of the human imagination. Hydrosols, I believe, are also inherently fractal.

I first saw the Mandelbrot set, perhaps the most famous fractal images, in the mid-1980s, when chaos theory was influencing people such as Brian Eno and other ambient musicians of the time. With the aid of a computer, I could move in, around, and out of the kaleidoscopic images, following patterns and threads that unfolded from within themselves. Hearing Severns speak, my mind flowed into the waters, seeing the same seemingly chaotic patterns, yet understanding that therein lay a much deeper order, far beyond my current understanding but integral to how the waters worked on the human body. The water has taken a new shape and form, carrying both the physical and vibrational image and dimensions of the plant and indeed of the entire universe through the plant. The fractal patterns of the body naturally responded to these subtleties, adding them to and absorbing them into its own healthy chaos. I was elated.

It is also worth talking about water here for a minute. I often joke that hydrosols are just water, as this is a refrain I have often heard since I began working with these substances five years ago. But they are not water, or perhaps more correctly, they are not *just* water. Hydrosols are amazing liquids with taste and smell and chemical makeup and therapeutic properties. They are not the same as herb teas or tinctures; they are not decoctions, macerations, or infusions; they are distillates, and they are as unique a product as any of the others I have mentioned. But they are also water, and that fact gives them a range of applications more diverse than those of many other phytotherapeutic substances. For more on water, turn to chapter 2.

WHAT ISN'T A HYDROSOL?

Now that we know what hydrosols are, let's look at what they are not. They are not distilled, spring, or tap water with essential oils added. Nor are they water and essential oils combined with a dispersant (alcohol or glycerin) to dissolve the oils in water. Water with fragrance oil or other synthetic compounds added to it is not hydrosol, nor are the cohobated distillation waters, with the exception of rose and melissa, which are virtually unavailable in any other form. (Cohobation means the hydrosols are recycled repeatedly through the plant material in the still to extract the maximum amount of water-soluble components.)

One product on the market called French Rose Water contains the following ingredients: aqueous extract of rose, imidazolidinyl urea, methyl paraben, carmine, and French rose essence concentrate. This is definitely not a hydrosol!

Many aromatherapy books describe ways to "make your own hydrosols" by mixing essential oils and water, but if you are not distilling plant material in a still, you are not making a hydrosol. No ifs, ands, or buts. A true hydrosol does contain both essential oil and water, but that is only a fraction of what is in it, and you cannot extract all the other ingredients, or the aroma, by combining water and oil. Besides, the water and oil don't mix. Distillation does not release any of the alkaloids that alcohol extraction draws out; therefore, tinctures mixed with water are also not a replication of hydrosols.

Every liter of hydrosol contains between 0.05 and 0.2 milliliter of dissolved essential oil, depending on the water solubility of the plant's components and the distillation parameters. However, the essential oils in solution in a hydrosol will, when analyzed, show a chemical profile different from that of the pure oil from the same run. Why? Because some of the chemicals in the essential oil are just too lipophilic (oil loving) to stay in the water and others are just too hydrophilic (water loving) to stay in the oil; therefore, are found only in the hydrosol. Furthermore, each product is unique. Hydrosols contain water-soluble substances from the plant material, such as those you would obtain in making a decoction or tea. These water-soluble components are not found in the essential oils and are made up primarily of water-soluble acids. Therefore, mixing plain water and essential oil gives you only half the story, at best.

The essential oils found in hydrosols are frequently *in solution,* meaning that they are not visible on the surface and do not separate out of the water. It is for this reason that a cohobated hydrosol is undesirable, since in cohobation the majority of the essential-oil microdrops will bind together and become big enough to separate from the hydrosol, improving oil yield but reducing the therapeutic ingredients in the water.

Finally, there is the key issue of pH. Hydrosols have a wide range of pH but are always on the acid end of the scale, ranging from a low of 2.9 to a high of around 6.5. Distilled water has a neutral 7.0 pH, and tap water can have an alkaline pH of up to 8.0, depending on where you live. Essential oils have a pH somewhere between 5.0 and 5.8; thus, in combination with water, they will have a midrange 5.0 to 7.0 pH, eliminating the particular benefits that very acid waters can provide.

FAKES AND ADULTERATION

Over the past few years, more and more people have begun selling hydrosols. This is wonderful news, since an ever increasing number of varieties are becoming available. However, I am constantly amazed by what I am offered in the way of fakes. Take jasmine, for instance. Jasmine is gorgeous, and I am not such a purist that I avoid solvent-extracted absolutes, as some French aromatherapists are known to do. However, there is no distillation involved in the production of jasmine absolute, which involves a purely chemical extraction process, and therefore there is no hydrosol. What is being sold as jasmine hydrosol is either a totally synthetic product or a mixture of water and jasmine absolute. Manufacturers in India do produce a unique product called attar of jasmine, which involves the hydro-distillation of jasmine flowers in a base of sandalwood oil. This production method, which has not changed for centuries, does produce a jasmine water, but it is not widely available and may never be. The samples I have received are very beautiful but retain much of the sandalwood personality. Perhaps one day we will have a real jasmine hydrosol; a recent sample has given me high hopes, but for now it is mainly a myth, and a chemical one at that.

Other common fakes are the citrus, for example, orange, lemon, tangerine, and grapefruit. These oils are cold-expressed from the zest or peel without distillation, and therefore no hydrosols exist for these fruits. I was shocked recently to read a paper by a well-known, highly qualified aromatherapist and M.D. that repeatedly mentioned citrus-rind hydrosols. Heaven knows what products the paper is referring to because they are certainly not true hydrosols. One intrepid distiller I know has managed to produce an orange-zest hydrosol from the dried peels of the Valencia orange, which is a most extraordinary accomplishment. So who knows what the future will bring, but for now you can be sure that most citrus waters are not hydrosols. Lime oil is occasionally steam-distilled, and I have encountered lime hydrosol once or twice, but as the provenance was unknown and commercially grown citrus fruit is heavily sprayed with chemicals, I opted not to use this hydrosol for therapeutic applications. What *is* available is hydrosol of citrus leaf, or petitgrain. The waters of mandarin orange, Clementine orange, and lemon leaves are particularly desirable and have profound appetite-stimulating properties that are very useful in treating eating disorders and appetite loss caused by pharmaceutical medication.

Then there is rose, sublime rose. Rose hydrosol does exist, of course, but many of the products on the market are synthetic and produced for use in the food and flavor industry. Also remember the subject of cohobation: there is a depth of flavor and scent to uncohobated rosewater that, once tried, is never mistaken, but it is hard to find and you must be willing to pay more for it. If rosewater is not cohobated during distillation the resulting essential oil is incomplete chemically, aromatically, and therapeutically, and the already infinitesimal yield further reduced. For these reasons uncohobated rose is very rare and most of us must buy the cohobated hydrosol—which in this case is not really a hardship! Some small distillers who do not have enough roses to produce essential oil are distilling their flowers only for the hydrosol, which is most exquisite, and because they are not producing oil, they do not cohobate. Rose is so much in demand, however, that much of the real rosewater available is now produced from dried rose petals or flowers. It is nice, tastes good, and smells sweet, but it pales in comparison to a distillate from fresh flowers. Rose petals are extremely delicate; the smell of dried roses compared with that of fresh *Rosa damascena* or *R. centifolia* will give you an idea of the difference in the water products.

So it seems that hydrosols are a bit of a tricky business. They are still a little hard to find, especially in true therapeutic grade, but then so are therapeutic-grade essential oils. There is still much less known about them than about the oils, and their primary use up to now has been in cosmetic products and aesthetic treatments. But hydrosols offer so much scope and benefit that they are worth pursuing, and I hope the information in this book will broaden their appeal for all their myriad applications.

In the meantime, let's examine our definition of what hydrosols are a little more closely.

THE DESIRED QUALITY PARAMETERS

I came to know hydrosols as a coproduct of the distillation of essential oils. Therefore the parameters that I have followed in selecting and judging quality in a hydrosol are the same as those that I use for oils.

I have always believed that anyone working with natural products must bear in mind environmental issues and, in fact, should cultivate a relationship with the living planet and the energetic elements: earth, air, fire, water, and spirit. The environmentalist David Suzuki, in his book

The Sacred Balance, devotes an entire chapter to each of the elements and another to love. From his point of view, we are the air we breathe, the earth from which our food and medicine come, the water from which we are born and of which our bodies are made, and the fire that is the spark that animates all life. I share this view and will talk about aromatherapy and hydrosols in the context of this same philosophy. Our health is inextricably linked to the health of the planet, Gaia, and we cannot isolate what we do and our pursuit of health into a merely personal experience; it is a global experience, a spiritual path, and a serious responsibility.

The following are the parameters that I have always adhered to in selecting and evaluating quality in aromatherapy products:

- One single, botanically specific plant

- Certified organic or biodynamic agriculture

- Chemical-free agriculture

- Sustainably wild-crafted and tested for chemical contaminants

- Distilled or extracted specifically for therapeutic use

- Stored and transported to maintain therapeutic values

One Single, Botanically Specific Plant

Plant-based products for therapeutic applications must be derived from one single, botanically specific source. If we look at peppermint, we see that it is just one of many mints, including spearmint, corn mint, pennyroyal, orange mint, apple mint, and so on. Botanically specific peppermint oil or hydrosol must come from a distillation of *Mentha piperita* alone. Weeds are contaminants, as are other kinds of mints, since they contain chemicals and aromatic compounds that affect both the smell and the properties of the final product.

There are also many varieties of peppermint, and each has different chemical structures. The country of origin, rainfall, temperature, altitude, insect and pest interaction, method of agriculture, and use of chemicals are factors that further influence these differences. Distillers of plants destined for use in therapeutic applications must be able to ensure not only that it is just peppermint that they harvest but that it is the desired variety. Most aromatherapists prefer *Mentha piperita* var. *Mitcham* for therapeutic use. Its fragrance is soft and sweet, and chemically it is low in the ketone menthone and the oxide menthofurane but high in the desirable alcohol menthol. Once available only from Europe, this type of peppermint is now produced in the United States.

Certified Organic or Biodynamic Agriculture

Ideally, certified organic plant material should be used in the making of hydrosols and oils. A second choice would be chemical-free plant material, sometimes called noncertified organic. Noncertified organic is becoming more widely available as farmers move toward organic certification but have not been chemical-free long enough to become certified, a process that takes anywhere from three to seven years, depending on the country.

There are now many recognized and respected organic certification organizations around the world, and they have strict guidelines that must be met before they will give out their seal of approval. Any legitimate dealer who claims to have certified organic products will provide the name of his or her certification agency and can usually provide copies of his or her certificates upon request. Most of the organic growers in Europe are certified by an independent body called Ecocert, but there are also soil associations in most countries and some government agencies that certify organic products.

The requirements for certification are many. The soil where the plant material is grown must be tested and confirmed to be free from chemical applications for a specified number of years (this differs from country to country and agency to agency). Seeds must come from organically cultivated plants and must not be treated with fungicides, pesticides, growth hormones, or other chemicals; in some organizations seeds from nonorganically grown but chemical-free sources are permitted. Cultivation of the plants from the moment of seed germination must be free of synthetic or chemical applications, and fertilizers must be natural composts or manures from (ideally) organically raised animals. Many distillers use the "muka," or waste, from the distillation as fertilizer, creating a natural cycle and returning to the earth that which was taken out. Weeding, which is achieved on most farms by the use of herbicides and weed killers, must instead be undertaken by hand and by the use of mulch. Plastic and fiber mulching sheets have been developed for just this purpose, and interesting discoveries about plant behavior have come from the use of these mulch sheets. Tomatoes, it appears, are highly competitive plants, and by using red mulch sheets under the plants, growers can use the tomatoes' competitiveness to promote the production of more fruit.

So you can see that not only is organic farming labor intensive and complex but the certification of these methods is also extremely difficult. Farmers pay a lot of money to receive their certificate; it is the only way that certification organizations like Ecocert, Demeter, and others can afford to operate. If the process did not pay for itself, certification agencies would have to turn to corporate or government financing, which might influence the process or criteria. Again, the cost of certification must be factored into the price of the final products.

There are also associations, like Demeter, that certify biodynamically grown plant material. The biodynamic growing process goes one step beyond organic growing in that every aspect of cultivation, from germination and planting to weeding, composting, mulching, and harvesting, is done in accordance with the natural rhythms of the earth, the planets, and the plants themselves. Some biodynamic farmers play music to the crops and talk to them to promote growth and, of course, ask permission before harvest. In the days before artificial fertilizers, herbicides, and pesticides, all plant material was either harvested from the wild or grown organically. It made sense to follow the cycles of the moon, the seasons, the rains, the movement of animals and peoples. In ancient Egypt the flooding of the Nile controlled the cycles of life; you simply couldn't plant when your farm was under four feet of water. But when the Nile receded, it left behind several inches of fertile mud on the fields, which helped not only to feed the crops but to retain moisture during the hot dry months that followed. The annual movement of the Nile was part of the very fabric of life, and even the pharaoh's power was judged on the abundance of the yearly flood. So biodynamics include the rhythms of human beings as well.

However, with the advent of modern agricultural techniques and the proliferation of chemical treatments for every aspect of plant production, organic and biodynamic practice all but vanished. Happily, for the last thirty years or so, movements in Europe and Australia have encouraged organic growing practices and the biodynamic cultivation of plants for food and health, and thousands of farmers in North America, both large- and small-scale, are also returning to these time-tested methods. In late June 2000, the U.S. Department of Agriculture closed its public comment period before announcing national standards and definitions for organic growing throughout the United States. A giant leap for humankind!

Although the use of chemicals on plant material designated for human consumption is regulated to some degree, many chemicals were approved decades ago. The Food and Drug Administration (FDA) in the United States admits that if applications for some of these chemicals were filed today, they would be turned down. But new chemicals are approved every year, and it is often only with the twenty-twenty vision of hindsight that we see problems of toxicity to the environment and ourselves. Fortunately, some of the most destructive chemicals have been removed from the market, and we are a little more careful these days. DDT is a case in point. Banned in 1978 in the United States, DDT was originally considered safe, although we now know how incredibly toxic it is to both humans and the environment. However, a recent major infestation in eastern Canadian conifers prompted some to suggest that DDT be brought back. Fortunately, the idea was rejected.

Chemical-Free Agriculture

Even if we assume that agrichemicals are safe, they are frequently used in ways other than those expressly indicated. For instance, in the early

1990s a survey of foods in the United Kingdom found that lettuces contained many times the allowable limit of chemicals, indicating that they had been sprayed just before harvest, although manufacturers' recommendations suggested that spraying be ceased at least seven to ten days prior to harvest. The chemicals did not have any time to leach out of the lettuce and were being consumed in nice healthy salads. Unpeeled carrots were also a danger for the same reason. Peeling the carrots was shown to remove the majority of the residual chemicals and thus render them fit for human consumption. There is no way to point the finger of blame, since farmers frequently do not understand the full implications of agrichemicals on foodstuffs and health, while manufacturers may not do enough to advertise the possible dangers, and the governments do nothing but talk.

In his book *Seeds of Change: The Living Treasure*, Kenny Ausubel states, "Eighty percent of the known health risks come from thirteen pesticides on fifteen crops and products. Of greatest concern are tomatoes, beef, potatoes, oranges, lettuce, apples, peaches, pork, wheat, soybeans, beans, carrots, chicken, corn, and grapes. Broccoli, whose crucial health benefits are well documented, is treated with fifteen separate chemicals and it can't be peeled. Apples can have up to a hundred different pesticides on them, seventy on bell peppers and a hundred on tomatoes."[5]

We know from clinical analyses that plant materials grown under modern chemical-farming conditions retain chemicals. When distilled, the plant material components are extracted and condensed, and therefore the chemical residue becomes concentrated. What may be acceptable levels in a plant could easily become highly unacceptable levels when concentrated in essential oils or hydrosols.

The Canadian Ministry of Agriculture and a number of universities are now working jointly on studies assessing the effects of organic versus conventional farming. In a paper titled "Effects of Organic and Conventional Production Systems on Yield and Active Ingredient Concentration of Medicinal Plants," researchers at Laval University "examined the influence of three organic production systems and one conventional production system on dry matter yield and active ingredient concentrations." Using thyme, *Thymus vulgaris*; horehound, *Marrubium vulgare*; and German chamomile, *Matricaria recutita*, "preliminary results showed that dry matter yield was higher with the conventional production system for all species and active ingredient concentration was higher in the organic systems for thyme and horehound. Higher active ingredient concentration in these two species was obtained in the organic-biodynamic system."[6] As the issue of standardized extracts and "active ingredients" becomes critical to the mainstream scientific acceptance of botanical products, it is most satisfying to note that organic and biodynamic systems can produce more of what we want from a plant than chemical farming can. Quality, not quantity, is what we get from organics.

Then there is the issue of the environmental effects of conventional agriculture. The earth is already very polluted; we know that all too well. The air, the water, the soil, from the Arctic to the Antarctic, even out in the middle of the oceans, is polluted. These contaminants are affecting our health both directly and indirectly. The rise in environmental sensitivities, asthma, allergies, eczema, psoriasis, chronic fatigue, colitis, and even cancer is being researched for possible links to pollutants. Pollution is killing us, and we cannot expect to use conventionally farmed products full of these same chemicals if we wish to benefit our health. So be nice to yourself and the planet: buy organic.

Genetically Modified Plants

Another reason to buy organic is the issue of genetic modification or engineering of foodstuffs. The hot topic as we move into the new millennium is "Frankenfoods," science's answer to modern agriculture's problems of supply and demand, or so it is said. The public backlash to genetic modification of food is in full swing. In an article from the *Manchester Guardian* in the summer of 1999, Joanna Blythman writes, "Recently, the Tories have intensified their efforts, demanding food labeling to be extended to cover all GM [genetically modified] ingredients (including derivatives, and additives); obligatory labeling on animal feedstuffs, so that GM ingredients cannot continue to be anonymously included in feed (as is happening at present);

statutory, not voluntary, regulation of field trials; and a public register of these trials. . . . All UK supermarkets and leading food brands have now deserted the sinking ship, and are pulling the plug on GM ingredients. What started as a steady trickle has become a flood, with recent high-profile defections including Nestle, Unilever, Cadbury."[7] The fast-food chain McDonalds removed over twenty genetically modified "ingredients" from its U.K. items in response to the public protest. However, these same GM products have not been removed in North America.

The most pertinent issue in genetic engineering seems to be the destruction of the natural biodiversity of the planet, particularly within food crops. Biologists warn of the potential problems: "Variety is not only the spice of life, but the very staff of life. Diversity is nature's failsafe mechanism against extinction. Any Banker recommends a diversified portfolio in case one stock fails."[8] Combine this with the increasing interdependence of chemical farming and the new bioengineered crops with a view to the bottom line and you have a complex problem for which there is no easy solution. It is not that farmers and agribusiness companies don't deserve to make a profit; everyone does. However, no one deserves to make a profit at the expense of whole nations or, worse, the earth herself. Genetically engineered food is patented. Farmers can be fined or sent to jail for keeping seed to replant the next year. The April 1999 issue of *Harper's* magazine reprinted a letter that agribusiness giant Monsanto sent to thirty thousand farmers the previous year. The letter warned farmers that "saving and replanting seeds from genetically engineered crops constitutes 'piracy.'"[9] Now consider that sales of Roundup Ready soybeans, a GM crop, have gone from one million acres in 1996 to over thirty-five million acres in 1999 and the predicament of farmers becomes clear.

The same article also mentions that Monsanto, "since 1996, spent $6 billion acquiring seed companies like Cargill International Seed ($1.4 billion) and DeKalb Genetics ($2.3 billion). Rival DuPont followed suit by spinning off its petroleum division, Conoco, and forming a $1.7 billion 'research alliance' with Pioneer Hi-Bred International, the world's largest seed company."[10] Tim Yeo, the U.K. agriculture minister, also quoted in the *Manchester Guardian,* says, "Far from GM crops being a way of improving food supplies, there is a risk that their introduction is intended mainly to enhance the market position of a small number of companies, I believe that both Britain and Europe could secure a commercial advantage if a completely segregated source of GM crops can be preserved."[11]

Of course, if you live in a tiny rural village in Indonesia where twenty varieties of rice have traditionally been grown, then the impact of both chemical farming and patented genetically engineered foods is even more extreme. These farmers can become permanently in debt to the owners of the seed patents, forced to buy seed that they can't afford every year, forced to buy the chemicals that this seed needs to grow; and

meanwhile they lose the natural biodiversity of their habitat and diet. The water, their drinking supply, becomes polluted with the chemicals. And either the pests develop some immunity to the chemicals over time or their natural predators, who would in most years keep the pests under check, succumb to the toxicity of the pollutants. It's a nasty, vicious circle.

It is, of course, the ultimate irony. As Garrison Wilkes of the University of Massachusetts says, "The products of agro-technology are displacing the source upon which the technology is based. It is analogous to takings stones from the foundation to repair the roof."[12] The problems of monoculture agriculture have been devastating for humankind since they began. Here is a partial list of the human, environmental, and economic disasters that have resulted from monoculture farming and the erosion of biodiversity in agriculture:

- 1840s: Irish potato blight; 2 million die in the famine

- 1860s: Vine diseases cripple Europe's wine industry

- 1870–90: Coffee rust robs Ceylon of a valuable export

- 1942: Rice crop in Bengal destroyed; millions of people die

- 1946: U.S. oat crop devastated by fungus epidemic

- 1950s: Wheat stem rust devastates U.S. harvest

❧ 1970: Maize fungus threatens 80 percent of U.S. corn hectarage.[13]

Is it worth the cost, both monetary and environmental, to pursue this line of research and thinking? Surely we can read the writing on the wall, and we must have the ability to respond, to be responsible, in a more appropriate way to the demands of the future.

Sustainably Wild-Crafted and Tested for Chemical Contaminants

If you can't find organic hydrosols and essential oils, the next-best choice is those that are sustainably wild-crafted. Sustainable means that the species can withstand harvesting and still proliferate. It does not mean we take all we can see of a species without thinking; remember the dodo!

The Canadian distillers with whom I work extensively on hydrosols hire only extremely skilled pickers, people who live on and with the land, to harvest their wild plants. Unskilled and cheap labor would not only pick any old plant but pick without regard to the health of the individual plant and the plant community. As with some animals, there is a critical mass to plant populations, and when the population falls below a certain point, it will become extinct. The Canadian distillers also discovered that although branches from trees felled for timber could be used in distilling, the branches needed to be cut by hand, not ripped from the trunk by the huge

stripping machines. The logging industry always wasted the branches, but the oil is unusable for therapy unless some individual care has been applied to the harvest. Mechanical stripping strips the therapeutic properties from the plant and also introduces pollutants such as lubricants from the machinery. There is more to wild-crafting than meets the eye.

Nature's balance is already under threat from pollution, destruction of biospheres like the rain forests and wetlands, destruction of natural biodiversity, genetically altered plant material that kills insects, and who knows what else. If we truly wish to sustain the balance while harvesting from the wild, it is indeed a craft that we must practice. Old friends of mine who have made a sustainable business from wild-crafting are owners of the Algonquin Tea Company. They express what we all feel:

> Wild-Crafters as Emissaries for Nature
> We feel privileged to be wild-crafters. Jokingly, we would say we're priest and priestess, bringing forth the healing spirit of the goddess Gaia for the people. Part of our inheritance, as keepers of the earth faith, is the responsibility to reciprocate. These days, with the dramatic increase in development, resource extraction, pollution, and climate change, it is debatable whether picking wild plants for commercial use should be legal. Here we make the practical and ethical distinction between wild-crafting and simply harvesting from the wilderness. The tradition of wild-crafting may be defined by two interlaced

practices. The first movement involves catching a surplus from the land's perennial tides of abundance. The other act is to aid in the earth's spontaneous regenerative cycles. In the harvest/regenerative relationship we must know when to go forward and when to back off; the ancient and reciprocal relationship of wild-crafting draws from, and gives to, the land.

Perhaps the most obvious benefit of wild-crafting is that it provides our huge urban family with the healing essence of the natural world. A less obvious part of the relationship is that in harvesting plants from wild areas we give "value" to these areas, ultimately helping to ensure the preservation of these sacred places. Another, perhaps even more subtle but essential, aspect of traditional wild-crafting is that it perpetuates and preserves our primal relationship with the healing deities of the plants and land. In working with a place and its plants, we reproduce the original healing experience. From this perspective, the aromatherapy tradition owes its healing abilities to our ancestral/primordial relationship with the land and its plant expressions of healing and regenerative energy. As humanity's gift and purpose may lie in our consciousness and role as earth stewards, the gift and purpose of the plant people is the healing and regeneration of the earth and all her children. As we reenter this circle of relations by using the harvested plant, we can experience the openness of desert sage, the comforting rush of a rich pine or

eucalyptus forest, or the sweet, mysterious musk of pond lilies in summer bloom. In the use of plant essences we evoke the earth's healing forces. In the traditional act of harvesting, we consummate our relationship with the plant. Wild-crafting is an art of sensitivity, care, and knowledge older than "agriculture." These practices, which are still being carried on by native people in remote areas, are based on an environmental ethic of give-and-take.

When we take from the land, it must be gently and reasonably; then we must give back, so the land can regenerate for future generations of life. To "take reasonably" we must be guided by our common sense and not greed. For example, if we find a plot of ginseng or goldenseal and know it takes three to ten years to grow roots of harvestable size, then reason tells us that at the very most, if the plot seems healthy and productive, we may take as much as one in three or as little as one in ten plants per year, depending on the rate of regeneration. Each plant in each case will dictate what should be taken. With some plants, like comfrey or mint, we may be able to harvest up to half the above-ground growth four to twelve times per year, on nine out of ten plants (always leaving 10 percent for seed).

An increasingly common situation, where dramatic harvesting practice may take place, is in areas of development or logging. It is very important to keep an eye on these locales and develop a relationship with the landowners and/or the workers. These situations may provide unusually large amounts of harvestable materials (as are generally needed for the production of essential oils). When trees are being cut or land is being cleared, everything from the branches down to undergrowth plants is plowed under, burned, or left to fry in the sun. In such cases tons of bark and/or leaf material may be gathered with little additional cost to the already dramatically altered ecology. We don't see this as mercenary but as wise use. The other side of relationships with "land developers" is twofold. If developers are outright abusing the land, you are there to call them on it or if necessary blow the whistle. Or you can use a more subtle means of influencing the "development." For example, a landowner told us about an area which had been clear-cut and where he thought blue cohosh grew in abundance. We identified the plant and potential harvesting area and then talked to him in order to get a picture of the land's history. Knowing that the cohosh that was inside the cut line (destined to be lawn) was doomed, we waited till mid-summer, when the plants had borne fruit and were starting to fade, and then harvested 100 percent of the plant. Where other plants survived in the forest shade, we scratched up some areas and seeded at least five times as much as we had harvested. Generally in a wild area you would harvest only one in five blue cohosh. The landowner in this case received 10 percent of the funds raised from the sale of the

plant material. The landowner may get from 2 to 50 percent of the harvest's value, depending on the abundance of the plant and the difficulty of harvesting and processing.

The next year the same gentleman phoned us again and asked if we were interested in mullein, which was now growing in the spot where the cohosh had been, healing the overexposed land. We went and harvested half the aerial leaves but left all the plants to flower and seed so that they could become part of the meadow culture which the owner had now been convinced might be more profitable and beautiful than a lawn.[14]

In many parts of the world wild-crafting is the only way to gather plants. Either land is too expensive, the soil is too poor, or the crop is not valuable enough to make farming an option. In Madagascar, for instance, much of the island is (or was) jungle rain forest, the population predominantly rural, and wealth unevenly distributed. However, Madagascar produces many unique plants and beautiful essential oils and has some very good distillers, so a mix of approaches exists. In 1998 one company began a special project with cinnamon leaf oil. The main impetus was not the value of the leaf oil, less than one-fourth of the value of the bark oil, but the desire to discourage the killing of the cinnamon tree. Cinnamon bark is valuable in any form, so valuable that it is common practice to uproot the tree and hack out the roots, which look and smell much like the bark and are used as a cheap adulterant of cinnamon bark products. Of course, this kills the tree. Madagascar rain forests are just as fragile as any other, and the widespread destruction of cinnamon trees and all that grew near them allowed severe erosion and other environmental damage to occur. The solution was to give value to something that only a living tree produced . . . the leaves. Now pickers can be convinced to harvest leaf and bark in a sustainable manner and leave the tree alive for future harvests. Further value has been given to the crop through the sale of the cinnamon leaf hydrosol.

It is this kind of professional integrity that we should look for in the producers of hydrosols and essential oils. Of course, many countries have a difficult history that makes environmental concerns regarding wild-crafted plants take on a whole new picture. Who can say what residue may exist in soil, water, and plants in war-ravaged or overindustrialized countries? Can modern testing methods ensure that the plant products from these regions are clean and truly health giving? Can people even afford the tests? When will the law actually regulate the use of chemicals and pollutants based on a belief that people and the planet, not just profits, must be protected? When will we start to consider the complex interaction of these elements in the products we choose to use for our health? The wings of a butterfly can change the weather; the choices we make today will determine our future.

> For millions of years, on average, one species became extinct every century. But most of the extinctions since prehistoric times have occurred in the last three hundred years.
>
> And most of the extinctions that have occurred in the last three hundred years have occurred in the last fifty.
>
> And most of the extinctions that have occurred in the last fifty have occurred in the last ten.
>
> It is the sheer rate of acceleration that is as terrifying as anything else. We are now heaving more than a thousand species of animals and plants off the planet every year.[15]

Distilled or Extracted Specifically for Therapeutic Use

Distillation is not a new art. Although the perfection of the process is usually credited to Avicenna (Ibn Sina) in the eleventh century, the art was known long before then. A clay still was found in Pakistan that dates back to the year 500 B.C. The Greek alchemist Zosimos described the three-legged still, or "Tribikos," of Maria Prophetissima, from the year 299 A.D. The Chinese were distilling plum wine into brandy in 500 A.D., using a boiling/condensing technique, long after the emperor Wang Mang (r. 9–23 A.D.), who made alcohol by freezing wine, nationalized the brewing and fermenting industries.

As early as 2600 B.C. the ancient Egyptians were boiling plant material in large pots covered with the shorn fleece of a sheep or a heavy cloth. The wool acted as a type of condenser, absorbing the aromatic steam and cooling it within the fibers so that it condensed. The fleece was then wrung out to extract the aromatic substances, which were allowed to separate in clay vessels. The wood extracts—sandalwood, cypress, myrrh, cedar, and pine—were important elements in many aspects of Egyptian life and death, including, of course, the expensive and lengthy process of embalming. In all these cases it appears that hydrosols or aromatic waters were produced and considered a valuable product of the exercise. Paintings of this process have survived to this day.

There are three main types of distillation for hydrosols. Steam-distillation, water- or hydro-distillation, and hydro-diffusion. I will discuss steam-distillation at length here, but the other two methods are also worth examining, as they are the subject of much debate among producers. There is a massive difference, of course, between industrial steam-distillation and all manner of therapeutic distillation. The yield from therapeutic distillation is usually about half that of industrial output.

In *steam-distillation,* today's techniques differ only slightly from those of the ancients. The still design remains quite simple, although there is magic in its measurements. Basically a still is a large pot with a grate in its bottom and a removable lid that can be secured to create a hermetic seal. The height of the pot should be greater than the width of the pot to prevent the steam from channeling up only one side or the center of the plant material. Obviously, it is important that the steam travel through all of the

plant material so that all of the oil can be extracted. The steam is allowed to enter at the bottom of the still in a trickle, wafting in like a light fog rolling over the land. The steam enters through a grid or cross of pipes with vent holes that face down to further slow the entry of the steam and to ensure that it fills every centimeter of the still body. Industrial distillation forces the steam into the still under pressure and in high volumes, but therapeutic distillation prefers this gentle trickle of steam. Sometimes it can take up to two hours for the steam to make its way through all the plant material and reach the condenser. The grid is placed above the steam pipes to keep the plants away from the steam until it fills the still completely.

It was the shape of the lid and condenser that Avicenna really perfected back in the eleventh century. His design became known as a Moor's head, for its resemblance to the arches and minarets of Moorish architecture. Originally, and even today in small stills, coiled condensers were used. That is, the pipe down which the steam travels as it cools back into water is coiled like the shell of a snail. Many alchemists believed that the angle and rotation of the coil should in fact be based on the torus, a specific spiral angle of rotation that exists in nature: shells, leaves growing along a branch, the spin of a maple key as it floats to the ground. Many believed that using the sacred geometry of the torus created a more natural flow, one that would enhance the energy of the material being extracted. But what modern aromatherapy distillers know is that many plants require specific condensing parameters, and some distillers have multiple condensers in different shapes and sizes so the most appropriate cooling and therefore separation can be chosen for the plant material being distilled. This knowledge is part of the art and science of the alchemy of distilling.

The condenser is cooled by running water that flows from the bottom to the top, surrounding the internal pipe with cold water, thus cooling the steam and converting it back into water and oil. That water is now a hydrosol. Most essential oils are lighter than water and will float on the surface of the hydrosol as it collects in the receiving vessel. For this reason distillers use a Florentine flask to collect the output from the still. This specially designed container has two outflows. One drains the hydrosol from the bottom of the flask, allowing it to flow out and be collected (which also serves to prevent the flask from overflowing) and leaving the oil inside. The second outflow is near the top of the flask and is used only after the distillation is complete, when the oil is decanted through this pipe, leaving most of the remaining hydrosol in the Florentine. Because distillation produces many times more hydrosol than oil, it is important that the two can be separated during the process. You couldn't make a Florentine large enough for all the water. This also allows distillers to collect only the most therapeutic portion of the hydrosol output, usually the first 30 percent of a distillation run, although this varies from plant to plant. The hydrosol produced near the end of the run has little therapeutic value, as most of the components coming over by this point are too lipophilic to remain in the water. If distillers add the end product to the more potent early hydrosol, the waters are diluted, reducing both their aroma and their properties. Other parameters relevant to collecting hydrosols can be found in chapter 3.

In *hydro-distillation* the plant material and water are combined in the still and the whole thing is then brought to a boil. The hot water draws out the oils, just as steam does, and it is carried to the condenser and cooled into hydrosol and oil. This method is one of the oldest and has both benefits and drawbacks. First, it takes a huge amount of heat energy to bring a still-size volume of water and plant to a boil. Just think how much longer it takes to boil a pot of potatoes than a kettle of water. Modern-day uses of this method are most current in countries where fire is used as the heat source or where electricity or gas are inexpensive. It is also the method used in India for the production of certain attars and ruhs, (the Indian name for hydro-distilled oils), notably from rare flowers like tuberose, jasmine, rose, and lotus. For attars, the receiving vessel contains sandalwood oil, which becomes infused with the flower essence; in ruhs no sandalwood oil is used.

Those who distill by this method say that it produces a finer, more complete product, as hot water is cooler than steam and shocks the plant material less. Also, there is less conversion of alcohols to esters in the chemical makeup of the oil, and certain other fragile and highly odiferous molecules may also be better retained. I have had many hydrosols produced by hydro-distillation and can say that for the seed hydrosols, as well as some root and bark ones, this method does indeed seem to produce a richer hydrosol product but a much lower yield. With these tougher materials, the still can be filled with the water and plant, then left to "stew" for twenty-four hours or more before distillation is begun. This seems to allow more of the water-soluble components to be extracted. For other plant material there seems to be much less difference in the products of therapeutic steam- versus water-distilling. There is still no agreement as to whether the life span is shorter or longer for hydro-distilled hydrolates versus the steam-distilled version.

Hydro-diffusion is an odd, if interesting, approach. In this case the steam inlet is at the top, above the plant material, and the outflow to the condenser is below. When you consider that steam is prone to flow up, not down, you can see what I mean by *odd!* The shape and dimensions of the still are different from those used in steam- or hydro-distillation, being wider than tall, in this case. This method has proved popular in countries where water is in short supply, as the steam is already partially cooled by its travel through the plants, so it requires less cooling in the condenser to be turned back into water and oil. Bear in mind that it takes a lot of water to keep a condenser cool, and many distillers heat their swimming pools, greenhouses, or homes by recycling this water. In hydro-diffusion, as in steam-distillation, the steam is created in an outside source, requiring less energy to produce than in hydro-distillation. Many countries in Africa are using hydro-diffusion, and their water scarcities are as legendary as their abundance of therapeutic plant material, so I am glad this method is available. The hydrosols and oils produced by this method are every bit as lovely as those produced by steam or water.

Distillation is such an art that you can count on your fingers and toes the number of truly great aromatherapy distillers in the world. They account for around 2 percent of the total global production of essential oils made each year. All the rest, whether organic or industrial, fall short by comparison. For this reason, and for the sheer fun of it, many aromatherapists today want to try distilling for themselves. We are all alchemists at heart, and distilling on our own provides a much deeper understanding of the plants and the oils and hydrosols they produce.

I take all my students to an aromatherapy distillery as part of their training; it is the only way to truly understand the level of work, commitment, and love required to produce our precious aromatics. This year they spent more than half a day deep in the forest, surrounded by black flies and mosquitoes, gathering just four hundred pounds of larch branches, tying them in bundles, and hiking them back out of the woods, fording streams and ditches. This four hundred pounds only half filled the still, and after nearly six hours of distillation we produced just 270 milliliters of the exquisite pale green oil. As one of the students remarked afterward, "I thought I understood the work involved, but this changes everything. I'll remember this for the rest of my life!" And I'm sure she will. Many tabletop distillers are now available (see the appendix for sources), and both science companies and aromatherapy companies offer distillation units for sale for the home experimenter. Even the Gaggia coffee company makes a still; it looks like a fancy cappuccino machine.

In large-scale distillation, the steam is usually created in an outside source, although ancient designs and home stills usually boil the water for steam in the same pot in which you place the plant material. Water boils at one hundred degrees Celsius and at this point changes phase to become a gas, or steam. If the water is placed under pressure, the boiling temperature can be changed, similar to the way that altitude can affect the boiling point. In therapeutic distillation the boiling point must be kept at one hundred degrees Celsius so the steam generator and still can operate under only atmospheric pressure. In industrial distillation the steam is generally superheated, meaning that its boiling point is raised under pressure. This has two main functions: First, the hotter steam extracts the volatile components from the plant material more quickly, and second, superheated steam moves more rapidly and under pressure can literally be injected into the stills at an accelerated rate, vastly different from the gentle trickle preferred for aromatherapy products. Thus, industrial distillation is shorter, more cost-effective,

and concerned only with the maximum output for the minimum cost.

Another practice that is more common in industrial distillation, although it has its place in therapeutic distillation as well, is cohobation. Cohobation means simply that the hydrosol or condensed water that comes off the still is recycled. The receiving vessel, called a Florentine flask, has an outflow that takes the water back to the steam generator, where it is reheated and passed through the plant material again. Cohobating the hydrosol means that any microdrops of essential oil that were dispersed in the water have an opportunity to coalesce into drops big enough to separate into oil, thus improving the overall oil yield of the distillation. Water, which as we know is a precious commodity, is saved and the cost of production further lowered. In therapeutic distillation, cohobation is used in distilling rose, where many of the four-hundred-plus chemical components are highly water-soluble and the yield of the rose so low that every drop is extremely valuable. Uncohobated rose oil is missing many of the plant's important therapeutic and aromatic compounds because they stay in the water, and therefore it has little value and is never seen.

Home distillation units frequently utilize cohobation because the tiny amount of plant material being distilled yields so little oil that the extra drops that cohobating can achieve make the process worthwhile. The downside of cohobation is that the resulting hydrosol is nearly useless from a therapeutic point of view, as it contains almost no dissolved essential oil, and the repeated heating of the water also seems to damage the water-soluble components in the hydrosol. But it still smells nice and is fun to play with.

Industrial distillation is perfectly acceptable when the resulting oil is to be used only for the extraction of specific compounds. The mono-terpene pinene in some pine oils is extracted for use in artificial apple flavors, sclareol from clary sage is in cigarettes, and the camphor in corn mint is used in cold remedies and liniments. However, the extreme heat and pressure of the steam have damaging effects on some of the chemical constituents in the plant material and can "burn" the plant, giving an off flavor or odor to the oil as a whole. Also, essential oils are volatile, so excess heat frequently "boils off" some of the delicate high notes that are desirable in aromatherapy.

Let's look at the production of lavender oil for a minute. Most of the lavender commercially grown in France and other countries is actually a hybrid lavender more properly called lavandin. There are many lavandins: *Lavandula hybrida* x *abrialis,* x *reydovan,* x *grosso,* to name a few. These are the plants that you see in the stunning photographs of the lavender fields of Provence. Lavandin produces a much higher yield of essential oil than does true lavender (*Lavandula officinalis, L. vera,* or *L. angustifolia*), usually three to four times the amount. But let's assume that we have true lavender plants to fill our still; what would we need to do to produce the most therapeutic oil possible?

If our still holds between 170 and 200 kilograms and we let it run for one hour, we would get approximately 1 kilogram of lavender oil. This would be true lavender oil, and if it was produced from organic plant material it could honestly be marketed as "certified organic lavender essential oil." This is what many people are buying. However, analysis of this oil would reveal that it likely did not contain the full range of therapeutic chemicals that we want for aromatherapy. Most notably the coumarins would be missing.

Coumarins are one of the main sedative components of lavender oil and are produced only after the first eighty to ninety minutes of distillation. Back to the still. If we leave the distillation to continue after that first hour, for say, another two to three hours, we will have a total oil output of approximately 1.1 to 1.2 kilograms. The first hour yields a kilogram and the next two hours yield only one hundred or two hundred grams, an increase of only 10 to 20 percent; it's hardly worth it . . . or is it? If we analyze the oil at the end of the three-hour run, we will find that the coumarin content of the oil is now around 0.25 to 0.3 percent. A tiny amount, but it is enough to impart the renowned sedative property to lavender oil. From a therapeutic point of view we must expect our oil to be complete and therefore contain this tiny percent of coumarins, but from a financial point of view we are virtually tripling the cost of the distillations, since the difference in overall yield is so minute.

Economics of Distillation

One of the ways a distiller can help offset some of the increased costs of therapeutic distillation is through the marketing of hydrosols. If the waters are not cohobated, distillation produces a lot of hydrosol—hundreds of liters, actually. Although not every drop produced throughout the distillation run is of therapeutic value, somewhere between twenty and thirty percent of the output can be used from an average large still. Although each liter sells for only a few dollars, even twenty liters per run times the multiples of runs can amount to a reasonable sum of money added to the value of the essential oils. The distillers I work with have told me that selling their hydrosols has made a positive difference in their yearly incomes, and they consider hydrosols a coproduct, not a by-product, of the distillation process.

Essential oils produced by therapeutic distillation are expensive; are extremely labor-intensive to produce; require the eye, hand, and heart of an artist combined with the mind of a scientist; and do not produce huge profits for the producers. However, they not only offer us healing properties but can help us commune with and access the actual "life force" and knowledge of the plant, and on a larger scale they connect us with the planet and each other in new and healing ways. Spending more to purchase these oils is an easy choice when you look at it like this.

Stored and Transported to Maintain Therapeutic Values

Once essential oils and hydrosols are produced, they must be treated with care and must remain in their perfect state until the moment they are used. It sounds easy, but this is the stage at which much of the tampering actually takes place. Essential oils are frequently adulterated, fractionated, or boosted by real or synthetic chemical isolates to "improve" odor or simply increase volume and therefore profit. Suffice it to say that even buying direct from distillers is not without pitfalls, and the large distributors and brokers of essential oils may be many hands down the line from an honest producer. It is the responsibility of individuals to train their nose, study their botany, read labels, know their suppliers, and truly understand their oils to determine and ensure that what they use are in fact real, authentic, whole, unaltered therapeutic essential oils.

Hydrosols, even more than essential oils, require great care after production. As they do not contain many of the antibacterial and non–water-soluble chemicals we find in oils, they have less natural preservative inherent in their makeup. Many of the distillers who keep their hydrosols instead of letting them run down the drain or into the field simply pour the waters into containers and put them on the shelf. The waters are not filtered, nor are the containers sterilized. Even if they were sterilized before filling, hydrosols come off the still quite slowly, and it can take many hours to fill a receptacle with hydrosol. During this time anything from bits of plant material to dust and insects can get into the vat. One company that sells over two tons of rose hydrosol per year recently told me they have even found gravel in their hydrosols during filtering.

What of adulterants? We know about adulteration of oils, but who would adulterate water? Unfortunately the practice is not uncommon. Water is the most obvious adulterant used, since we're talking about water anyway, but diluting a hydrosol with plain or distilled water not only dilutes its effects but drastically shortens its life span. Alcohol is another common adulterant of hydrosols. Alcohol, like water, is undetectable by smell if it is in low-enough concentrations, and it increases volume as well. But alcohol does cost money and is mainly added as a preservative, greatly increasing a hydrosol's shelf life by killing organisms and bacteria that may be present. In countries of the European Union, hydrosols that are sold for cosmetic/aesthetic purposes must now by law contain alcohol, a minimum of 12 percent by volume. The fact that this renders the hydrosol almost useless for cosmetic purposes, since true hydrosols are alcohol-free options for skin care, did not seem to influence the lawmakers. However, the alcohol *has* been effective in preventing contamination and lengthening shelf life, even allowing hydrosols to be safely kept at room temperature in retail stores with no worry of spoilage—but more on this later.

THE ODOR FACTOR

Hydrosols are aromatic compounds, and it is important to consider this when working with them. One of the frequently quoted rules of aromatherapy is that you don't use an oil on someone if the person finds the smell unpleasant. The rationale is that a disliked odor will have detrimental effects on the health of the patient that far outweigh the beneficial effects a particular oil would have for the individual concerned. If healing has as much to do with state of mind as with medical intervention per se, then a different approach to this problem may be in order.

If someone intensely dislikes the aroma of *Eucalyptus globulus* but has a bad chest cold with lots of congestion and phlegm, a mild headache, slight fever, and general body aches, there are two options: use other oils with similar therapeutic properties to effect an improvement in condition; or take the time to explain just how eucalyptus would help, validate your choice, give the individual options on how to use it (in a bath, in inhalations, topically, or internally), and help the person to understand why it would be worth putting aside his or her dislike of the odor for a short period in order to "get better faster." You will find most people not only respond but also understand the argument on many levels, including the unconscious and subconscious, and you also plant a seed of deeper understanding in the psyche that can have its own benefit to the healing process. You can apply this same process when using hydrosols.

Hydrosols smell. Some are strong, others mild. Some smell nothing like the essential oil, while others are very similar to the oil. However, hydrosols never smell *exactly* the same as the oil or plant from which they are extracted. In some instances the hydrosol is so markedly different that you might not instantly recognize it by smell alone. This may be disappointing to some, but there are reasons for it.

Hydrosols contain only very small amounts of essential oil, and the oil in them is often not complete. GCMS (gas chromatography, mass spectometry) analysis shows that some of the most non–water-soluble components of the essential oil extracted directly from the plants do not appear in the essential oils extracted from the hydrosols. Certain trace compounds may also be absent, and some chemicals may appear in a slightly different form. Thus the odor of this solution-extracted oil is not exactly the same as that of the whole essential oil. Then there are the completely water-soluble components that will never show up in the essential oil but are plentiful in the hydrosol. These lend their own fragrance and qualities to the water, further altering the odor.

The smell of the mixture running off a still is sometimes quite unpleasant. The sweetness of lavender doesn't develop for days, often several weeks, after separation, and it takes even longer for the fragrance character of rose to fully develop. Fresh essential oils resemble hydrosols in that they exhibit a certain wetness and a slightly vague, not quite defined aroma that can

be confusing. Indeed, essential oils need time to rest and coalesce after distillation before they are ready for use. Hydrosols require time to mature as well. They begin to settle several days after distillation and will be aromatically stable four to five weeks later, with the aroma peaking anywhere from two to five months after distillation and remaining that way until degradation begins.

Some hydrosols are definitely an acquired taste! If you maintain the view that you don't use smells you don't like, there will be many hydrosols that will never make it to your cupboard. If you can take the step of acknowledging that even some not-so-pleasant smells can offer a world of benefit, then you are on your way. And your life and health will be richer for it. Let's look at some of these odd characters.

Not-So-Sweet Smell of Success

Yarrow is a complex essential oil. Depending on the country of origin and the plant's botany (either diploid or triploid), yarrow oil can range from bright, sapphire blue to a haylike green-yellow in color. The smell of the blue essential oil is potent, intensely herblike, sweet but with a sour edge like old balsamic vinegar; somewhere in the middle of the smell you can tell it comes from a flower, but it is not floral and it reminds one of wild places and open fields in summer. Yarrow hydrosol is . . . well, it's a bit stinky, really. One client described it as puppy breath. There is absolutely nothing flowery in the odor, but if you can bring yourself to get past its scent, yarrow hydrosol is one of the most versatile tools for regaining and maintaining health. It has broad applications for most of the body, including the digestive, endocrine, and circulatory systems, is incredibly purifying, and works wonders for skin and hair care.

Consider also Greenland moss, sometimes called Labrador tea *(Ledum groenlandicum).* Around one thousand kilograms of wild-harvested Greenland moss are required to make one kilo of oil. It grows in peat bogs in out-of-the-way places and even well north of the snow line. This certainly contributes to the power of its effects. The smell of Greenland moss oil is divine: the savage garden, the sweetness of spring rain, and peace—deep, profound, and lasting peace that touches the soul. If Gaia chose a perfume, it would be this. The hydrosol is flatter, slightly musty; you will recognize it as *Ledum,* but if you adore the oil, the water will disappoint. However, its therapeutic benefits make it worth using, and it is a specific for the liver that is incomparable among hydrosols.

So what do you do when you don't like an odor? Have a little conversation with yourself, rationalize it, then do what you do with your oils: blend. There are many sweet and yummy hydrosols to play with, and even yarrow can be disguised with a little mixing and matching. Just bear in mind the physiological properties of your combinations so you know what to expect in the way of effects.

Not all hydrosols smell bad, of course. Most don't; they just smell different. And like smelling an oil for the first time, your senses have to integrate the information carried in the aroma (and taste) before you really get to know a hydrosol. Although aromatic, hydrosols are not oils; they are aromatherapy in the broadest sense of the word. When using hydrosols, you use the smell, the taste, and the chemistry of the substances to achieve your therapeutic goals. Neroli water works as a perfume, but it also deals with stress, anxiety, and too much coffee. Yarrow would never be a choice for cologne, but it will stop the itching of eczema and psoriasis almost on contact. We must go beyond what we already know when we work with these healing waters, and we must be willing to learn, adapt, and listen to what they have to say.

OILS VERSUS WATER

"Why use hydrosols when we have essential oils?" To answer this question, let's again take a look at potency. An essential oil is highly concentrated. Some plants, like German chamomile, produce only a few drops of oil per kilo of plant. Others contain extremely potent chemicals that are needed in only small amounts to exhibit their anti-infectious effects. If we are trying to fight a staphylococcus infection, we might combine oils like oregano, thyme CT thymol, and palmarosa. One dose used internally would be only one or two drops taken three or four times a day. This is really a tiny amount of oil, but it will have a large effect on the infection. However, these tiny doses add up and actually amount to the ingestion of a very large amount of plant material. Depending on the problem, we may or may not need that kind of potency, and in extreme cases, our bodies just can't handle it.

If a person suffering from real starvation is given a big meal, the body will reject most of it, since it can no longer process either the volume or the content of the food. It appears the same thing may be true with severely immune-depressed people. In this case the body simply cannot handle a large dose of medicine, especially medicine designed to enhance the immune functions. Research is showing that a depressed immune system may, if overstimulated, just shut down under the strain of responding to the medicine. Essential oils are known immune modulants, and because they are so concentrated, it is reasonable to assume that, in certain cases, some oils may be too strong for some systems. The body may try to respond to the chemical cues to increase activity, but if it is unable to do so there is the potential for a negative reaction. This is not healing.

The same is true for infants, whose immune systems are still developing and whose senses, especially smell, are highly sensitive. Would you give a baby a kilo of chamomile to help it sleep? Of course not. Now think how concentrated German chamomile oil is; how much plant is in a drop? Even lavender, which is much less concentrated, is stronger than necessary for undiluted use on an infant. Lavender oil will take varnish off a table; why use it neat on a child? If you can smell it, it's too strong for your baby, is a good rule of thumb, and that's just from an olfactory point of view. The chemistry also dictates that infants, children, and invalids respond equally or better to lower doses. Less is more in every case.

Enter the hydrosols. Already significantly milder than essential oils; water-soluble for ease of application, absorption, and ingestion; and dilutable down to homeopathic proportions, they are the obvious choice for these special conditions. Everything about them is gentle—the smell, the chemistry, and the potency—but they remain highly effective.

Of course, you do not need to be a baby or have a depressed immune system to benefit from hydrosols. They are powerful, healthy supplements that we can use in the same way we use vitamins, minerals, and herbs,. Although they do not replace essential oils, hydrosols work exceptionally well in synergy with oils for any aromatherapy protocol. This book will also show that hydrosol therapy is a viable practice in its own right.

~

TWO

Wholly Water!

Water will not stand still. It is always off to somewhere else;
restless, talkative and curious.

Tom Robbins, *Jitterbug Perfume*

It would be impossible to talk about hydrosols without addressing the issue of water. Water is one of the most critical elements in health and wellness, and unless we recognize its value and the relationship between water and hydrosols, we will be missing half the point!

Water and the control of water supplies made the Egyptian and Roman empires great, and some historians attribute the fall of the Roman Empire to the use of lead water pipes that slowly poisoned the population. Water is now regarded as a commodity to be harnessed for its power or sold for its cleanliness. The temporary contamination of the Perrier springs in France several years ago, and the resulting recall of millions of bottles of springwater, was a national catastrophe causing great economic turmoil. The global policy of damming and diverting lakes, rivers, and other waterways is changing the face of the world and our weather. When phase one of the James Bay dam in Canada was opened, it caused a shift in the earth's crust, and over a million acres of fragile environment was permanently flooded. The damage we have done to water all over the earth and the problems of supplying adequate quantities of high-quality drinking water are two of the biggest issues facing us as we move into the twenty-first century. Consider the distribution of water on earth (see chart on the following page).[1]

The bulk of our water is in the oceans, ice caps and glaciers, and groundwater. Over 97 percent of the water on earth is salty and therefore unusable by us, and 90 percent of the fresh water is unavailable, being deep underground or frozen. "Only about 0.0001 percent of fresh water is readily accessible."[2] We have managed to pollute most of it in some way, and especially high concentrations of poisons are being found at the polar ice caps, where they have been building up for many years. Of the available fresh water on the

LOCATION	VOLUME (KM³)	PERCENT OF TOTAL
Oceans	1,322,000,000	97.2
Ice caps and glaciers	29,200,000	2.15
Groundwater (below water table)	8,400,000	0.62
Freshwater lakes	125,000	0.009
Saline lakes & inland seas	104,000	0.008
Moisture in soil (above water table)	67,000	0.005
Atmosphere	13,000	0.001
Stream channels	1,250	0.0001
Total liquid water in land areas	8,630,000	0.635
World Total (rounded off)	1,360,000,000	100.0

earth, nearly one-quarter is in the lakes and rivers of Canada, which has 98,667 cubic meters per person, compared with the United States with 9,277 and Russia with 30,298 per capita.[3] Sadly, most of this fresh water is in the Great Lakes and their watershed, an area of land that has become contaminated with some of the most toxic chemicals known, including huge amounts of PCB (polychlorinated biphenyl).[4]

Such are the problems of accessing fresh water that the city of Tampa, Florida, is looking to desalination of seawater as an option in supplying the ever increasing demands of that region. Jerry L. Maxwell, a leading proponent of the desalination project and general manager of Tampa Bay Water, was quoted in a front-page story in the *New York Times:* "We are where we are because of the travesty of development in Florida." The first problem is demographic. The area has seen a fivefold increase in population in the past fifty years. The second is environmental: "depleted aquifers, dry wetlands and fallen trees, all casualties of pumping water from the ground to supply rapidly growing communities, often carried out with little heed for the consequences."[5] It is just this kind of situation that illustrates the complexity of managing water supplies.

Water is life. The adult human body is about 60 to 70 percent water, depending on the amount of body fat; the approximate water content in various parts of our bodies breaks down as follows:[6]

Saliva	95.5	percent
Lymph	94	percent
Blood	90.7	percent

Plasma	90	percent
Bile	86	percent
Brain	80.5	percent
Lungs	80	percent
Spleen	75.5	percent
Muscle tissue	75	percent
Liver	71.5	percent
Red blood corpuscles	68.7	percent
Cartilage	55	percent
Bones	13	percent
Teeth	10	percent

We lose around two and one-half liters of water per day just sitting still. Activity and climate can increase this water loss dramatically. Racing-car drivers sweat out several liters in a single race. "Basically, each of us is a blob of water with enough macro-molecular thickening to give us some stiffness and to keep us from dribbling away."[7]

WATER AS MEDICINE

Despite its importance to our health, many people just don't like to drink water. They didn't grow up drinking water and find it impossible to imagine consuming a liter or two in a single day. In fact, a liter is just short of thirty-two ounces, and what we actually need is closer to two and one-half liters, or eighty ounces, per day.

Of that two and one-half liters, close to one liter will come from the foods we eat, but that still means that we must drink at least one and one-half liters of pure water daily if we are to avoid dehydration and keep our body in balance. Modern substitutes like soda pop; teas, whether herbal, green, or black; coffee; and the endless variety of fruit juices and other beverages are not a substitute for water. Most of these drinks are actually diuretic, meaning they take water out of the system; they may contain preservatives, artificial colors and flavors, and the equivalent of several spoonfuls of sugar or, worse, corn syrup. Drinking nonwater beverages only increases your body's need and desire for the real thing.

Water is truly a medicine. For thousands of years "plain old water" has been used to treat health conditions ranging from fevers to allergies, dermatitis to migraine, nervousness to indigestion, colds and flu to pain and swelling. Water was *the* cure for centuries and was used hot, warm, or cold, depending on the condition. Water was also heated to become steam and frozen to become ice, as these changes in the form and temperature could treat a whole new range of health issues. Natural mineral and hot springs were centers for spiritual practices, and many of the great cultures of history were founded on rivers and lakes, from the Tigris and Euphrates to the Nile, the Yangtze, and the Amazon. Water has been combined with herbs, massage, and heat. It has been used in baths, compresses, dips, and sprays; in fact, hydrotherapy is perhaps the oldest "profession" in the world.

WATER QUALITY

For those who do drink water, the current choice becomes one of source. Do we drink tap, spring-, filtered, or distilled water? Bottled water is popular these days, as we are forced to address our concerns for health and worry about the ability of modern water processing to successfully remove all the pollutants from our municipal supplies. But not all bottled water is created equal, as we shall see. In the spring of 2000, the town of Walkerton, Ontario, experienced an outbreak of *E. coli* in its drinking water. At least eleven people died, and a number of other deaths may have been linked to the outbreak. Hundreds ended up in hospitals and doctors' offices, and the ongoing investigation indicates that at least some levels of government were warned of the problem months, perhaps years, before it hit the critical point. In the United States, the EPA (Environmental Protection Agency) has reported that much of the tap water does not meet minimum quality standards, and some sources suggest that drinking water may contain a wide variety of pharmaceutical drugs passed on from humans through their urine, as well as toxins seeping in from agricultural sources. There is even an urban legend in circulation that Seattle's water supply is now caffeinated due to the enthusiastic coffee consumption of that city!

Cryptosporidium is a waterborne parasite that lives in animals and can be passed into water sources through their waste. It has been found in rivers, lakes, reservoirs, and other types of surface water. In 1993 cryptosporidium in the water supply caused four hundred thousand residents of Milwaukee to become ill with flulike symptoms, and some of the very young and very old victims died. Later that year, a failure of Washington, D.C.'s filtration process caused elevated turbidity (particulate matter in the water) and an increase in gastrointestinal complaints. No wonder people are turning to bottled water.

Bottled water may come from underground aquifers, springs, wells, and other deep-water sources that are protected from the environment and tested for purity. These waters are the product of hundreds of thousands of years of natural filtration and purification by the planet and are the most desirable waters for health purposes. Bottled water may also be taken from surface, subsurface, or shallow groundwater; lakes and streams; or approved municipal supplies. Water from these sources is subject to purification processes according to government regulations. The Centers for Disease Control (CDC) in Atlanta recommends reverse osmosis, one-micron absolute filtration, ozonation, and distillation as the preferred methods for purifying municipal and surface water. As far as shelf life is concerned, in some countries it is two years from the date of bottling, regardless of whether the packaging is glass or plastic. Plastic bottles have been suspected of releasing toxins (pthalates) into the products they carry, but most of the data find no problem with water in plastic, owing to its generally nonreactive nature.

Clean water and where to find it is the big problem. The questions remaining are: How safe and effective is modern water filtration? How reliable are the tests being done? Trihalomethanes (THMs), the best known of which is chloroform, are suspected of being carcinogenic and can be created when chlorine is added during water treatment and it interacts with organic matter in suspension. Areas where the municipal water sources are surface or subsurface, such as lakes, rivers, and shallow groundwater, contain the highest quantities of organic matter and are the most likely to develop THMs. The more time there is between water treatment and delivery, the more the concentration increases, and it continues to increase as long as "free chlorine residuals" are present—a case of more chlorine than is necessary being added to the water. High pH levels and warm temperatures also increase formation of THMs, which means that summer months show higher counts in drinking water and that hot water is more likely to contain these toxic chemicals.[8] Researchers in California have linked a likelihood of miscarriage with high THM counts in drinking water, and the studies have been repeated in Canada with similar findings on both miscarriages and stillbirths, reported in the professional journal *Epidemiology*.[9]

Supply and Demands

Regarding water supply and availability, Sandra Postel, director of the Global Water Policy Project in Massachusetts, writes, "Many major rivers now run dry for large portions of the year, including the Yellow in China, the Indus in Pakistan, the Ganges in South Asia and the Colorado in the American southwest. Worldwide, one in five acres (two hectares) is damaged by a build-up of salt that is slowly sapping the soil's fertility. The number of people living in water-stressed countries is projected to climb from 470 million to three billion by 2025."[10] As Postel points out, the pollution of land through lack of adequate water is a huge problem and is compounded by the fact that much of the water that does percolate through the soil has a negative effect because of pollutants, rather than the cleansing effect one would imagine.

American Scientist published a twelve-page article titled "Impacts of Industrial Animal Production on Rivers and Estuaries" that focuses on North Carolina, the second-largest hog production state in the United States and an area of complex environmental regions, including many coastal floodplains and watersheds. These areas are where many of the CAOs, or concentrated animal operations, are located, and their effects and demands upon the local environment have been devastating. In 1997 the North Carolina General Assembly placed a two-year moratorium (recently extended for a third year) on the construction of new concentrated animal operations as a result of the pollution and waste-lagoon spills from these facilities.[11]

Blue Babies

Not only did toxic waste spills from these CAO farms damage local waterways for up to a hundred miles, but they also killed tens of thousands of fish and other water life, deposited toxic silt in riverbeds that can continually repollute any time the silt is disturbed, and created seepage into ground- and well water used for human consumption. A 1995 study in the area found "ammonia-N concentrations up to 300 mg/L and nitrate-N up to 40 mg/L in wells downslope of unlined swine waste lagoons. Wells upslope had ammonia-N concentrations of 0.2 mg/L and nitrate-N of 3.3 mg/L or less. The EPA's drinking water standard for well water is 10 mg/L of nitrate or less, a limit designed to prevent an infant blood disorder known as 'blue baby syndrome,' or methemoglobinemia. In the body nitrate is reduced to nitrite, which converts hemoglobin to methemoglobin, making red blood cells unable to carry oxygen."[12]

There are endless statistics on the plight of the world's water, and it is a major agenda item for the United Nations, the World Health Organization, the governments of most countries, and the political platform of every environmental and humanist organization around. It is also an issue for every human being and for Gaia herself. We need water; we must start valuing and respecting it before it's too late. But I don't mean to be all doom and gloom. Water does wonders, and there are some truly wonderful waters out there. Even more interesting is that research into the healthy effects of certain water treatments has found no difference in efficacy between spa waters and regular tap water. All is not lost!

DRINK, DRANK, DRUNK

If you have health problems and drink less than two liters of water per day, you may be suffering from dehydration. Before or along with any other form of treatment, increase your water intake until you reach the two-liter mark. This may take several weeks or months, depending on how much water you are drinking currently. As with any change in diet or lifestyle, an increase in water intake should be done slowly. The kidneys need time to adapt and relearn how to process all this fluid. Usually you will begin to notice improvements in overall health as soon as you have been drinking more than four or five large glasses a day for at least a month.

If you want to start drinking more water but don't like the taste, you could try adding hydrosols; they are, after all, a good flavoring agent as well as being therapeutic, and unlike most flavorings, they are free of salt, sugar, and additives. Start by spritzing very small amounts into each glass of water you consume. Vary the hydrosols so that the health properties specific to each one are not overwhelming. You will soon notice a positive difference in how you feel. Convince yourself that you're drinking iced tea by adding a spritz of melissa combined with clary sage. Neroli and rose are really good on their own. Bay leaf, sage, and rosemary are nonsweet options and make highly refreshing beverages, but avoid sage if you have high blood pressure.

It will soon become a pleasure to drink "flavored" water, and you may find that the occasional glass of unflavored water becomes more appealing over time. Before you know it you will be downing water by the liter, with or without hydrosols, and your body will love you for it. The consummate water drinker can feel the fluid as it enters the stomach, then the bloodstream, and can describe its progress throughout the arteries, cells, and tissues as surely as you can describe the flow of any river.

You may find it easier to drink large quantities of water if it is at room temperature or barely cool rather than ice-cold. Research has shown that ice water can cause spasms in the stomach owing to the temperature shock. While there are times when cold water is desirable to reduce temperature rapidly, a sufficient quantity of neutral-temperature water has the same effect and will not cause abdominal cramps. Warm or hot water can be used to stimulate peristalsis in the bowel, or if drunk in very large amounts (with or without sea salt), it can work as an emetic, causing vomiting.

The prime times for drinking water are morning and evening. First thing in the morning drink two large glasses thirty minutes before breakfast or your usual morning beverage. This stimulates elimination and acts like an internal shower, waking up the body and preparing it for activity. In the evening, drink a large glass about thirty minutes before retiring, which will allow you time to relieve yourself before sleep. Additional water should be consumed before rather than during meals to improve digestion, make the appetite more stable, and facilitate elimination. If the water is drunk before eating, it also helps dilute the hydrochloric acid in the stomach, making the food bolus less acidic when it passes into the small intestine. Drinking during a meal means that the food itself will absorb the water and swell, contributing to the overstuffed feeling so many people experience after eating. Water should also preface any physical exertion or a gym workout and is highly beneficial for those working in environments lacking fresh air, such as closed-system office buildings.

Supplying the body with adequate water to prevent dehydration is critical, and the immediate perceivable effects include increased energy, improved digestion, enhanced mental function, balanced metabolism and sometimes weight loss, improved circulation, healthier or younger-looking skin, and for some, an increased libido. The effects of dehydration from chronic water shortage in the body include fatigue, poor digestion and constipation, stressed liver and kidneys, headaches, muscle spasms and cramps, uric acid buildup, and gout; even arthritis has been linked to dehydration.

If your blood is 90 percent water and each red blood cell is 68 percent water, imagine the stress on your heart as the blood becomes dehydrated and thickens because of its decrease in volume. If the lymph, so integral to the immune system, is 94 percent water, how strong is your immunity to the flu when dry winter air and central heating dehydrate your entire being, including the lymph? If the liver is nearly 72 percent water, no wonder you get a hangover when you drink dehydrating alcohol and don't rebalance the organ with pure water. Thirst and a dry mouth are not the first messages the body sends, and it is only when we start rehydrating ourselves that we begin to realize what we have been missing.

Water Therapy

Drinking water is the first essential to maintaining health, but there are many more ways to use water therapeutically. Bathing is one of the nicest and, at least in North America, one of the most forgotten. I often ask my clients if they bathe, and the usual reply is, "I have a shower every morning." Showering is not bathing. Showering is washing, and although they are a part of health maintenance, showers can be more healthy if you end with a blast of cold water or use jet streams and the like. However, a shower is still not a bath. Bathing involves submersing every part of the body, from neck to feet, simultaneously.

Bathing

In India the practice of therapeutic bathing extends back thirty-five hundred years, and the sacred Ganges River has been used by humans since the beginning of time! The Romans prescribed baths for chronic liver and kidney problems; the Chinese for cramps, convulsions, and syphilitic ulcers. Various cultures have used bathing for gout, kidney stones, rheumatism, dropsy, and melancholy. The British city of Bath is named for the facilities built around the curative waters of the river Avon, discovered in 860 B.C.[13]

In 1920 the American physiologist H. C. Bazett observed that "a marked diuresis, or increased urinary excretion, was one of the most characteristic effects of such baths on healthy men. Further study demonstrated that whether the water was cold, tepid, or warm made no difference in this effect, but full immersion of the trunk of the body did. Partial immersion of the limbs alone, or even the shallow immersion of a home bathtub, did not cause increased urination. Sitting up to the neck in a pool for a few hours, however, clearly increased the excretion of water, salts, and urea, the chief components of urine."[14]

These results have been repeated in many studies. Total immersion can stimulate the body to excrete as much as two liters of sweat and urine during a treatment. In cases of edema, phlebitis, and kidney problems, this can bring significant relief. Hepato-renal failure, late-pregnancy toxemia, cirrhosis of the liver, and high blood pressure have all responded well to deep-water immersion in clinical trials in the United States, Britain, and Russia. Total immersion in tepid or cool water is still used to treat typhoid and smallpox and is based on theories developed by a Scottish physician, Dr. James Currier, working in the early 1800s.[15] The same treatment can be used for high fever, coupled with the consumption of three or four large glasses of room-temperature water.

Swimming is often the first exercise recommended to people who have suffered an accident or injury. It is a gentle, low-impact, low-gravity activity providing a level of resistance that benefits muscle tissue and provides cardiovascular exercise as well. Even racehorses get exercised in swimming pools as part of their training and injury-recovery program. When we immerse ourselves in seawater, the water from a mineral spring, or any water enhanced with natural salts and add products like hydrosols and essential oils, we create synergies that have additional positive effects. The Dead Sea is famed for its health-rejuvenating properties, as are spas. A new appreciation for the healing properties of water is steadily growing, and hydrosols are a key element in the search for the benefits of hydrotherapy.

You will find more information on how to use hydrosols in chapter 5, but remember: Any hydrosol that is to be used for internal consumption must be absolutely fresh and free of contamination. It should not contain preservatives, alcohols, or additives. Like water, it must be pure, clean, and alive.

A PLACE IN HISTORY

In the beginning of humankind's love affair with odor was the issue of survival. Smelling danger, smelling what was good to eat or drink, smelling a healthy potential mate, smelling weather . . . these were the aromatics that helped humankind survive and evolve. Then we discovered fire. Smoke from burning aromatic woods developed mystical powers. Teas, infusions, decoctions, and macerations in both oil and water followed, and fire helped us produce these mixtures.

As was mentioned before, distillation seems to have appeared at odd, seemingly unconnected intervals prior to its perfection in the eleventh century. Archaeological investigation indicates that water—hydrosol, to be precise—was the product coming off these early stills. It is also important to remember that the development of herb "gardens" began a very long time ago. Aromatherapy is, after all, an herbal or *phyto-*therapy, and it is the connection with and the power of the earth that were accessed through the plants. Distillation was just another step in our quest to access that magic, that *quinta essentia* that is the power of nature. It is estimated that humans started saving and planting seeds some ten thousand to twelve thousand years ago. The Egyptians were planting herbs, trees, and sacred flowers for religious, health, and aesthetic uses over four thousand years ago, and Roman chamomile *(Chamaemelum nobile)*, has been identified as one of the main ingredients in the embalmed mummy of Ramses II (d. 1224 B.C.). The Romans already occupied an area from Turkey to France by the time Theophrastus wrote his herbal *Historia Plantarum* in 300 B.C., and plant material from all the corners of the empire were exchanged and planted in gardens for their myriad properties. The early Christians based their monastic gardens on the designs of the Egyptians, Syrians, Persians, and Romans; "when Saint Benedict founded the Benedictine order at Monte Cassino in Italy in 540 A.D., gardening was second only to prayer in the monastic regime."[16]

It seems perfectly reasonable—when one considers that plants and spirituality or ritual have been inextricably linked since the evolution of humankind—to return to that thinking today. Science does not have all the answers to the magic properties of the plant realm, and if we are truly to call ourselves aromatherapists, herbalists, naturopaths, or any similar title, we must surely recognize and embrace the spiritual and energetic aspect of our work with the natural world. The earth itself was once recognized as a goddess, Gaia, and honored for its gifts. The recognition of Gaia has returned, starting with the scientists of today. In Islamic traditions the rose has its origin in a drop of sweat from the brow of Muhammad. The word *baccalaureate* came from the Greek practice of crowning graduating doctors with the *bacca laureus,* a garland of bay leaves.[17] And even sixty thousand years ago we used plants as part of the rites of burial. In the grave of a Neanderthal man found in Iraq in the 1970s, the body was surrounded with flowers, including yarrow, still widely known for its therapeutic properties.

Manufacture and Use

For those early distillers who could barely grow enough roses or produce as much hydrosol as was demanded by their wealthy clientele, the issue of storage was unimportant. Let us assume that the hydrosols either were used quickly so they never had time to "go off" or were stored, like foods, in cellars or cooler environments and in clay vessels, since evaporation through the clay would help keep the contents cool. The waters, being far less expensive than the oils, became the product that filtered its way into general use. One of the ways they were used was in cooking. Desserts were heavily fragranced with honey, spices, and waters of rose and orange blossom. But again, in these times we must assume either that the waters were produced and used so quickly that spoilage was uncommon or, and perhaps more correctly, that even if they developed bacteria or "went off" they were used anyway. Modern research shows that large quantities of ground clove bud added to contaminated meat can render it completely safe for human consumption while not destroying its palatability.[18] But except for a few hydrosols like rose, neroli, sage, and oregano, interest in the waters and their value waned as the value of the oils was recognized.

The end of the nineteenth century saw the discovery of the germ. Science entered our lives, and essential oils proved themselves worthy of study not only as substances that could kill these germs but as compounds of interest in the pursuit of chemical knowledge. Much of the first research in biochemistry was done with essential oils. They were already highly refined, and it was easier to isolate their parts than those of the whole plant. During the modern renaissance of aromatherapy, the oils naturally became the first substances to regain popularity. For all the same reasons that they were desired in the past, oils came to mean aromatherapy, and vice versa. But as with any renaissance, as time goes by, interest broadens and people seek greater understanding and more diversity in knowledge. Now, at the end of the millennium, we see the rebirth of interest in plant waters, and one day they may be a form of aromatherapy completely independent of the oils.

PHYTOTHERAPY

The Holistic Approach

The issue of the "terrain," as the French call it, or "constitution," in homeopathic terms, is particularly relevant to hydrosols. It is also a basic tenet of holistic health. All disease is an imbalance, and although in treatment the symptoms are considered, the character of the individual is just as important. The premise is that when you rebalance the terrain, disease will disappear.

In France much of the way essential oils are used is as "phytomedicines," in the modern pharmaceutical sense. The aromatogram is a case in point. Modeled on a scientific test used to determine the efficacy of antibiotics on specific organisms, the aromatogram is exactly the same test but uses tiny disks impregnated with essential oils instead of antibiotics. The aromatograms show the "kill zone" of each substance tested and can be used to design treatments for a huge variety of pathologies, including those that may be antibiotic resistant. However, in vitro is not the same as in vivo. It is not completely uncommon for the oils that work in an aromatogram to have less than the expected effect when given to the person in question, and vice versa. *Why?*

Sometimes essential oils may be too strong for a person. Sometimes they just don't work, for no apparent reason. So the constitution, or terrain, must be addressed. Galen and his formulaic approach is out and Hahnemann comes in. The aromatherapist will then try to rebalance the individual, choosing oils like lavender, rose, sandalwood, and vetiver that address issues of emotional, spiritual, and psychological health. Sometimes rebalancing the terrain is enough; the immune system kicks in and the pathology will disappear. Sometimes rebalancing the terrain creates an environment of healing, and the individual's body will then allow the oils to do their work. Just think how effective hydrosols must be on this level of healing. Hydrosols really are the next aromatherapy. A constitutional aromatic. Eureka! as they say.

When I first realized that neroli water would stop caffeine jitters, a colleague told me my evidence was too anecdotal to be accepted. Why would just a few sips of water with this hydrosol have such an effect? The aroma of the hydrosol alone does not do it, and it is not the rehydrating effects of the water, since just a few sips work. But I couldn't prove my finding scientifically; I just realized this was a constitutional reaction by the body to the tiny amount of hydrosol in the glass and the copious amounts of espresso in my system. So next time you have too much caffeine or, for that matter, really bad stress, reach for the neroli and see for yourself. Aromatherapy has over four thousand years of anecdotes to fall back on. Does science—or the lack of it—make this history any more or less true? I think not.

Homeopathy and Hydrosols

Homeopathics are the vibrational, or subtle, edge of the spectrum of holistic healing. Treatment follows many of the concepts of Ayurveda and traditional Chinese medicine in that the client is considered a whole and sickness is seen as an imbalance of the terrain as opposed to a disease to be eradicated. So it is that I look at hydrosols as the equivalent of a homeopathic version of essential oils. Gentle and safe in their pure state, highly effective in extremely low dilutions, and with few contraindications or safety precautions, hydrosols are the subtle, constitutional form of aromatherapy.

Although homeopathy was originally conceived of as a constitutional healing mechanism, it has been some years since the concept was "invented," and there are now as many schools of practice in this modality as in aromatherapy. It is interesting to note that Hahnemann, in "proving" some of his remedies, turned to essential oils. For him the only viable method of ingesting sufficient quantities of plant material to elicit the symptoms he wished to cure was to ingest oils. The analogy between hydrosols and homeopathy can be drawn further. Modern homeopathy allows for both the constitutional and the prophylactic or treatment-oriented use of remedies. For example, bronchitis is an imbalance in the system but it is also an infection, and there are many remedies that will "treat" bronchitis as an ailment while simultaneously balancing the constitution. So it is with hydrosol therapy. For bronchitis, *Inula*, *Eucalyptus globulus* or *E. polybractea*, rosemary CT verbenone, oregano, tea tree, or winter savory hydrolates would all be appropriate. Chosen wisely, and considering the nature of the individual, any of these could address the bronchitis while stimulating the body's natural immunity and overall function. In other words, the hydrosols act both constitutionally and specifically on our health.

Hydrosol Remedies

Homeopathic remedies are prepared by repeated dilution and succussion (banging) of standard tinctures in 60 percent alcohol or high-proof vodka. The more diluted and succussed the remedy, the stronger its potency. Alcohol is the chosen medium because it contains water, which can best hold and expand the medicinal vibration of the remedy. The alcohol also acts as a preservative and antibacterial agent.

Hydrosols can be used in the same way as the tinctures in homeopathy. Single drops can be diluted in quantities of distilled water and succussed to distribute the energy of the hydrosol throughout the water. If we follow Hahnemann precisely, we dilute one drop of hydrosol in ten drops of water, bang (succuss) the bottle on the table one hundred times, and thus have a remedy of 1c. If we do this six separate times we will have a 6c remedy; if we dilute the 6c twenty-four more times, we will have an infinitely stronger 30c remedy, and so on. Laborious and time-consuming as this may be, it seems to work just as well with hydrosols as with tinctures. And remember, the more you dilute, the stronger your remedy.

My experiments in this area stem as much from my homeopathic experiences as from the problem of ingesting Greenland moss *(Ledum groenlandicum)* hydrosol. It works well; in fact, it works a little too well. Greenland moss is so efficient and rapid a detoxifying substance that some clients just find it too strong at the standard dilution of thirty milliliters in one liter of water. Even when the dose is cut in half (fifteen milliliters per liter), which I now recommend as standard with Greenland moss, some clients still seem to be "proving" the effects. Nausea, vomiting, bile reflux, and diarrhea were all symptoms that these people experienced; yet usually these were some of the symptoms that cleared up during a detoxification with *Ledum.* The clients associated the smell and taste so strongly with the effects that even a whiff of the hydrosol thereafter could make them run for the bathroom.

So I diluted the *Ledum* until I thought it was imperceptible, that is, one drop in one liter of water. One client still reacted, however. Now the problem was twofold. This woman had responded so violently to the original dose that even the thought of *Ledum* now elicited nausea. How could we get over the fear reaction and

enable her to use the remedy? At one drop per liter the smell was virtually undetectable—but not, apparently, if you were looking for it. I then diluted one drop in thirty milliliters of water, succussed it thirty times, then repeated the process two more times and told the woman it was a different hydrosol. She did not experience any of the previous negative symptoms, felt a moderate overall improvement along with some significant detoxification, and said that she would have preferred a more flavorful hydrosol! Unfortunately, it was not possible or ethical to keep up the pretense, and once told that it was *Ledum,* she did not wish to continue the treatment, reaction or no. Fortunately there were other hydrosols to turn to, and a combination of yarrow, sweet fern, and a small amount of rosemary CT verbenone eventually did the trick, clearing her liver, solving chronic constipation, and helping her reduce dependence on a number of drugs and other remedies.

I continue to make tests of dilution, but it will require much more experimentation, perhaps by qualified homeopaths, to fully determine whether hydrosols offer a viable option to remedy preparation by tincture. What I do know is that hydrosols work, even in extremely low dilutions such as those prepared for homeopathy. They also work very powerfully when used by the single drop (see the section Shiatsu and Acupuncture in chapter 5 for more information).

Probably the biggest drawback to this kind of treatment is the delicate nature of hydrosols. Tinctures will stay viable and free from bacteria for fairly long periods, thanks to their alcohol content. Homeopathic remedies, which are diluted in alcohol, also benefit from this preservative action. Not so with aromatic waters. Hydrosols ideally contain no preservatives and must be packaged in sterilized containers and stored carefully to avoid degradation. Any aroma-homeopathic remedy made in the manner described will either require the addition of alcohol or have a short life span suitable only for immediate use; these problems can be circumvented somewhat if the clients are willing to prepare the dilutions themselves.

Hydrosols and Herbs

With this in mind, the tinctures that my colleagues and I have prepared in the last three seasons were made using 95 percent ethyl alcohol diluted to 60 percent with the hydrosol of the tinctured herb. This was then poured over the herb and left to macerate for about two weeks. The tincture was then strained and filtered through fine cheesecloth and diluted down to the appropriate level of alcohol by volume with more hydrosol. I call these products Aromatic Tinctures, a trademarked name. They smell and taste quite remarkable—unlike traditional tinctures, which smell only of alcohol. They also contain both the alcohol-soluble (complex sugars, alkaloids) and water-soluble (acids, aromatic and carbon molecules) components of the plants.

I have now made Aromatic Tinctures of melissa, *Ledum, Echinacea,* Saint John's wort,

German chamomile, and yarrow. Some of the tinctures were succussed after the hydrosol was added, some were not; personally I find that succussing or banging the Aromatic Tincture before every use is the best method. The efficacy of the tinctures seems to be enhanced by the hydrosol, and they certainly smell and taste much better than most tinctures. It is too early to know exactly how different they are in physical effect, but they "feel" more active and have yielded some exceptional results with adults, children, and pets. I believe the addition of hydrosols will be a recognized way to prepare tinctures in the future. I have replaced all my flower remedies with Aromatic Tinctures.

We are also working with tinctures by adding complementary hydrosols. German chamomile water added to melissa tincture creates a more sedative nerve relaxant. Melissa tincture with neroli hydrosol is for states of high anxiety, panic, and exam jitters; and then there's Saint John's wort tincture with linden hydrosol, which is a real knockout. The possibilities are endless, and in this case shelf life is not an issue because of the high alcohol component of the tincture.[19]

Herb Teas

We can also compare hydrosols to herb teas. For literally thousands of years herbs have been used for health in the form of tisanes. A small amount of herb is steeped in hot or boiling water and the resulting tea is consumed for specific physical or mental conditions. Chamomile tea relaxes the body, calms the mind, and aids sleep. Linden treats stress and anxiety and also aids sleep; peppermint helps indigestion and wakes us up. Ginger root gives warmth and eases a cough or motion sickness. There are hundreds of herb teas with "accepted" or "proven" properties. In fact, the German government's Commission E has approved medical uses for many tisanes, including peppermint, fennel, linden, German chamomile, and melissa.

The average tea bag weighs two grams. Depending on the herb, this equates to approximately four to eight grams of *fresh* plant material per bag. We might add anywhere from 100 to 150 milliliters of water and brew the mix for ten to fifteen minutes, depending on the desired strength of the tea we are preparing. The result is a ratio of maybe 0.08:1 herb to water. Hydrosols, depending on the plant material, are at the very least 1:1 plant to water and more frequently 3 or 4:1. If herbal teas work, can't we assume that something so much more concentrated will also work? Diluted (thirty milliliters in one liter of water), hydrosols are still as strong as, or stronger than, herb tea. In fact, considering that they are made with steam, we could perhaps think of them as "herbal espresso," the supercharged version of herb tea.

There is also the issue of fresh versus dried plant material. We know that some of the volatile and fragile components of herbs are lost during the drying process. Drying techniques are, in fact, one of the biggest problems facing herb growers. I recently saw an innovative drying container for organic herb production. The fresh plant material is spread on a net suspended three feet in the air in an enclosed room, and both fans and heaters circulate warm air through the material. The temperature is controlled to ensure optimum speed of drying with minimum loss of volatile components for each type of plant and plant part being dried. In this manner one hectare of German chamomile flowers can be dried in less than a day. However, we know that most herbs on the market are not dried so carefully and many are not organic. Recent studies in the United States and Canada on herbs imported from China showed that these "medicinal herbs" contained large amounts of chemical contaminants in the form of pesticides, herbicides, and so on and also contained far less than the expected concentrations of active therapeutic compounds. If we were to make a tisane from such herbs, what medicinal value would it have and what concentration of active ingredients would be in each dose?

When plant material is distilled for essential oils and hydrosols, it is often put into the still in a fresh or only slightly wilted state, rarely if ever fully dried. If we are buying from certified organic producers, we are getting not only a contaminant-free product but also one in which the fragile and volatile components remain in the plant material being processed, thus delivering a more therapeutic finished product. Ultimately the effectiveness of hydrosols must be significantly higher than that of herbal teas, regardless of dilution rates.

There are, of course, varying qualities in

waters, as in oils, and just because a hydrosol is certified organic does not make it good. I was sent some certified organic rosewater last spring, but neither the taste nor the fragrance was very rich. The internal effects seemed minimal and that "feel-good feeling" I associate with drinking rose was missing altogether. When I called the supplier, I asked if the distillation was just for hydrosol or for oil as well. The supplier informed me that, like many others, the company distilled rosewater from dried roses year-round to keep up with demand. There was no oil produced from the distillation and the plant-to-water ratio was 1:1. That may work in baklava but not for menopause.

On the other hand, a shipment of cinnamon hydrosol from leaves wild-harvested in the Madagascar rain forest was a feast for the senses. Distilled by local people in very basic conditions, the water had a richness of scent, flavor, and effect that was superb. As well as being delicious, this hydrosol was particularly energetic and helped a severely stressed woman get through a lengthy and nasty court battle, focused and with a smile on her face, without filling the prescription for Prozac that her doctor had given her.

Traditional Chinese Medicine

Traditional Chinese medicine (TCM) has developed over millennia, and there are four-thousand-year-old Chinese texts that list herbs and uses that are still relevant today. It is important to remember, however, that many of the herbs are specific to the geographic region of China and either do not grow in the West or are just now being explored for their agricultural potential. Some, like ginseng, are already big business in North America; others, like dong quai and ma huang, are now test crops for organic farmers in appropriate climates, but many Chinese plants are simply not suitable for our geography. If you wish to use hydrosols to replace certain Chinese herbs, you must get a really good materia medica to ensure that the botanical species of the hydrosols are the same as those of the herbs. Some substitutions are possible, and in the aromapuncture treatments we are testing (applying single drops of hydrosol to acupuncture points), the Western attributes of the hydrosols are also applied.

Most Chinese "remedies" are mixtures. In fact, there are very few single-herb treatments. Hydrosols lend themselves to being blended, as we have already seen. Also, as anyone who has used TCM knows, a Chinese remedy often consists of a bag of herbs with detailed instructions on the remedy preparation. I once had a treatment that involved boiling the herbs for one hour the first day, then reboiling for twenty minutes every day for three days thereafter. The mixture had a ferocious odor, and my neighbors began to doubt that "aromatherapy" had any benefits at all. How much simpler to just blend your hydrosols, which have already been "boiled," and drink that as your remedy.

There are TCM practitioners in several countries exploring hydrosols and essential oils.

This is another area where I believe we will see some exciting developments in the years to come. There is more on the use of hydrosols in acupuncture, acupressure, and shiatsu in the section on esoteric use in chapter 5.

PRODUCTION AND TRANSPORT

Following are the desired parameters for producing and transporting hydrosols:

- ⁌ Sterile containers to receive the hydrosols at the still

- ⁌ Distillation or best-before date noted on each batch

- ⁌ Controlled temperature for storage at the source

- ⁌ Rapid shipping methods

- ⁌ Controlled temperature storage at the end

- ⁌ Filtration for particulate matter

- ⁌ Inert storage containers

The first point of concern in maintaining the shelf life of hydrosols is where and how they are produced. Most stills producing therapeutic-grade essential oils are not in pristine laboratories or modern factories. Stills are located in sheds, barns, open fields, forests, deserts, and so on. Usually the deciding factor is the location of the water source, as distillation requires large quantities of water, both to produce the steam and to cool it in the condenser. Plant material, although bulky, is more easily transported to the site of the still than is water.

As we know, water, at least clean water, is a rare and valuable commodity. Not everyone has an ancient aquifer or pristine spring in his or her backyard. Although distillers who produce certified organic products have their water sources tested as carefully and frequently as their plants and oils, some distillation is done with water that might not pass this exacting standard. Now, although this is still a major concern, distillation purifies water, and even nonpotable water can be made safe if distilled; nevertheless, we want as pristine a source for our distillation water as possible. So let's assume that we start with really clean water and that the distillate that runs off the still comes out in a totally pure form, free of contamination, free of bacteria, and containing only those additives that it has gathered from the plant material in the kettle. Why, then, is there a problem?

Sterile Containers to Receive the Hydrosols at the Still

The average flow of a distillate is three to five liters per hour, although this obviously varies from plant to plant. It therefore takes from four to seven hours to fill a twenty-liter container. If the still is in an open space, everything from insects to dust to plant parts and, of course, bacteria can enter the jug along with the hydrosol during this time. Even if the container is sterile to start with—and your hydrosol is sterile by nature—by the time a lid is put on the jug, the contents are no longer guaranteed sterile. Even a modern, clean factory environment will have dust and airborne materials, if only from the kilos of plant material being moved around. But how bad is this? It depends on where you are and what you're distilling. Some hydrosols seem more prone to bacteria growth than others. But one thing is certain: how the waters are treated once they are bottled is a key factor in their life and preservation.

In my experience hydrosols that are produced in the middle of the desert or jungle are difficult to acquire. Blue tansy *(Tanacetum annuum)* hydrosol is one I have long sought, but as I was told by the director of the Moroccan essential-oil producers' organization, I am unlikely ever to get it. This oil is most frequently made in mobile stills that are taken to sites where the plant material grows. It is not worthwhile to bring the water back, and as this is a low-yield blue oil from a region without excess water, experiments with cohobation are now becoming common. I would argue that hydrosols of low-yielding, rare, or expensive plants actually have greater value both for the distiller and for the end user. Rock rose is a case in point. Rock rose oil is made from the resin that forms on the leaves of a wild plant that has a tiny yield and is laborious to gather. No matter what price is charged for the oil, it's not a big moneymaker for producers. Now factor in the hydrosol. Therapeutically it is extraordinary and has the lowest

pH of any hydrosol. If you add the sale of forty to fifty liters of hydrosol to your oil revenue, production becomes slightly more rational.

Most, though thankfully not all, of the distillers who keep and sell hydrosols are working from some kind of fixed site, or if the still is mobile, it is not in the back of beyond. Thus the actual quantity of particulate matter that enters the waters is somewhat reduced. Rose may be an exception, as mentioned previously; even gravel has been found in drum-size containers and more than once I have filtered out insects and significant quantities of floating plant parts. I am working with distillers on a number of control measures for hydrosols, including placing the receiving vessels in a sealed area and using fine mesh screens over the mouth of the jugs, and this year we will experiment with a special food container that will vacuum-pack the waters. I believe that these measures have resulted in higher-quality products with a longer natural shelf life and are well worth the effort they require.

Distillation or Best-Before Date Noted on Each Batch

Once produced and in bulk containers, each batch of hydrolate should be labeled with the distillation date and all other information necessary to track production. Good distillers may even be able to tell you the field or location that the plants came from by the batch code. This helps identify not only products and sources that are different in quality but also products that are different in effect. Calamus *(Acorus calamus)* root grown in Europe or Asia contains high levels of the toxic ketone beta-asarone. The Canadian variety is completely beta-asarone–free and therefore safe for use in therapeutic applications. Just as with essential oils, we must know all we can about the hydrosols we use.

Controlled Temperature for Storage at the Source

The distillers of hydrolates must be willing to care properly for the waters if they are to have value as a therapeutic commodity. Cool, constant temperatures with minimal or no light and sterilized dark or opaque containers are the best choices. Of course, cold storage is not always easy, but most distillers have some cool, dark facilities for their oils. The ideal temperature for the waters is around ten to thirteen degrees Celsius (fifty to fifty-five degrees Fahrenheit), and the consistency of the temperature range is important in preventing condensation inside storage vessels. Usually the dilemma becomes one of space. If you have only enough room for your oils in the cold store, are you really going to keep the waters? Is there enough value, both monetary and therapeutic, in hydrolates to justify the extra care they require? For many the answer is already yes, and for others it soon will be.

Rapid Shipping Methods

Transportation of the waters is the next issue in preserving their shelf life. Depending on where you live and what you are buying, hydrosols may come from very near or very far away. Australia and New Zealand, for instance, are very far from anywhere except each other. For this reason, it is extremely difficult to obtain hydrosols from that part of the world. The cost of air transportation is very high, and hydrosols are heavy; like water, one liter weighs one kilogram. Surface transportation means shipping by boat. This is exceedingly slow, and unless you are willing to find and pay for temperature-controlled shipping, it is out of the question, as spoilage is sure to occur in the weeks or months at sea. I have begged one Australian distiller on countless occasions to ship me some of his unique hydrosols, explained that I would assume all the risks of spoilage, and arranged air cargo, but to no avail. He, like many others, has had bad experiences shipping the waters in the past and is reluctant to try it again. For this reason most of the eucalyptus hydrosol on the market comes from Portugal, where a high-quality oil is being produced.

It is a fact that at least 20 percent and up to 60 percent of the cost of a hydrosol is in the transport. Air transport is the only viable method, since any shipping means that there are no controls over temperature and storage conditions. Hydrosols are fragile, and if they are left in a hot warehouse or boat for weeks on end, the likelihood of degradation skyrockets. Even air transport means the hydrosols are not temperature controlled for at least a few days. I once shipped product to Banff, Alberta, in the middle of January. Sent priority courier overnight, they arrived frozen solid but were quite fine when thawed very slowly. It is only with prolonged exposure to unsuitable conditions that the problems really begin.

It is worth taking care and spending what needs to be spent on transportation. There is no way to guarantee how the hydrosols have been treated prior to shipping, although you do your best to buy reliably. But you do have choices in how the products are treated after you receive them, and storage is critical.

Controlled-Temperature Storage at the End

Once the hydrosols arrive, get them to cool storage as fast as possible. I have found that a constant-temperature environment that fluctuates no more than two or three degrees Celsius in either direction is as important as the baseline temperature. Ideally, hydrosols should be stored in an area that is kept around ten to thirteen degrees Celsius. This is slightly warmer than most refrigerators, but refrigeration certainly does them no harm and is the easiest method of temperature control for smaller quantities. A cold room is the perfect option for large amounts, and if you are considering handling hundreds of liters per year, this option is worth investigating. Cold rooms protect your investment and protect your customers.

Filtration for Particulate Matter

It is advisable to filter very large containers of hydrosol upon their arrival. First, this will remove any particulate matter, reducing the substances that can carry bacteria, and second, you are more likely to notice any contamination, molds, and the like that may already be present.

The many methods of filtering waters are described later in the book, but at the very least a paper filter, such as an unbleached coffee filter, should be used. Paper filters are easily sterilized by a very short blast in a microwave oven. Microwave them for only one or two seconds at a time until you know what your oven's power is like. I prefer not to use microwaves at all, but as a means of sterilizing things they have some use.

Inert Storage Containers

If the hydrosols are shipped in metal containers, you will want to decant them immediately. Water causes metal to rust. Although aluminum flasks with a phenol-resistant coating are acceptable, they are expensive and are rarely used for hydrosols except in small retail quantities. Unlined aluminum is unacceptable since, like essential oils, hydrosols may interact with the metal. Most often hydrosols are shipped in plastic containers. The best plastic containers are made of Nalgene. This is a totally inert plastic available in a variety of densities, but it is quite expensive. I have never had any problems with leaving the hydrosols in Nalgene in storage. You can also fit taps to these containers, making decanting easier and circumventing the necessity of frequently opening the vessels to pour off small amounts. Rigid plastics are better than softer plastics, as they are less likely to react with the contents. Many bottle suppliers have a good range of high-quality, phenol-resistant plastics that are suitable for shipment and storage of hydrosols. Glass is the ideal medium for transporting hydrosols, and hydrosols seem to do best in cobalt glass. However, at some point cost must be factored in; weight is a consideration in shipping, and glass is breakable, heavy, and expensive. Users must make their own decisions.

I recommend selling small quantities of hydrosol in glass. Anything over five hundred milliliters (one-half liter) should be packaged in a high-quality rigid plastic, and I usually advise customers to decant into glass if feasible. Generally, if you are storing in plastic other than Nalgene, you should try to keep your stock rotating. An option is to bottle into plastic to order, minimizing the concerns. Remember, we are not talking about oils here. Hydrosols do not contain the chemical constituents of oils that can melt plastic, Styrofoam, varnish, or paint. No hydrosol is that concentrated, and the percentage of oil that hydrosols contain is too small to worry about. So in most cases, the danger of storing hydrosols in plastic is only marginally greater than storing a mineral water in plastic.

BOTTLING, SALES, AND HOME STORAGE

The desired parameters for the bottling, sales, and home storage of hydrosols include

- Minimal handling and smelling of product prior to packaging
- Only sterilized packaging components
- Proper labeling
- No added preservatives
- Storage after packaging
- Shelf life and marketing

Minimal Handling and Smelling of Product Prior to Packaging

It's difficult. A big jug of your favorite water or, even worse, a new one you've never smelled before arrives at the door. All you want to do is take off the lid and smell it. I used to do it all the time, and I watch every buyer of hydrosols do the same. Scents are addictive. However, smelling directly from the container risks contaminating the whole shipment. It is preferable to decant a small amount into a clean glass to judge flavor, aroma, color, and clarity and to reseal the large container immediately. Try using a wine glass, then get your nose in it. Use a teaspoon and taste it straight. Hold it up to a light and see if there is a tint of color or a faint milkiness. Look for suspended particulate matter or anything unusual. There are a host of qualities to appreciate, and you will soon learn to read the signs and understand what they mean. After you have examined the pure hydrosol, add a little to a glass of water and taste it again. It is always astounding just how strong pure hydrosols can be and how soft they become when diluted in water.

If you intend to resell your hydrosols, it is worth providing testers. People don't know the waters like they know the oils and will often buy something only if they have the chance to smell or taste it. Testers should have screw-cap lids so the nose test can be undertaken, and they should be replaced with fresh hydrosol every few weeks or more frequently if heavily used. Although they will last longer if kept cold, I often leave my testers at room temperature so the full aromatic qualities can be appreciated. Cold, their aroma is weaker, and people find it much harder to appreciate their differences.

Only Sterilized Packaging Components

When bottling hydrosols for your own use or for resale, it is imperative that you use only clean, ideally sterilized, containers. Bottles are not clean when you pick them up from the warehouse; at the least they are dusty. Whatever method of cleaning you use, wear gloves. Some of the sterilizing liquids, like ethanol, are hard on your hands, and if you touch a clean area with bare skin it will no longer be "clean." If you are bottling for home use and will be using up the

hydrolate in two to three months, you may find it sufficient to wash the bottles in very hot soapy water and rinse them in a mild vinegar solution or to run them through your dishwasher. For more efficient home cleaning, wash the containers, then dry them in a five-hundred-degree oven for twenty minutes. Bottling for resale requires that you use 95 percent ethyl alcohol (ethanol), hydrogen peroxide, or a more efficient sterilization procedure than washing and drying. If you are using plastic caps, do not put them in the oven but do ensure that they are thoroughly dry before bottling begins. Plain water added to a hydrosol shortens its life, and tap water may contain a number of chemicals or bacteria.

Spray bottles are the best choice for small quantities of hydrosol. The sprayer unit can be disassembled quite easily, and ethanol or hydrogen peroxide can be used as a sterilization liquid. Boiling sprayer parts may work, depending on the brand of sprayer; you will have to experiment if you wish to try it. However, boiling will not kill all bacteria, and if you are bottling for resale, ethanol is the best choice. Never use anhydrous alcohol, as this has been chemically treated to remove the water content of ethyl. Food-grade hydrogen peroxide is another viable choice if you cannot obtain ethanol. Both the bottle and the sprayer units can be sterilized with peroxide in the same manner as with alcohol, but be sure to use food-grade peroxide and not the topical hydrogen peroxide used for wound cleaning and bleaching. Be careful; peroxide is very strong.

Ethyl alcohol has an advantage over peroxide in that it evaporates very rapidly. Thus, once rinsed, any residue left behind will totally evaporate in a minute or two. I have found it difficult to dry out the drips of hydrogen peroxide fast enough to feel that no recontamination occurs under nonlaboratory conditions. The best method with peroxide is to rinse the items with the peroxide, then dry the parts in a hot oven. Aseptic bottling of foodstuffs often uses this process, although it is automated in those cases.

The protocol we use at Acqua Vita is easy and quite effective. We sanitize just the number of bottles we intend to use immediately. All sprayers are separated into their components and placed in a sealed container of alcohol (sealed because the alcohol evaporates so readily). The bottles are then filled and rinsed with alcohol. The large containers of hydrosols are removed from the cold store only long enough to fill the bottles so that the overall temperature of the bulk quantity does not change. Some bottling is done in the cold store. The sterile bottles are filled with the hydrosol; the sprayers are removed from the ethyl, quickly dried off, and reassembled; and the lids are put on. We set up a little assembly line, and although it is slightly labor-intensive, the benefits justify the effort.

Proper Labeling

Labels are applied immediately, or even before bottling, as it is impossible to differentiate between a hundred blue bottles without removing the lids. The beauty of spray bottles is that once on, the lid never needs to be removed. From the day of bottling to the day the bottle is empty, you can dispense your hydrosol without risking contamination through frequent opening and closing of the container. Even when bottles are labeled STERILE CONTAINERS, DO NOT OPEN, I watch people walk over, unscrew the lid, and hold the bottle to their nose. I know they just can't help it, but really . . .

If you buy hydrosols to resell, you should include the distillation date, the expiration or best-before date, or both on your labels. You should also include the plant's country of origin as well as common and Latin names. The labeling requirements for hydrosols should be no less than those for oils.

No Added Preservatives

In my definition of hydrosols, I state that they must not contain additives or preservatives. This is a purist's definition; ultimately it is a matter of personal choice. If you do forego preservatives, the information about pH will help you monitor your unpreserved waters. Ethyl alcohol, a good sterilization medium, can be used also as a preservative, as it is in commercially available witch hazel, which is actually a hydrosol. *Hamamelis virginiana* is distilled only for its aromatic water, and this is the true witch hazel. However, the witch hazel you buy at the health-food store or pharmacy contains no less than 1 percent and up to 30 percent alcohol by volume. Witch hazel hydrosol is only moderately stable, and as it is sold in such huge quantities in so many outlets, something must be done to stabilize the product. Since witch hazel is often used as a "sports rub," adding ethyl alcohol to it is not considered a problem. However, as you will read under the profile of *Hamamelis,* there is much that it is good for, and many of these properties, such as its beneficial effect on varicose veins, are diminished by the addition of alcohol.

Another preservative being explored is grapefruit-seed extract. This natural compound has antioxidant properties and some bactericidal effects. However, it makes many hydrosols foamy, changes the pH, and is highly bitter, so only the debittered variety is appropriate for our purposes. If you are using hydrosols only topically, the bitterness is less of an issue, but I don't know anyone who doesn't want to drink rosewater or neroli or chamomile or bay or . . . There is also the issue of organics with grapefruit seed. Citrus fruit is heavily sprayed with chemicals from flowering to maturation. It is difficult to believe that none of these chemicals are found in the seed. Although I'm not in favor of its use at all, anyone seriously wishing to pursue this option should look for both debittered and organic grapefruit-seed extract.

After alcohol, chemicals are the most commonly used preservative. If asked to choose, I would take the alcohol over the chemicals any day. However, in the cosmetics industry, where many products contain hydrolates, chemicals are the standard procedure. Products made with preservative-free hydrosols do have a much shorter life,

and this would not be acceptable for a large commercial company.

Storage after Packaging

Storage of hydrosols after sterile bottling should be the same as for bulk storage: a cool or cold and constant temperature, away from heat and light. Treat hydrosols like you would milk or a bottle of mineral water. If you drink half a bottle of mineral water and then leave it in the car for two weeks, do you want to drink it again? It's just common sense. Treat hydrosols with a little respect and they will stay fresh for at least eight months and for up to two years or more from day of distillation.

Shelf Life and Marketing

Most products have a shelf life, and certainly all-natural products, particularly those without added preservatives, have a shelf life—usually a short one at that. Why, even Budweiser beer, which is preservative-free, has a shelf life of only 110 days. Why is it, then, so difficult for us to understand that hydrosols are the same? Perhaps it is because we are so spoiled by the longevity of most essential oils, which can have a long or even indefinite life span. Many improve with age like fine wine. Is this what has skewed our expectations of hydrosols?

Yet many aromatherapy exams include specific questions regarding the citrus and conifer oils because they have a relatively short shelf life.

It is considered good training to be aware of this and know how to deal with it. Oxidation of these monoterpene-rich oils can happen any time, and if it does, the oil is usually thrown away or used for household cleaning because of the increased dermocausticity.

Shelf life is a fact of life. Many of the carrier oils used in aromatherapy have short shelf lives: rose hip seed, avocado, hazelnut, macadamia, borage, evening primrose—the list is endless. Even long-life carrier oils like sesame, olive, and real sweet almond oil will go off eventually. So, although hydrosols *do* have a short life, many of the products we already incorporate into our aromatherapy practice actually have shorter lives. Perhaps our fears should be placed in perspective, where we can see that they are born mostly out of lack of knowledge and information and are not the final word on these wonderful products.

HYDROSOLS IN THE MARKETPLACE

Throughout this book are constant references to the subject of contamination and degradation of hydrosols, but for the most part, if you buy good products from a reputable supplier, care for the waters as directed, use them on a daily basis (it's the best way to see and feel the effects), and don't leave them where they will be damaged by high heat or bright lights, you will rarely have a problem with spoilage. Unfortunately this is of no benefit to those who wish to mass-market hydrosols.[20]

A Question of Scale?

The funny thing is that small-scale distribution and handling of hydrosols is easier than large-scale. Unless you gear up to transport and store everything in refrigerated trucks, put coolers at the retail outlets, and package only under sterile conditions with adequate filtration, you are creating the ideal conditions for problems to arise. Now, if hydrosols were treated like a foodstuff, or even beer (remember Bud?), then they would be handled in just this manner, but they are usually treated as cosmetics. The public treats very few cosmetics with this kind of elaborate care. However, most aestheticians will tell you that you should never put your fingers in a jar of cream because you introduce bacteria that will happily grow in that nice rich base. But do you use a little spatula to scoop your cream or face mask from the jar? Most people don't. So, for the mass market, a real change in thinking must occur if a hydrosol product is ever to become commercially viable.

Enter the grocery store. In the past three years a whole range of healthy beverages have been launched to capitalize on the juice-bar and health-food phenomenon. These drinks contain real fruit and a range of supplements like spirulina, wheat grass, ginseng, Saint John's wort, ginkgo, and so on. They contain no preservatives and have a short shelf life. It is not uncommon to see them in the cooler right beside the soda pops and iced-tea drinks. These products are changing the way people think about their beverage choices. For many, especially the hip young, the health conscious, and the upwardly mobile, it is these new drinks that fill the shopping cart. And these consumers pay attention to the dates, and they do drink them quickly, which means they also buy more. These beverages cost more, but that is to be expected of a natural-health product. It is quite a shift in consumer buying habits, and it has happened in a relatively short time.

Food, Not Fluff

Greg Farrell, reporting in *USA Today* in an article titled "Bottling Botanical Essences," states that in 1998 "these products racked up sales of $4 billion." A three-year-old company, South Beach, "which infuses all of its SoBe beverages with these herbs, projects sales of $180 million this year [1999]." Snapple Beverages also launched a healthy-drink product line called Elements, "peppered with new-age ingredients such as ginseng," reports Farrell. Marian Salzman, chief trend watcher at advertising agency Young and Rubicam, says, "Herbal everything is now. I think we can look for herbal helpers in everything from breakfast cereals to tea bags, from enriched waters to smart yoghurts." John Bello, the founder of SoBe, says, "There's an emerging health consciousness. It's a cultural shift and it has spawned a huge and growing industry."[21]

The mistake made with hydrosols has been to expect them to be sold in the same manner as essential oils or commercial body-care products. Why not take the idea from the health-juice companies: Create little custom fridges, beautifully decorated; splash freshness dates and instructions all over the labels and advertising; and promote the freshness, fragility, and purity of these fabulous substances. One practitioner I know doubled sales of hydrosols by putting a small glass-front fridge in her waiting room; it works!

And there's more to market with hydrosols. First, we're talking water here. Today around 30 percent of people carry bottles of water wherever they go. This is a new consciousness in plain view. Water is chic. Water is in. Water improves overall health, and people notice the difference. And hydrosols are water! Even better, hydrolates taste best when diluted in water, and they have definite healing properties. It's water that works and tastes like a health drink. And hydrosols are no more expensive than those little four-ounce "green drinks." And isn't linden blossom or wild ginger as exotic as mango and lichee?

Accessibility

In late 1999, nearly 50 percent of aromatherapy stores, distributors, and practitioners surveyed sold and/or used some hydrosols. Every new aromatherapy book at least mentions hydrosols, and every year new waters come into the marketplace. Interest is exploding, and the uses for hydrosols are no longer primarily as an additive to cosmetic or beauty products. We are seeing the birth of a new paradigm in the world of aromatherapy.

The renewed interest in the waters is partly the result of an increase in the variety now available. There is also a greater interest in the broader therapeutic possibilities of this new aromatherapy. Aromatherapists are not just aestheticians or just bodyworkers; they are holistic health practitioners. Educational standards in aromatherapy everywhere have been greatly improved, and professional, peer-reviewed organizations exist. Conferences, seminars, and educational opportunities abound, and professional insurance is mandatory. We are considering ourselves professionals in the field of health maintenance and care and we would like the public to consider us professionals as well.

The increase in professionalism also means that aromatherapists are seeking higher and higher standards in the quality of the products they use. A health professional wants a professional product, and today that means essential oils produced specifically for therapeutic use. The public is also catching on to this new standard, and the demand for quality products is starting to explode. As with any move forward, one finds that a level of information and education lies underneath. The quality issue was raised by the shift in the scope of practice and the surging popularity of aromatherapy. The information demands, which both created and resulted from these shifts, mean that most new books and the majority of aromatherapy companies now highlight quality as their biggest selling point: quality of information, quality of sources, quality of products, quality of practice. Only the best is good enough. And as was discussed in chapter 1, it is not a moment too soon. We can't treat health with polluted products.

Economics

But there is a finite amount of therapeutic-quality product available. Every year there is more, but demand is outstripping supply, and as with any natural product, there are no guarantees on yearly output. Nineteen ninety-nine saw a major harvest crisis in *Helichrysum italicum*, the herb known as immortelle. The resulting shortage caused the price of immortelle oil to nearly triple. This drastic situation coincided with a huge surge in consumer and practitioner interest in the oil and hydrosol, which has extraordinary health properties. The result is that immortelle may now sell for the same price as jasmine absolute.

Perhaps it is also because of the economics, at least in part, that hydrosols are becoming better known. As was discussed earlier, the sales of hydrosols can provide significant added income for a distiller. If the revenue from the sale of hydrosol is added to the income from the sale of the essential oil, even in a year of low yields distillers will be able to offset some of their losses on the oil with the income from the water. The distillation business is hard work, a labor of love requiring skilled employees for every aspect, and not everyone makes a good distiller. I like to compare it to wine production: Anyone can make wine, but not everyone makes Chateau Lafitte.

MAKING HYDROSOLS

While there is a body of knowledge, both written and oral, on essential-oil distillation, there is much less knowledge about the coproduct hydrosols. My own conversations with distillers reveal that making hydrosols differs quite a lot, depending on both the size of the still and the quantity and type of material being distilled. It also varies from year to year, just as the parameters for oil production vary depending on the amount of rainfall, length of season, hours of sun, mean annual temperature, geographical location, and so forth. In a wet year, such as 1998, the plants contain more water, and this greatly affects both the oils and the hydrosols. In fact, the 1998 crop of hydrosols was very prone to bloom, had significant variations in pH, and had the shortest life spans of any I have dealt with thus far.

There are some basic rules for collecting hydrosols. Generally the still is allowed to run for a period before the distillate waters begin to be collected. This is a bit complex to explain. First, the steam may actually run for some time before distillate begins to flow. In a still that holds five hundred kilograms of plant material, it may take from as little as thirty minutes to as long as two hours before the steam travels through the charge (plant material packed into the still) and makes its way to the condenser. At the receiving end of the condenser is a vessel known as a Florentine flask. As was explained earlier, the Florentine allows the hydrosol to flow out, once the flask is full, while the precious essential oils remain within the flask. A neat bit of design.

When the distillate water begins to flow from the condenser, it is rare for there to be any oil in the first few minutes. A small still with a high-oil-volume charge may produce oil within one to two minutes after flow commences; a larger still or a lower-oil-volume plant material may not produce oil for quite some time. Some distillers believe that the hydrosol should be collected only from the moment that oil droplets start appearing. Others believe you should take it from the beginning of the run.

Then there is the question of when to stop collecting the distillate. It is widely agreed that you do not collect all the hydrosol from a run. The chemicals that come over in the oil at the late stages of distillation are primarily non–water-soluble, large, and heavy molecules; as these would not have an appreciable water-soluble component, the hydrosol at this point is becoming more and more waterlike and could in fact dilute the hydrosol collected from the early stages. But what is the cut-off point? Here the alchemy and knowledge of the distiller are trump cards. However, there is a scientific component based on the changing chemistry of the distillates as the process happens and the pH changes. As a rule of thumb, no more than two-thirds of the distillate waters, frequently as little as 20 percent, is generally kept for use as hydrolate; the rest is allowed to flow away or is returned to the fields and the plants that were its source.[22]

Home Distillation

Home distillation kits are becoming the rage. This is happening both for the fun and experience of the process and because people are moving from cheaper commercial oil to expensive organic and authentic oil. It is natural to assume that you can make your own oils, and there is a certain cachet to distillation. However, as pointed out earlier, not everyone makes great oil, and some plant material contains so little oil that even a big home still is too small to produce usable quantities of plants like chamomile, rose, and angelica. However, home stills will produce hydrosol and can easily be used for this purpose.

Generally speaking, hydrosols are of better quality when essential oil is also produced in the distillation process. If you are not getting oil, it means one of two things. First, the oil is not being adequately extracted from the plants or is being lost during the process. Remedying this will require modifications to the still, steam source, or distillation parameters. Second, the oil is all in solution in the hydrolate. Now, depending on how much you want the oil, this may or may not matter to you. Although there is never very much oil in solution, it usually averages around 0.05 to 0.2 milliliter per liter. This can add up to a significant amount over several liters of hydrolate, and for this reason most home stills cohobate the waters. If you want your hydrosols to have maximum therapeutic value, you should not cohobate, but you will lose oil yield as a result. A few years ago I rigged up a home distiller for hydrosols; whenever I processed

oregano there was not a drop of oil to be seen, while sage and other plants produced both lovely oil and water. The oregano hydrosol was one of the strongest I ever had and I believe that was because of the quantity of the oil in suspension.

Remember also that we do not all live in the right climate for certain oil-bearing plants. Rose geranium, for instance, is African in origin, and although it will grow well outside in northern summers, it does not produce the same wonderful aroma. And, of course, we don't all have cinnamon trees in our yards. The home distillation enthusiast must be prepared for surprises and lots of experimentation.

GOOD CLEAN FUN

I should add one last thing here. Hydrosols are not only for health but also for pleasure. They can be played with, consumed, bathed in, washed with, poured in fountains, mixed with champagne, used on your pets, fed to your plants, and more. You can do whatever tickles your fancy with hydrosols, and you can afford to do it all. Hydrosols are not expensive. Even organic, top-quality hydrosols are reasonably priced, and they are virtually harmless. One mother I know puts her two boys in the tub armed with plastic spray bottles of diluted lavender hydrosol, then she leaves them to it. They have serious water fights and are graduating to hydrosol-filled water pistols! But it's just good clean fun, and they sleep like babies afterward. She can rest assured that as long as one doesn't bonk the other with the sprayer, the hydrosols will never hurt them.

If you make your own hydrosols, therapeutic or not, you have a wonderful aromatic "goodie" to enrich your life in winter, summer, spring, or fall. Cook with them, in sweets and savories. Pour them into shampoos, creams, lotions, or any body-care product, just for the smell of it. Iron your clothes with hydrosols; the French do. Spray your bed linens each night before retiring; pour some hydrosol in the rinse cycle of the washing machine or the dishwasher. The sky is the limit here, and after all the talk about contamination, storage, and filtering, the bottom line is that hydrosols really are fun, easy, and safe to use.

So go crazy, and let the living waters of distillation go with you.

THREE

The Monographs

Such flippant rejection of many millennia of accumulated knowledge has its price, as does the rejection of traditional medicine from foreign cultures.
Robert and Michele Root-Bernstein,
Honey, Mud, Maggots, and Other Medical Marvels

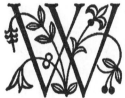hen I initially put together this chapter I divided it into two sections. The first covered those hydrosols that I had accumulated a large amount of data about, had spent time working with in my practice, and had received feedback about from my clients and other practitioners who also explored the waters. The second section covered those hydrosols that were still relatively unknown, at least to me, or those for which only a small amount of data and little or no clinical experience was available. After feedback from a couple of my diligent proofreaders, I decided to combine the two sections, listing all the monographs together. This means that you will find the known beside the unknown, large amounts of data followed by the briefest of descriptions.

It is an interesting thing that once you start exploring a subject, in this case hydrosols, the subject seems to come to you. So it is with the waters. In the time it has taken to write this book, no less than fifteen completely new waters have landed on my desk. The plants want to be heard, they have messages for us, and so their voices are combined, large and small, and I, for one, am impressed by their variety. The information has been compiled over four and a half years from many sources. Some scientific data does exist, but other information is the result of aromatherapy practice on real clients and the anecdotal evidence of people who work extensively with this new aromatherapy.

METHODOLOGY

So how did I arrive at my conclusions? Obviously it was a lengthy process. I began by considering the properties of the essential oil equivalent to the water, comparing the effects and eliminating those that did not appear to transfer to the hydrosol, and making notes on the "new" properties that seemed to be unique to the water. However, I realized there were too many possibilities that I could be missing, so I devised a new method. For each hydrosol, I made notes that listed therapeutic properties ascribed to the plant in all its various forms. The properties list covered herb (fresh and dried), tincture, decoction, infusion, tea, macerated oil, essential oil, homeopathic remedy, local and traditional applications, and in some cases Ayurvedic uses and Chinese medicinal properties. The lists were huge! But by going over them carefully I found obvious overlaps, properties that appeared in every form and others that appeared frequently enough to be noteworthy.

Gallons of hydrosols have been consumed in the past few years by myself, clients, colleagues, our families, and our animals. The process of elimination has yielded some of my findings. When the importance of the pH values became clear, they too were incorporated into my lists, and I know they are significant factors. For instance, Dr. H. C. Baser, in his presentation at the Third Aromatherapy Conference on Therapeutic Uses of Essential Oils, said that chemical analysis of oregano hydrosol showed no indication that it has antiviral or even marked antiseptic properties, yet my experience says that it has both. But by looking at the pH and thinking about the bacteriostatic properties of a substance with a 4.2 pH, we can see that even if the chemistry doesn't indicate antiseptic properties, the pH does, and this probably gives the hydrosol its in vivo effects. There is still so much to learn.

Of course, there were more than a few surprises, and in some cases the waters act like one particular therapeutic form of the plant, be it the homeopathic, the fresh herb, or the oil. But when there are still too many unanswered questions, I have called the uses experimental. Is this data written in stone? I hope not. Unlike so much of the information in aromatherapy books, this is all pretty new. We've been compiling our data on the oils for a very long time, and science has added its own dimension to our knowledge. Unfortunately, this isn't so for the waters. I am sure that over the next few years new research will come to light, and I look forward to the information explosion. I want to continue learning about these incredible aromatic waters. As I said, this information is not carved in stone, but it is a basis to work from, a starting point, and at the moment that's what we need.

CHEMOTYPES

Since we are dealing with the therapeutic properties of hydrosols, we must be as specific as possible concerning the origins of the waters. When it comes to the subject of chemotypes, there is still much confusion and misunderstanding in aromatherapy circles. I have seen articles printed in the journals of reputable organizations that completely confused chemotypes and functional groups (the chemical groups in essential oils and hydrosols), which is really a shame, because this promotes confusion, not education and growth.

A chemotype (CT) occurs when a plant of a specific genus and species produces a particular chemical in a higher than normal amount because of geographic location, weather, altitude, insect and environmental interactions, and the like. A chemotype is not a different species or genus, nor is it a type of chemical; it is merely a chemical anomaly within the plant that occurs naturally. A case in point is thyme, specifically the genus *Thymus* and the species *vulgaris*. Thyme produces at least six different recognized chemotypes. At least four of these are available from good aromatherapy suppliers. Commercial purveyors of oils tend to refer simply to red thyme and white thyme, indicating those that are potentially dermocaustic, red, versus those that are not dermocaustic, white. This may be of some help to the practitioner, but it is not the whole story. Red thyme could be thyme CT carvacrol or thyme CT thymol, while white thyme could be thyme CT linalol or thyme CT geraniol.

Thyme CT thuyanol contains an alcohol (alcohols are a functional group) that has as much "killing power" as a phenol (another functional group). It could, therefore, be considered red thyme by some, but others might consider it white thyme, since thuyanol causes no dermocausticity even undiluted but is strong enough for the most nasty infection. Then there is thyme CT paracymene, a monoterpene chemotype (monoterpenes are a functional group) that one

would probably consider white thyme, since monoterpenes are not particularly dermocaustic unless oxidized. However, thyme CT paracymene may cause skin irritations in sensitive people, and therefore it might just as easily be labeled red thyme. Thus, to refer to thyme in simplistic terms can only increase confusion and a fear of using the oil. This is not healing.

In understanding the complexity, using thyme becomes easier. By being specific, the user can choose the most effective treatment and remove a good part of the guesswork. So, a fungal infection on the skin could be successfully treated with an alcohol chemotype like thyme CT linalol, while a chronic condition of this type may respond better to a stronger phenol chemotype. As this is a dermal infection requiring topical applications, you could use thyme CT thymol but only in low dilution owing to its dermocausticity, or you could turn to the unique thyme CT thuyanol, since it is not irritating to the skin but acts like a phenol. A blend to treat this kind of condition could contain both thyme CT linalol and thyme CT thuyanol for maximum efficacy.

I refer to separate chemotypes of hydrosols so that the users of this book can look for the best possible choice from the many options available. Also, it is the sign of good distillers and/or suppliers that they offer chemotype-specific hydrosols. In all likelihood, this means they are producing aromatics specifically for aromatherapy purposes only.

PROTOCOLS

The standard dilution rate for the internal use of hydrosols for therapy is thirty milliliters (two tablespoons) of hydrosol diluted in one liter (thirty-two ounces) of water. If you wish only to flavor your water, use the smallest amount necessary to give the desired intensity of taste. Of course, using only a tiny amount of hydrosol does not mean that it does not have an effect on the person. Hydrosols are very powerful, physically and vibrationally. I have already discussed the homeopathic comparison, so do bear this in mind if you flavor your water on a regular basis. Never choose a hydrosol with properties that may be inappropriate to your body or mind. You will often be drawn to what you need, but it is always important to check the properties of any given hydrosol before you start using it.

In holistic health, treatments are often given on a three-week basis. You use the remedy, oil, herb, or preparation every day for three weeks, then stop for one week. This is an important part of natural healing. The body needs time to register, process, and then incorporate changes. By taking time off, you allow the changes and adjustments that the treatment has made to be assimilated. You allow the health to come to a new balance, a new homeostasis. After seven days without treatment you will be able to reassess the health condition and make a better decision on what else is needed, if anything. If you keep making changes without cease, the body does not have time to catch up, and you may continue treatment longer than is necessary or advisable. Use respect: Less is more.

The Three-Week Internal Protocol

In the three-week protocol, thirty milliliters (two tablespoons) of hydrosol dissolved in one liter of distilled water or springwater is to be consumed throughout the day. This is repeated daily for twenty-one days, then stopped for seven days. (In the case of Greenland moss *[Ledum groenlandicum]*, use fifteen milliliters [one tablespoon] of hydrosol, not thirty.)

This protocol is most useful when addressing specific health concerns and issues of a constitutional nature. For instance, lymphatic congestion that is causing swollen lymph nodes could be treated with a three-week protocol of bay laurel. If the swelling in the nodes disappears in the first few days, it is still worth continuing the treatment, as this helps create an environment in which the symptoms are less likely to reoccur. However, if the nodes are still clear after the seven days off, you would know that you do not need to resume the treatment.

A constitutional predisposition to asthma attacks in stressful conditions could also be treated with the three-week protocol. In this case we would aim not at dealing with the asthma but at treating the stress response. Hydrosols of lemon balm, Saint John's wort, and neroli are a few options; they could be combined or used individually. If the body is less likely to become stressed, then the attacks are less likely to happen. This also helps break the learned stress response. If a certain situation no longer stresses you during the three weeks you are consuming the hydrosol, it is less likely to stress you in the future. In this case the week off would determine whether another three-week cycle should be undertaken based on the reoccurrence of the asthma attacks.

HOW THE MONOGRAPHS ARE PRESENTED

The profile on each hydrosol is given in three sections: "Aroma and Taste," "Stability and Shelf-Life," and "Properties and Applications." I have listed the hydrosols in alphabetical order by their Latin name, but below I have provided a chart of common names and pH values arranged alphabetically by common name so you can reference the Latin names and find them in the book. This is done for reasons of clarity and because plants have correct names just as people do, and they appreciate it greatly when we bother to learn them.

The abbreviations *flos, ec, z,* and *fe,* that sometimes appear after the Latin name refer to the flower, bark, zest, and leaf, respectively.

CONTRAINDICATIONS

AVOID means what it says; don't use it under the specific conditions listed. Contraindications are rare with hydrosols, so if they are mentioned, it's for a reason.[1]

Table of Common and Latin Names and pH Values

ENGLISH NAME	LATIN NAME	pH
Angelica root	*Angelica archangelica*	3.8
Artemesia	*Artemesia vulgaris*	3.8–4.0
Balsam fir	*Abies balsamea*	3.8–4.0
Basil	*Ocimum basilicum*	4.5–4.7
Bay laurel	*Laurus nobilis*	4.9–5.2
Black currant	*Ribes nigrum*	3.6
Black spruce	*Picea mariana*	4.2–4.4
Calamus root	*Acorus calamus*	4.6
Cardamom pod	*Elettaria cardamomum*	4.5

Cedarwood	*Cedrus atlantica*	4.1–4.2
Cinnamon bark	*Cinnamomum zeylanicum* (ec)	3.3
Cinnamon leaf	*Cinnamomum zeylanicum* (fe)	3.9
Clary sage	*Salvia sclarea*	5.5–5.7
Clementine petitgrain	*Citrus clementine* (fe)	4.3–4.4
Coriander/cilantro	*Coriandrum sativum*	3.5–3.7
Cornflower	*Centaurea cyanus*	4.7–5.0
Cypress	*Cupressus sempervirens*	3.8–4.0
Elder flower	*Sambucus nigra*	4.0–4.2
Elecampane	*Inula graveolens*	4.7–4.9
Eucalyptus	*Eucalyptus globulus*	4.1–4.3
Fennel seed	*Foeniculum vulgare*	4.0–4.1
Fleabane	*Erigeron canadensis*	3.9
Frankincense	*Boswellia carterii*	4.7–4.9
Geranium/rose geranium	*Pelargonium x asperum/P. roseat*	4.9–5.2
German chamomile	*Matricaria recutita*	4.0–4.1
Goldenrod	*Solidago canadensis*	4.1–4.3
Green myrtle	*Myrtus communis*	5.7–6.0
Greenland moss	*Ledum groenlandicum*	3.8–4.0
Immortelle	*Helichrysum italicum*	3.5–3.8
Jasmine	*Jasminum sambac*	5.6
Juniper berry	*Juniperus communis*	3.3–3.6
Larch/tamarack	*Larix laricina*	3.5
Lavender	*Lavandula angustifolia*	5.6–5.9
Lemon verbena	*Lippia citriodora*	5.2–5.5

Linden/lime flower	*Tilia europaea*	6.3–6.5
Melissa/lemon balm	*Melissa officinalis*	4.8–5.0
Neroli	*Citrus aurantium* var. *amara* (flos)	3.8–4.5
Orange mint	*Mentha citrata*	5.9–6.0
Oregano	*Origanum vulgare*	4.2–4.4
Peppermint	*Mentha piperita*	6.1–6.3
Purple bee balm	*Monarda fistulosa*	4.1–4.3
Purple coneflower	*Echinacea purpurea*	3.9
Rock rose	*Cistus ladaniferus*	2.9–3.1
Roman chamomile	*Chamaemelum nobile*	3.0–3.3
Rose	*Rosa damascena*	4.1–4.4
Rosemary camphor	*Rosmarinus officinalis* CT1	4.6–4.7
Rosemary 1,8 cineole	*Rosmarinus officinalis* CT2	4.2–4.5
Rosemary verbenone	*Rosmarinus officinalis* CT3	4.5–4.7
Sage	*Salvia officinalis*	3.9–4.2
Saint John's wort	*Hypericum perforatum*	4.5–4.6
Sandalwood	*Santalum album*	5.9–6.0
Scarlet bee balm	*Monarda didyma*	4.2–4.4
Scotch pine	*Pinus sylvestris*	4.0–4.2
Seaweed	*Fucus vesiculosus* and others	N/A
Sweet fern	*Comptonia peregrina*	3.8
Sweet gale	*Myrica gale*	3.7–3.8
Tarragon	*Artemesia dracunculus*	4.2
Thyme geraniol	*Thymus vulgaris* CT1	5.0–5.2
Thyme linalol	*Thymus vulgaris* CT2	5.5–5.7

Thyme thuyanol	*Thymus vulgaris* CT5	4.6–4.8
Thyme thymol	*Thymus vulgaris* CT6	4.5–4.6
Tea tree	*Melaleuca alternifolia*	3.9–4.1
White sage	*Salvia apiana*	3.6
Wild carrot seed	*Daucus carota*	3.8–4.0
Wild ginger	*Asarum canadense*	5.4
Winter savory	*Satureja montana*	4.1–4.2
Witch hazel	*Hamamelis virginiana*	4.0–4.2
Yarrow	*Achillea millefolium*	3.6–3.9

The information provided in this section refers only to hydrosols. Never substitute essential oils for hydrosols. They are much stronger, are not water soluble, and should not be used in the same manner as hydrosols.

THE HYDROSOLS

Abies balsamea/Balsam fir
pH 3.8–4.0

Aroma and Taste A woodsy taste and fragrance. Slightly musty and simultaneously wet and dry in smell. The taste is slightly flat and better in warm, sweetened drinks than in cold beverages.

Stability and Shelf Life Stable; good for fourteen to sixteen months, although the aroma starts to fade around twelve months.

Properties and Applications Balsam fir is the best-known "Christmas" tree and comes into its own in the dark months of winter. Recommended primarily for external applications, although some internal use is fine, but I do not recommend the three-week internal protocol.

A good general system tonic, balsam fir is antiseptic and seems to boost the immune system. It is of great benefit to sufferers of SAD (seasonal affective disorder); just smelling it can lift me from the winter gloom! Add it to the bath or shower (put the plug in); use one-fourth to one-half cup two or three times a week. A significant improvement is usually noticed after the first week. It is an excellent addition to bath or foot soaks at any time of the year, being neither heating nor cooling but still able to stimulate the system.

Balsam fir is both mucolytic and expectorant for the respiratory, renal, and reproductive systems. Use in inhalations, saunas, steam baths, humidifiers, and compresses. It is a good gargle or tea for winter. Mildly diuretic, it can also help remove fluid from joints and is a good topical compress for rheumatic, arthritic, muscular, and joint pain. It is gently stimulating to circulation while calming the mind, being energetically expansive and opening.

For chest congestion, use balsam fir in a compress, on its own or in combination with essential oils. Follow with a rub of essential oils including balsam fir; wrap up the chest with a warm, dry cloth and go to bed. This can be repeated several times a day.

For joint or muscle pain, use hot or cold compresses according to the individual and the condition.

Achillea millefolium/Yarrow
pH 3.6–3.9

Aroma and Taste   Strongly aromatic but not particularly pleasant; has been described as "puppy breath." Absolutely not floral in aroma or taste. The flavor is better than the smell but not by a lot, and it tastes better in stronger dilution than in weaker ones.

Stability and Shelf Life   Stable to very stable; can last up to two years, although it may develop a gray color and fine particulate matter after about fourteen months. Check the pH if you have any doubts.

Properties and Applications   One metric ton of yarrow flowers produces less than five hundred milliliters (one-half liter) of oil, so this is perhaps one of the more potent hydrosols. It is a good digestive aid and is significantly detoxifying, but in a gentle manner. A three-week course will improve digestion, increase elimination, and calm gastric spasms and rumbles and is recommended as part of a cleanse or weight-loss program. It improves digestion of fatty foods and seems to have hepatostimulant and/or cholagogue (bile releasing) properties, since it can quickly relieve indigestion and heartburn caused by overindulgence. Yarrow is antispasmodic for the digestive, reproductive, and muscular systems, used topically or internally. Cooling, it

helps reduce fever and eases aches and pains in association with flu and colds. It is anti-inflammatory and can be used as a compress with cypress for varicose veins and in a sitz bath for hemorrhoids and excessive or painful menstrual periods or postpartum healing.

A great balancer both physically and mentally, yarrow stabilizes body fluids and gets rid of excess water without being overly diuretic. Use it in a compress on its own or in combination with goldenrod for fluid in joints and rheumatic pain or for any area of swelling where fluid has accumulated. A mild antibacterial and antiseptic, it helps with problem skin, acneic conditions, and dermal infections, and as an anti-inflammatory it helps heal damage from sun and wind. Effective for cleaning wounds, it helps stop bleeding and could be used as an aftershave for its styptic properties, although, because of its odor, you may wish to blend it with other, more pleasingly aromatic waters. Yarrow is a good ingredient to use in a douche or sitz bath for endometriosis, in synergy with *Cistus*. This condition is quite serious, but hydrosols and oils can greatly reduce the severity and pain of the condition. This can reduce the need for opiate-based pharmaceuticals, which are commonly the only option.

Yarrow is a very effective water for use on

animals, as they like the smell. Skin problems and digestive issues will benefit particularly. For some the aroma is off-putting. In this case, combine yarrow with other hydrosols and essential oils that improve its fragrance. This water provides mental calm and can help one find peace. Like the oil, it is highly energetic and good for spiritual or distance work. Combine it with juniper berry for cleansing the aura, crystals, and work spaces.

Acorus calamus/Calamus Root/Sweet Flag
pH 4.6

Aroma and Taste   Highly unusual. One of the strangest odors you will ever encounter and a case of love it or hate it for most people. It is a peculiarly masculine aroma, and certainly it's preferred by men more than by women; perhaps that's why it's used in perfumery, to attract men!

Stability and Shelf Life   Stable.   Easily lasts eighteen months, probably reliably for two years.

Properties and Applications   Canadian calamus contains none of the hepatotoxic ketone beta-asarone, making it completely safe for use in aromatherapy both internally and externally. European and Asian calamus contain high levels of beta-asarone and should not be used for aromatherapy.

Calamus is a specific for the liver and can be used with Greenland moss in topical compresses and poultices for liver infections and dysfunction and hepatitis. French aromatherapy experiments by Dominique Baudoux with both topical and internal use of these two essential oils have yielded some very promising results in treating tumors and cancers in the liver, and the hydrosols are worth further exploration. A seven-day test of Aromatic Tincture of milk thistle and calamus-root hydrosol worked wonderfully well in detoxifying the liver and gallbladder, and it is certainly nicer and easier to take as a treatment than the better-known lemon and olive oil gallbladder cleanse and appears to be similarly effective.

Calamus is best known in perfumery, where it is used as a fixative and base note. The hydrosol makes a gently astringent aftershave on its own or combined with sandalwood, cedarwood, or bay laurel. My father reacted more positively to calamus than to any other aroma I have ever offered him; he practically grabbed it out of my hand and declared, "That's what I want in an aftershave!" He got it.

Angelica archangelica/Angelica Root
pH 3.8

Aroma and Taste Unusual. The first aromatic impression is reminiscent of dirty socks, but it is quickly followed by the dry, sweet, green herbaceous scent of the plant and oil. The flavor is slightly fruity, strongly earthy but not earthlike, with a hint of green floral tones, a really lovely taste. Diluted it becomes quite mild and retains the fruity-floral edge. There is also a hydrosol from angelica seed.

Stability and Shelf Life Unknown, but certainly twelve months or more.

Properties and Applications Experimental. Distinctly sedative, grounding, and calming to the nerves and very useful for anxiety states or high stress. A mild digestive, although not nearly as effective as the oil, perhaps because the hydrosol lacks the bitter principals to the same degree. It is warming to the system and can be used to increase appetite and tone the digestion.

Energetically, angelica is said to bridge heaven and earth, connect the seventh chakra to the first, and still have a grounding effect. When dowsed with a pendulum, both the oil and the hydrosol exhibit a phenomenal energy field, and so intention of use becomes a contributing factor in its applications for vibrational healing.

Artemesia dracunculus/Tarragon
pH 4.2 (variable)

Aroma and Taste A distinct licorice/anise scent but with the complex overtones of fresh tarragon; really lovely if you like tarragon. The flavor is very potent, almost overpowering when undiluted, but it softens considerably at normal dilution. Delicious, unusual, and hard to find reliably.

Stability and Shelf Life Unknown; at least twelve months.

Properties and Applications Significant digestive aid; relieves gas, bloating, colic, gastric spasms, and hiccups. Seems to have a relaxing effect on the nervous system, calming stress-related physical symptoms.

The essential oil is used in asthma treatments for its significant antispasmodic properties, and the hydrosol also seems to have pronounced antispasmodic properties, at least for the digestive tract. It is worthy of further investigation in respiratory conditions like asthma, whooping cough, and spasms of the diaphragm.

Absolutely delicious in cooking, and if you like tarragon, the hydrosol makes a wonderful beverage. Take it when traveling to keep the system working despite time zones and stress.

Artemesia vulgaris/Artemesia
pH 3.8–4.0

Aroma and Taste The French variety of artemesia is quite different from the variety grown and distilled in North America. It is much softer in smell, decidedly herbal, but not too green. The taste is herbaceous, bitter, and astringent, very drying in the mouth when taken undiluted. In dilution, the flavor softens significantly and has a more warming feel.

Stability and Shelf Life Moderately stable; lasts around eighteen months.

Properties and Applications This is one of the hydrosols used by Nelly Grosjean, in conjunction with her frictions, for both the digestive and circulatory systems.

A circulatory-system stimulant, artemesia seems to affect the capillaries and improves peripheral circulation. Artemesia can be used as part of a cleansing program to clean the blood, detoxify the liver, and improve overall digestion, especially in the spring or at the change of seasons. It greatly aids antiparasite treatments of all kinds, especially when combined with Roman chamomile hydrosol and oregano, cinnamon bark, clove, and tarragon essential oils,

which can be made into capsules with some bentonite clay. Its bitter and astringent qualities make it beneficial to the renal system. Try an Aromatic Tincture of dandelion and artemesia hydrosol.

I have found artemesia useful for respiratory complaints, particularly those of an allergic nature. It exhibits antihistamine, antitussive, antiinflammatory, and mild expectorant effects, although I do recommend a patch test or internal test dose before using it on people with multiple sensitivities and asthma. Internally, it is restorative for the reproductive system and can help rebalance the menstrual cycle when discontinuing oral contraceptives. Topically, it can be of benefit in a compress or bath for stiff, sore, or aching muscles caused by overexertion, especially when combined with black spruce and/or Scotch pine.

Very energetic, it is useful in rituals, vibrational healing, and working with the elemental and spirit world.

Note: There are many varieties of artemesia and some are best avoided. Ensure the correct botanical name of the hydrosol you purchase. See also another *Artemesia* under tarragon *(A. dracunculus)*.

Asarum canadense/Wild Ginger/Canadian Ginger
pH 5.4

Aroma and Taste   The fragrance is incredibly mild, almost faint; there is no hotness to it, rather a sweet, not quite spicy note, with only the barest resemblance to real ginger. The taste is even milder, so mild I often double the dose if I drink it just for flavor, and the flavor is just gorgeous. It is delicate, gentle, and closer to a flower than a root, neutral or perhaps on the cooling side instead of heating like the oil.

Stability and Shelf Life   Despite its pH, this hydrosol seems to have a long shelf life, eighteen months or more. I have one batch at two and one-half years that is still totally stable.

Properties and Applications   Native Americans drank a tea of wild ginger for treating arrhythmia and heart pain. The cardiotonic properties of wild ginger are mentioned in several herbals, and I have found the hydrosol useful in calming and balancing people prone to anxiety attacks, type A personality, and illness-related stress states. The powdered root boiled into a tea was used as an antimicrobial by several First Nation tribes, and based on this I have also tried the hydrosol on respiratory infections with some success, taking one tablespoon undiluted every hour for as long as necessary in cases of bronchitis and severe chest colds. One woman claims it cleared up her chest in three days with no other remedies.

Wild ginger also has traditional uses as a digestive and carminative, reducing gas and abdominal bloating, especially when caused by stress. Its effects on the nerves has also led to its use for neuralgia, sciatica, and headaches, including migraines. It was used by the Pomo Indian women of California to balance the menstrual cycle and so may affect the endocrine as well as nervous systems.

Chinese medicine uses wild ginger to open the meridians and improve the movement of chi, and it can be used in vibrational healing for balancing energy, with good results. I have consumed as much as three hundred milliliters of this hydrosol in one day and felt quite fantastic afterward.

Highly energetic, this tiny plant with its barely belowground creeping rhizome has been overharvested to extinction in many places. It is important, therefore, to buy only from sources that you are sure do not upset the balance of nature by unscrupulous wild-crafting.

Boswellia carterii/Frankincense
pH 4.7–4.9

Aroma and Taste Extraordinary. The scent is sweeter than the oil but unmistakably frankincense. Slightly resinous, like the conifers can be, the odor is also a little warmer than the steam-distilled oil, reminding me more of the CO_2 extract. The taste is quite bitter when undiluted but not unappealing. Diluted, it is divine and loses all the bitterness, becoming soft, warm, and very dry.

Stability and Shelf Life Unknown. Estimated at eighteen months.

Properties and Applications Experimental. The first effect is of energetic expansion. Taking a drop or two undiluted gives the distinct sensation that the "energy body" is expanding outward, rapidly, from the solar plexus. Try it before meditation, in ritual work, with crystals, or any form of energy healing. The oil is known to deepen and expand breathing and open airways, and the hydrosol seems to retain that property and can dry up excess mucus in the lungs and help expel phlegm. In "aromapuncture" treatments, one drop of frankincense on the lung points elicited a deep breathing that manifested an altered state almost on contact. Quite astounding and worth further exploration.

Internally frankincense is diuretic and very drying, and it should be explored for use in conditions where pus or discharge is present. It may be particularly beneficial in mouth or gum infections as a gargle, perhaps combined with immortelle, as well as for infections of the reproductive and urinary systems, in combination with sandalwood or *Cistus*.

Topically frankincense is fantastic on the skin. Mist over the face and leave it to air dry and your skin will have a noticeably finer texture almost immediately. Of great value where summer heat is combined with high humidity. Frankincense can be used in face masks for an instant lift or combined with rock rose and others for daily wrinkle treatments.

Cedrus atlantica/Cedarwood/Atlas Cedar
pH 4.1–4.2

Aroma and Taste   A light fragrance; dry, woody, almost sawdustlike, with sweet overtones. Reminds one of a cold sauna or cedar closet, although these are usually made from the wood of North American cedar (*Thuja* sp.), not the mountain or Mediterranean cedar (*Cedrus* sp.). Quite different from the pervasive aroma of the oil.

Stability and Shelf Life   Very stable. The odor begins to diminish after eighteen months, but the properties seem to be consistent up to two years or more, depending on the source.

Properties and Applications   This hydrosol is primarily used for topical applications. I do not recommend it for internal use except for specific pathologies, as it is extremely diuretic.

Cedarwood is the first choice for hair care. It has been used successfully as a treatment for thinning hair, some types of hair loss, scalp itch, and dandruff and to add shine and luster to dry, damaged, or treated hair. The French use it to soften and detangle hair as well as for dandruff. Shampoos can be diluted by 50 percent with the hydrosol, and conditioners by 30 percent or more. Cedar blends very well with rosemary CT cineole (for all hair colors) and both sage (for red and dark hair) and chamomile (for blond hair), although sage can easily overpower the cedar aroma.

This is also the hydrosol for animal fur. Its delicate aroma makes it well suited to use on cats to get rid of dander and help deter fleas. For dogs it can be used as a final rinse to be left on the coat after a bath for fleas, and it certainly makes them shiny and sweet smelling. Use in a spray bottle and add two or three drops of cedar oil for a daily flea spray in summer and autumn. Dogs seem to have a predilection for certain smells, and cedar is one of them.

Some skin conditions respond well to cedar, particularly weeping and cracked skin, some types of psoriasis, peeling and sweaty feet, dermatitis, allergic rashes, chicken pox, cold sores, and inflamed acne. Usually compresses of the straight hydrosols, or a strong dilution of 50 to 70 percent hydrosol and cool springwater, are the best option in treating skin. Cedarwood also combines well with yarrow hydrosol if intense itching accompanies the condition.

This hydrosol is wonderful in the bath, especially cool summer baths when the humidity is high. I put it in a kiddie pool and both my dog and I emerge greatly refreshed! Try it in the sauna; it is safe to sprinkle it directly on the rocks and it will help release mucus and phlegm from the lungs, or use it in a foot soak for tired hot feet after you've been standing all day long.

Centaurea cyanus/Cornflower/Bachelor's Button
pH 4.7–5.0

Aroma and Taste An extremely delicate scent. When the hydrosol is cold, the odor is almost undetectable; warm, it becomes vaguely floral. The flavor undiluted is also delicate, a little green, neither particularly floral nor herbal, with a slightly bitter aftertaste but nothing unpleasant. Diluted, the flavor almost disappears, and one smells more than tastes it.

Stability and Shelf Life Unstable to moderately stable; shelf life twelve months.

Properties and Applications Almost interchangeable with sandalwood hydrosol in topical treatment of skin conditions. One of only four hydrosols recommended as an eyewash (the other three are Roman and German chamomile and green myrtle). This probably has the widest application as an eyedrop substitute, and users who wear contact lenses say it works very well for them, although it should probably not be used while the lenses are in the eye. Topically, use cornflower as a compress for tired, swollen, or itchy eyes or for the effects of pollution or long hours at the computer.

Renowned for its cosmetic applications and cool feeling on the skin, cornflower is used to tone crepey skin and firm delicate and mature skin of the décolleté. It is also wonderful for dry and devitalized skin and can be added to masks, lotions, creams, toners, and makeup removers or used on its own before the application of a moisturizer. Combine it with rose geranium to combat very dry climates, on airplanes, or to give a dewy complexion. Daily compresses on the eye area, particularly when combined with rock rose, will visibly diminish fine lines and tone the tissue. Combine with witch hazel or lavender for cleansing cuts and wounds and compressing bruises. Cornflower is a good choice for diluting shampoos and conditioners or massaging into the scalp; it gives hair shine and highlights and is less drying than chamomile for blond hair.

A general system tonic, cornflower was once used as a tea against the plague. Why, I don't know, except that plague victims probably tried everything. Mildly diuretic and digestive, its bitter principals make it supportive to the liver and gently astringent. On its own or in combination with juniper, cypress, or tea tree, it makes an effective douche for urinary tract infections and is gentle enough not to irritate sensitive tissue. Internally and topically it can be used to reduce fever, particularly in infants, as its delicate odor is well tolerated. Research indicates that it may contain phytohormones, and it is certainly worth trying for hot flashes, both topically and internally.

AVOID during first trimester of pregnancy because of potential presence of phytohormones.

Chamaemelum nobile/Roman Chamomile
pH 3.0–3.3

Aroma and Taste   Extremely sweet, honeylike aroma and taste. Even more apple overtones than the oil has but softer, more delicate. Occasionally it will have a greener, more haylike aroma, but this appears to be a consequence of the distillation parameters and to me indicates an inferior product.

Stability and Shelf Life   Very stable, easily lasts for two years or more, although it is so popular that stock rarely lasts that long. I have some chamomile that is four years old and still quite fine.

Properties and Applications   One of the best all-purpose waters, right up there with lavender and melissa.

Roman chamomile is the number-one choice for baby care. It can safely be used right from birth, in bath water and as a soothing mist for bedding. Mothers can use it diluted to wash the breast area, and in addition to helping prevent cracked and sore nipples, its calming properties will make feeding time even more relaxing. Babies will soon associate the aroma of chamomile with Mummy and yummy. When child care is required, the handover is easier if the caregiver uses chamomile as well, as the child will feel that Mother is near. Diaper-rash redness and pain can be soothed with dilute chamomile, or use neat applications of a 50:50 blend of Roman chamomile and lavender waters to compress the tender skin. New mothers can use it in a compress or a sitz bath for postpartum relief. Homemade wet wipes for babies and young children should always include chamomile.

When teething starts, add two or three drops to a bottle of water to help calm diarrhea and stomach upset. Rub the gums with diluted chamomile frequently to reduce inflammation, swelling, and pain and to help soothe the associated crankiness. Children adore the flavor of sweet chamomile and will soon ask for it as they recognize the relief it brings. Spritzing a light mist over the blankets or in the air of the child's room will help children sleep.

Because of its effect on the nervous system, chamomile is a useful aid in stress reduction, depression, relaxation, insomnia, and aggravation. Combine it with melissa or one of the tree waters if alertness is required and to help calm road rage. It can be mildly euphoric, instilling a feeling of well-being. Use as a bedtime tea or bath for reducing stress, for physical relaxation, and for a restful night.

Chamomile is wonderful for skin care, for calming rashes, sensitivities, rosacea, acne, heat rash, and redness. Use it like lavender for burns and sunburns. It is the best all-in-one makeup remover, skin cleanser, and toner. Chamomile is fairly astringent owing to its very acid pH; do not use it singly or long-term on very dry skin, windburn, or similar conditions. Combined with neroli it is good for acneic conditions and oily skin; combine it with witch hazel for mature skin and with lavender or geranium for very dry skin.

Roman chamomile is one of only four hydrosols recommended as an eyewash, with German chamomile, cornflower, and green myrtle being the others. Compress eyes and wash them frequently with this and/or German chamomile for conjunctivitis. It is a good daily eyewash for soothing the effects of pollution, computer burn, and general redness.

Its very low pH makes chamomile a suit-able addition to a douche or bidet, and it will calm itching and noninfectious inflammations. It can also be used in combination with oregano or savory hydrosols in treating vaginitis and thrush. Men will find it useful as a wash for jock itch and general hygiene.

Pets, like babies, can derive great benefits from chamomile, which can reduce stress before travel, after a fight, during a storm, or even when visiting the vet. Teething, especially in puppies, can be as much of an ordeal for owners as for pets; use the same treatment for teething animals as you would for teething babies.

Basically, Roman chamomile is a must-have hydrosol.

Cinnamomum zeylanicum (ec)/Cinnamon Bark
Cinnamomum zeylanicum (fe)/Cinnamon Leaf
Bark: pH 3.3   Leaf: pH 3.9

Aroma and Taste   The leaf hydrosol is a candy: sweet, yummy, just like the best cinnamon sweetie you ever tasted. The bark hydrosol has a deeper cinnamon scent, with that intense edge one finds in the oil—candy for grown-ups. The flavor is also more intense but not at all hot, just wonderful. Both hydrosols are powerful but quite delicious undiluted and retain their flavors well even in microdilution.

Stability and Shelf Life   The leaf hydrosol seems very stable; I have a batch currently at two years with no sign of fading. The bark hydrosol is also stable and probably lasts eighteen to twenty-four months.

Properties and Applications   It took me three years to find cinnamon water, and then I got both leaf and bark within six months. Drink them for sheer pleasure, add them to coffee for a wonderful touch, or combine cinnamon, coriander seed, and cardamom pod hydrosols with hot water for an aromatherapy chai.

The leaf has a strong affinity for the

autonomic nervous system, balancing dramatic fluctuations and providing profound relief in states of extreme stress. One client has been using it almost continuously for a year while dealing with a particularly nasty court case and claims it has given her clarity and the ability to cope unlike anything else.

The bark is quite stimulating to the mind and body, excellent when one is tired and concentration and focus are required, much better than coffee and delicious *with* coffee. An amazing digestive, it relieves bloat and colic pains very quickly. The bark oil is famous for its ability to kill infections of the digestive tract without damaging the beneficial flora; it appears that the hydrosol has similar, if slightly less potent, effects, and using the two in synergy can achieve pretty remarkable results. Combine cinnamon with yarrow—yes, it overpowers yarrow's odor—to redress the balance of the entire digestive system, from appetite to elimination.

AVOID spraying directly on the face.

Cistus ladaniferus/Rock Rose
pH 2.9–3.1

Aroma and Taste   Described variously as "the smell of an old Rolls Royce belonging to a maharaja" and "dirty laundry." In other words, some people like it, others do not. It is an unusual fragrance reminiscent of the oil but lacking the complexity and depth, and those who love the oil may be disappointed. Herbaceous, quite dry, and warm in both scent and flavor, it's difficult to describe, but I like it.

Stability and Shelf Life   Very stable. Generally rock rose has a long life, two years or more without problems, but it seems to be greatly affected by seasonal variations from year to year.

Properties and Applications   Oral use is recommended for specific conditions only. This is because of the extremely low pH and cicatrisant (wound- and scar-healing) properties.

Rock rose supports all types of medicines and treatments and is a good postoperative choice for speeding internal healing and preventing bleeding; it can also be used as a supporting treatment for bleeding ulcers, ulcerative colitis, and Crohn's disease, especially when combined with basil, yarrow, or perhaps angelica. Highly astringent, cicatrisant, and styptic, rock rose hydrosol will stop bleeding almost on contact and is good for cleaning wounds, as a compress for hematoma with bleeding, and for the treatment of new scar tissue.

Rock rose is a powerful antiwrinkle treatment when misted on the face two times a day or compressed around the eye area and used in masks and lotions. It seems to exhibit microcluster behavior in the way it plumps cells, smoothing fine lines. Rock rose is a yang fragrance and makes a good aftershave, on its own or combined with German chamomile, calamus, and/or green myrtle.

One of the most important applications may be in the amelioration of endometriosis. This condition causes severe pain and discomfort, and rock rose is an excellent and powerful douche, especially when combined with *Helichrysum* and yarrow, but to be effective it must be used in a consistent daily program (see the recipes in chap-

ter 6). *Cistus* taken internally can also benefit endometriosis and heavy menstrual bleeding. Take thirty milliliters in one liter of water daily for five days before the start of the menstrual cycle and continue throughout the period, then stop. Monitor the effects and make notes so you can adjust the dosage to your particular needs and your body's response. Use more or less as you feel is appropriate—you know your body best.

Rock rose is powerfully energetic in its sphere of activity and is healing to mind, body, and spirit in times of emotional distress and shock. It is one of the ingredients in the Bach flower Rescue Remedy.

Citrus aurantium var. *amara* (flos)/Neroli/Orange Blossom
pH 3.8–4.5

Aroma and Taste Sublime, floral, fruity, refreshing, sexy, and luscious. One of the most complex-smelling hydrosols, and when it's great it is every bit as nice as the oil; in fact, some people prefer it to the oil. Wear it as a perfume. The flavor is sweet and, again, both floral and fruity, with a hint of greenness. Undiluted, the flavor is almost too perfumed, overwhelming the senses; diluted, it is unbelievable and must be experienced. Delectable.

Stability and Shelf Life Very stable; easily lasts two years or more, although the rather large variable in pH in samples tested has shown that the

lower the starting pH, the longer it will last. I kept one sample of a 3.9 pH neroli for over three years without its growing a bloom or developing particulate matter, but this is the exception rather than the rule.

Properties and Applications Neroli is a major antistress and calming agent, and it is mildly sedative to the central nervous system without causing sleepiness. It stops caffeine jitters and the effects of overindulgence rapidly, although the mechanism is undetermined. This is the choice for hysterics in children, babies, and even adults and is a wonderful treatment for sudden shock. It is also quite effective in children with hyperactive attention deficit disorder (ADHD) and can be used both topically and internally for this purpose. Give babies their own bottle to use as they feel the need.

Neroli is supportive for the physical and emotional bodies during detoxification programs and abstention or when quitting a habit or addiction like smoking. It is a digestive aid, stimulating bile release and relieving heartburn and reflux. It also seems to calm spasms in the digestive tract and valves and, in combination with basil water, has shown some promise for hiatal hernia. Misted on the abdomen or applied to acupuncture digestion points, it relieves stress-related bloating, gas, cramps, and constipation. Antispasmodic, antibacterial, and antifungal, it is good in a douche for leukorrhea or thrush, especially when combined with thyme or oregano and rock rose.

Neroli is a wonderful treatment for delicate, sensitive skin and for oily skin, because it is so astringent. Avoid use on very dry skin or use only 20 percent in combination with lavender, rose, and/or geranium. A superb toner on its own or combined with rock rose, it clears acne and irritations. Use it in face masks with clay and honey for the ultimate in luxury. Wear it as a natural perfume that won't aggravate the scent sensitive.

This is an affordable alternative to the pure essential oil, which is expensive and frequently adulterated or synthesized. It is delicious in all sweets and beverages, with fruit, or in jams and preserves.

Citrus clementine (fe)/Clementine Petitgrain
pH 4.3–4.4

Aroma and Taste   Quite close to the oil without the sharp, eau de cologne top note. Green, with a citrus bent, slightly wet, and clearly from a leaf. The flavor undiluted is very soft but leaves an orange peel–like aftertaste in the mouth, and in fact fills the mouth with an intense citrus zest/leaf aroma. Diluted, it is very delicious and highly aromatic, making it a wonderful beverage or blending ingredient.

Stability and Shelf Life   Unstable, twelve to fourteen months maximum. Must be closely monitored; check pH monthly.

Properties and Applications   Extremely effective and a very, very powerful appetite stimulant. The first time I drank this I was obsessed with food within an hour and had a stomach growling so loudly I could have chewed off my arm! The effect is most extraordinary, and even a very small amount diluted in water creates the desire to eat . . . lots . . . right now! It is being tested on people with eating disorders and the appetite loss associated with some drug therapies. It has shown highly significant results with cancer patients who suffer from drastic weight loss owing to loss of appetite; in these cases even tiny amounts added to drinking water have achieved appetite increase sufficient to effect weight gain in a very short time.

Other than the feeding frenzy, the overall effect when clementine is used internally is calming without being sedative. Topically it seems most appropriate for oily or combination skin, as it is slightly drying. Other petitgrain hydrosols do exist, for example, bitter orange and lemon, but this is the only one I have had experience with in therapeutic use.

Comptonia peregrina/Sweet Fern
pH 3.8

Aroma and Taste A mildly fruity, very green and dry herbal scent with an unusual undertone. The taste undiluted is herby sweet, with a strong taste of bitter cherries, really yummy. Diluted, the cherry fades and the herb moves forward. All in all a truly delightful and delicious drink.

Stability and Shelf Life Unknown. Certainly lasts one year or more, and based on the pH and initial trials, probably two years or more.

Properties and Applications Moderately antibacterial and astringent; use undiluted as a mouthwash for toothache, sore gums, and cankers; it works amazingly well—even better when combined with immortelle. Like bay laurel, sweet fern clears the lymphatic system, and I would choose this over bay for internal use in cases of malignant lymph nodes or tumors. In cancer treatments, combine with sweet gale and use at 50 to 70 percent dilution topically as a compress,

or internally take up to sixty milliliters per day diluted in water, in combination with any other treatments being used. There are a number of reported cases of cows being cured of tumors after grazing on sweet fern. Of course, in cases of cancer, please do tell your doctor about any natural treatments you are using.

The plant is actually a subshrub, not a fern, and it shows up in areas of depleted soil that have been lying fallow some years, helping revitalize the soil with its nitrogen-fixing roots. Historically it was used for poison ivy, which grows in similar locations, and also as a topical compress to draw out boils and abcesses. For poison ivy or poison oak, apply neat tea tree oil all over the area, then bind with cloths soaked in sweet fern hydrosol. It is imperative not to scratch poison ivy or it will go systemic and affect the entire body, including mucus membranes, which is highly unpleasant.

Coriandrum sativum/Coriander Herb-and-Seed and Coriander Seed
pH 3.5–3.7

Aroma and Taste Dramatic difference between the herb-and-seed variety and the seed-only variety, as one would expect. The herb-and-seed variety smells and tastes so strongly of cilantro that one has to look hard for the seed flavor underneath. Even diluted it is very intense and tends to bulldoze over any subtle flavors, although it blends well with the strongly herbaceous hydrosols like fennel or basil if used in a low percentage. The seed-only variety is much softer, with a very delicate nondescript odor but a sweet and intense flavor much like the ground seeds. Diluted, the flavor is very nice.

Stability and Shelf Life Unknown.

Properties and Applications An excellent overall digestive tonic. The seed variety works better on gas, bloating, and mild constipation resulting from poor eating habits. The potential for the herb-and-seed variety is in the area of chelation therapy. Fresh cilantro herb has been shown to chelate heavy metals, particularly lead and mercury, from the body. I would like to see some testing on the effects of the hydrosol in removing heavy metals, as this would be an amazing and inexpensive way to achieve this therapy.

Cupressus sempervirens/Cypress
pH 3.8–4.0

Aroma and Taste The aroma is quite delicate, somehow dry and warm smelling. Taste is bitter and dry, more green than woody, almost a little soapy when undiluted.

Stability and Shelf Life Moderately stable; usually good for up to fourteen months but can last longer.

Properties and Applications Very diuretic both topically and internally; use for treating water retention in tissue and in joints. Moderately astringent and styptic, it has a tightening effect on tissue and is useful in skin care for some acneic conditions, thread veins, and couperose skin. Cypress supports the venous system and improves circulation, both in topical and internal use, and may be applied to varicose veins, used undiluted in a compress, or diluted in a sitz bath for hemorrhoids in combination with witch hazel and/or chamomile. Combine with rosemary CT cineole or sage and spray on tired or heavy legs for relief and energy or add to a foot bath to reduce swollen ankles. It seems to have a balancing effect on blood pressure, but this may be due to its ability to balance fluid levels in the body as a whole.

Cypress and juniper berry are two of the most important hydrosols for cleansing and detoxifying the system and will greatly increase the excretion of urine. If you do a three-week course of this water, be prepared to run to the bathroom many times a day, particularly in the first week, as the body will release lots of retained fluid. Stimulating to the liver and kidneys, cypress is useful for gout, arthritis pain, cystitis, edema, phlebitis, and the effects of overindulgence. For these conditions, both topical and internal applications should be combined on a daily basis for at least one three-week cycle, after which time the condition should be reassessed

and the protocol repeated only if necessary. I have one client who found her psoriasis improved dramatically after a three-week course of 50 percent cypress and 50 percent juniper berry hydrolates taken internally; however, this requires more testing. Women may find that drinking cypress in the week before their period helps prevent some of the hormone-related water retention and moodiness associated with PMS.

The respiratory system will benefit from cypress's antitussive and expectorant qualities, even more when it is used in combination with *Inula* (elecampane). Use when there is much fluid or mucus in the system, in inhalations, internally, and by sniffing a few drops at a time into each nostril, then blowing it out. It is mildly analgesic undiluted, but for nasal use dilute it 50 percent in distilled water.

In the kitchen, use cypress in recipes and sauces for venison, game, and lamb or in marinades, where it adds a flavor better than any hickory smoke.

AVOID in the first trimester of pregnancy or in cases of kidney or renal disease, because of its diuretic and detoxifying properties.

Daucus carota/Wild Carrot Seed
pH 3.8–4.0

Aroma and Taste   On the mild side, as with all seed hydrosols. Warm, earthy, almost sweet in a bitter-chocolate kind of way. A comfort-

ing, human-type, musky aroma that appeals to men and women alike. The taste is on the dry side but with the same earthy warmth found in the scent, particularly appealing and complex.

Stability and Shelf Life   Very stable; should be good for two years or more, although some reduction in aroma intensity will be evident before that time.

Properties and Applications   Wild carrot seed will cleanse and support the liver, gallbladder, and kidneys, being mildly diuretic and specific to these organs. Use as part of a detoxification or cleanse; combine with clay to clean the bowels and use as part of an illness recovery, especially after viral infections or gastrointestinal complaints. Carrot also makes a good addition to colonics, being beneficial to the overall flora balance and healing and calming to irritations in the smooth muscle tissue.

It soothes skin rash, inflammation, and damaged skin; is calming for eczema and psoriasis; and is wonderful combined with yarrow, both for the synergy of the properties and for carrot's ability to mask yarrow's odor. Carrot seed is healing to the face after extractions, dermal abrasions, or peels and promotes the growth of healthy new skin cells. Combine it with lavender and apply it both before and after sugar or wax hair removal, or use it on its own for razor burn; men love it as an aftershave.

An overall tonic and restorative, carrot seed can be used to help the body adapt to the changes of the seasons, perhaps by virtue of the fact that it comes from a seed and so is specifically attuned to the rhythms of the earth's cycles. Delicious in soups, juices—especially vegetable juice—salad dressings, and sauces.

Echinacea purpurea/Purple Coneflower
pH 3.9

Aroma and Taste   Very fresh and bright; it literally zings in the nose at first sniff. This is followed by a deep, dark, haunting odor and finally a slight salty licorice smell with a bitter edge. The taste is also fresh and definitely alive. Very mildly bitter and green but somehow simultaneously honeylike, with the same undertone of salty licorice as in the aroma. Unique and very palatable.

Stability and Shelf Life   Unknown. Seems stable at one year or more.

Properties and Applications   Experimental. This hydrosol was made from the whole plant in flower, including roots. German research into *Echinacea* indicates that certain sugars (polysaccharides) present in tinctures and alcohol extracts of coneflower give it the immune-boosting properties for which it is chiefly known. Kurt Schnaubelt and others suggest that the sesquiterpenes found in the essential oil from the root and whole plant (up to 43 percent germacrene-D) also have immune-boosting properties, and the matter is being hotly debated among the chemistry fraternity. All I can say is that when you put this in your mouth, there is an immediate cellular resonance throughout the entire body that is very distinct and happens within seconds of ingestion. Whatever the chemists decide, the human body has already voted; it likes this a lot, thank you very much!

Elettaria cardamomum/Cardamom Pod
pH 4.5

Aroma and Taste   Quite a strong odor, sweet and full of aromatic subtleties, just like the freshly ground seedpod. The flavor undiluted is strong and sweet but not overpowering, a common trait among the seed hydrosols, which tend to be more delicate. Diluted, it is quite lovely, and it is exceptional combined with cinnamon hydrosol. Made from white cardamom pods; it would be interesting to acquire some made from the black or green pods to compare.

Stability and Shelf Life   Unknown. At least one year.

Properties and Applications   Quickly calms spasms and bloat in the digestive tract, as one would expect. It also appears to be mildly sedative or at least very relaxing and with a little honey makes a wonderful bedtime tea. I have been reliably informed that it has distinct aphrodisiac properties, which makes it extra good as a bedtime tea!

A delightful ingredient in both savory and sweet dishes; the flavor is very bright and will not overpower other ingredients.

Erigeron (or *Conyza*) *canadensis*/Fleabane
pH 3.9

Aroma and Taste Uninteresting and rather weedy smelling; a pervasive odor that lingers. The taste is also rather weedy, and as many hydrosols that taste better have some of the same properties, this is not a hot contender for internal use.

Stability and Shelf Life Stable. Lasts eighteen to twenty-four months.

Properties and Applications Experimental. Topically use as an anti-inflammatory for muscular and joint pain and for edema. Internally its main interest is as an antibacterial for intestinal complaints, diarrhea, or traveler's tummy; as a hepatic and pancreatic stimulant; and as a diuretic in renal infections. The essential oil has been explored for phytohormone properties, particularly in both late-onset and early puberty. Of course, medical research would say it can't af-

fect both, but with plants you never know. Researchers are investigating its use in treating perimenopausal symptoms and report some positive results.

The herb is known to have good insect repellent properties, hence its common name, fleabane, but the essential oil is too expensive to use in this manner. However, the hydrosol, applied liberally, frequently, and undiluted, functions quite well against both blackflies and mosquitoes, even in Canada, and this is worthy of further exploration.

Currently fleabane is being researched in veterinary medicine as a treatment for high blood pressure, as an anti-inflammatory for pain relief, for its ability to lower body temperature and reduce fevers, and for its use in insecticidal and flea preparations.

Eucalyptus globulus/Eucalyptus
pH 4.1–4.3

Aroma and Taste The smell is definitely eucalyptus but not as instantly camphoraceous as the oil. A bit unpleasant, particularly when applied neat to the skin, where it leaves a most disagreeable odor after it dries. Taste is strong, very bitter at first, with a powerful eucalyptus aftertastè; sweeten with honey for children.

Stability and Shelf Life Unknown, but appears stable; assumed to be eighteen months.

Properties and Applications Eucalyptus hydrosol is available for several of the different species, including *E. globulus, E. radiata, E. polybractea* and *E. dives* among others. Each has its own particular benefits and applications, just like the oils. I have not yet found hydrolate of *E. citriodora*.

Like the oil, eucalyptus hydrosol is the first line of defense against respiratory problems and infections, coughs, colds, chest infections, and hay fever–type allergies. It makes a good gargle, mouthwash, or cough syrup on its own or combined with essential oils at the rate of one drop of oil to one tablespoon of hydrosol per dose. At the onset of a cold or flu, take one teaspoon in a small amount of water every two hours on the first day that symptoms appear. It works even better if you combine it with "living embalm-ing" two or three times a day, using palmarosa or ravensara essential oils.[2] If a respiratory infection takes hold, take the bihourly teaspoon dose in addition to drinking fifteen milliliters of eucalyptus and fifteen milliliters of *Inula* hydrosols dissolved in one liter of water per day. The hydrosol can be coupled with oils in inhalations, and oils may be applied topically to the entire thoracic area and the tops of the feet.

Very mildly diuretic, eucalyptus seems supportive to the hepatorenal system, enlivening both liver and kidney functions, improving excretion, and giving a general feeling of lightness. A Polish researcher is using it to tone and invigorate the pancreas.

Japanese research has shown eucalyptus to have reasonably strong antioxidant properties in both topical and internal use. An immune booster, it can be used in a prophylactic manner by practitioners who are in constant contact with clientele during flu season. Gently stimulating to both the mind and the body, *E. globulus* is useful when you're feeling low or sick but must keep going.

AVOID undiluted topical or internal use for children under four years. Other species of *Eucalyptus,* such as *E. radiata,* are more appropriate for children.

Foeniculum vulgare/Fennel Seed
pH 4.0–4.1

Aroma and Taste   Strong licorice odor with a sweet, almost sugary edge, although some are sweeter than others. Has been described as "anise and almonds." Taste is very pungent; undiluted, the sweetness is almost undetectable, but it becomes more apparent the more it is diluted.

Stability and Shelf Life   Moderately stable but variable. I have had some last for fourteen months or more and others that bloomed after only eight months—probably a result of distillation parameters and handling, as it is not that widely available.

Properties and Applications   A powerful digestive, acting to relieve gas and bloating, stimulate peristalsis, reduce spasms and gripe in the intestines, and soothe nonspecific stomachaches. It has a general purifying effect on the entire digestive system but does not counteract all forms of heartburn and reflux, although this may be a function of the product variability.

Grosjean suggests drinking fennel hydrosol for cystitis, claiming relief can be achieved in just a few hours. Although fennel is not recommended during the first two trimesters of pregnancy, it is useful for new mothers after the birth, as it promotes lactation and can also help combat infant constipation. Spritz a little hydrosol on a tissue and place it near the baby, but do not spray it directly on the infant. The proximity of the aroma is usually enough to prompt a bowel movement.

Fennel has an interesting effect on the respiratory system. In some people it acts as a powerful decongestant and expectorant and may benefit allergy sufferers, smokers, and those prone to bronchitis and similar conditions. Perhaps combined with the known respiratory benefits of tarragon, with which it shares a licorice flavor, this may prove to be a useful allergy treatment and prophylactic.

Do not use it in cooking, as it is totally overpowering, although one drop can be interesting in strong-flavored dishes.

AVOID long-term use. For children under six years of age, do not give more than one drop at a time, and dilute it in water.

Fucus vesiculosus, F. canaliculatus, Laminaria digitata, and Other Species/Seaweed

Aroma and Taste   Seaweed and salt water multiplied by one hundred!

Stability and Shelf Life   Unknown.

Properties and Applications   Experimental. The species listed are just three of the known varieties that have been distilled for essential oil and hydrosol. Depending on the country of origin, the species will differ. Two other hydrosol lovers have mentioned this one, so it seems there are people experimenting. The only variety I have had came from Corsica, and the dramatic contrast between the smell of the oil and the smell of the hydrosol was truly surprising. The oil was much more pleasant, less fishy, although the hydrosol was certainly interesting. An obvious choice for future trials on hypothyroid and endocrine-system imbalance. Also, it seemed powerfully diuretic and would have potential benefits in cellulite treatments, both topically and internally.

Hamamelis virginiana/Witch Hazel
pH 4.0–4.2

Aroma and Taste   Very delicate herbaceous scent, with a slight woody edge. Smells plant-like without being overly green. Taste is rather dry and nondescript, except undiluted, but it is not recommended for use in this manner. It has a powerful astringent effect in the mouth and is slightly bitter. Smells nothing like commercially available witch hazel.

Stability and Shelf Life   Moderately unstable; lasts eight to twelve months and is prone to bloom but is easily maintained if the pH is monitored closely.

Properties and Applications   Primary use is topical. Use only real witch hazel hydrosol, not the "witch hazel" sold in pharmacies and health-food stores because they contain between

1 and 30 percent alcohol by volume. The alcohol is an effective stabilizer and preservative and may have benefits in witch hazel's use as a sports rub, but it makes it inappropriate for the uses described here and precludes all internal applications.

Witch hazel is possibly the strongest antioxidant hydrosol. In topical applications it reduces redness, rashes, itching, swelling, and scaling of skin. Heals cracked or blistered skin and is extremely good for soothing eczema and psoriasis, alone or combined with yarrow. It is powerfully anti-inflammatory and cicatrisant and is an effective wound wash and antiseptic. Can be used to calm bites and stings and is very synergistic in combination with one of the chamomiles. I react badly to mosquito bites, and this really works. Famous for its healing effects on varicose veins and hemorrhoids; use in a compress or sitz bath two or three times daily, even during pregnancy. Diuretic even in topical applications like compresses, it reduces edema and rheumatic and arthritic pain. Also makes an effective gargle for sore throat or hoarseness and can be combined with cypress oil as recommended by Schnaubelt.

Along with rock rose, witch hazel should be considered one of the most important antiaging substances and antioxidants. Add it to any skincare product, or spritz it on the face and décolleté morning and evening after cleansing and before moisturizing. Although it is astringent enough for teenage skin, it is eminently suitable for mature or damaged skin

AVOID commercial witch hazel; although it is a hydrosol, it always contains preservatives.

Helichrysum italicum/Immortelle/Everlasting
pH 3.5–3.8

Aroma and Taste   Unusual. For some it is like honey on warm toast, for others, dusty old clothes! I would say dry, warm, herbaceous, and haylike, with an edge of hot summer and dusty hilltops, and decidedly Mediterranean. The flavor is strongly bitter, almost soapy, with no hint of the sweetness evident in the scent.

Stability and Shelf Life   Stable. Usually lasts for two years, although it is so effective for so many things it gets used before it fades.

Properties and Applications   A strong anti-hematoma, although less dramatically analgesic than the oil. Applied in a compress to bangs and bumps or old aches, it can even bring subcutaneous bruises to the surface, exposing hidden damage. Wonderful as a sports rub after a workout or physical labor because of its powerful anti-inflammatory and mild analgesic properties. Used in synergy with the rather expensive immortelle essential oil, it can reduce the amount of essential oil needed during a long-term healing, such as for broken bones, where there is a lot of bruising and swelling. Significantly anti-inflammatory and cicatrisant for all wound and tissue damage.

Combine immortelle with rock rose in a douche for endometriosis, fibroids, and painful periods. Regular use, especially in combination with essential-oil treatments, can significantly ameliorate these conditions, and in some cases fibroids can be cured altogether (see the recipes in chapter 6). Immortelle is a must for aftercare in any surgery, speeding the healing of incisions and needle wounds, reducing swelling and bruising, and also detoxifying the liver of anesthetic. It is also a wonder for cleaning and healing tattoos or body piercings.

Use as a mouthwash after dental work. For gingivitis or receding gums, use one tablespoon neat or mixed 50:50 with water as a mouthwash two times daily every day for six months and watch your dentist be amazed. It is also of use in combination with herbal treatments supporting the liver, such as milk thistle, black radish, and artichoke, yet another bitter. Internal use of the hydrosol in a three-week protocol can speed recovery after a long illness, particularly if combined with Greenland moss, another liver supporter. Use two parts immortelle to one part Greenland moss and drink thirty milliliters diluted in a liter of water daily.

In skin care it can help heal scar tissue and is good in synergy with the essential oil and with rose hip seed oil and other hydrosols like carrot seed, sage, and frankincense. One client used it constantly throughout the day in light mists after a car accident, and her quite severe bruising disappeared in a matter of days. It is good for sensitive, mature, or congested skin and helps heal ingrown hairs.

Hypericum perforatum/Saint John's Wort
pH 4.5–4.6

Aroma and Taste The odor is very dry, green, strongly herbaceous, and slightly flat. The taste undiluted is much sweeter than one would think, but the aftertaste is more like the aroma and very dry, almost tannic. Diluted, it tastes like a curious herb tea, something familiar and yet mysterious.

Stability and Shelf Life Unknown. Seems fairly stable at twelve months.

Properties and Applications Experimental. Saint John's wort is now the subject of much study and research since the confirmation of its antidepressant properties. However, plants never do just one thing, and Saint John's wort is no exception. The hydrosol has shown some antidepressant or, perhaps more precisely, mild euphoriant properties and is worthy of clinical trials. It is very effective in cases of asthenia and seasonal affective disorder (SAD); try keeping a glass of water with Saint John's wort hydrosol beside the bed and drink it upon rising in the morning in winter; by the time you've had your shower you'll feel great.

Quite astringent and possibly tannic, it acts on the digestive system, cleansing, calming, and reducing colicky spasms and in some cases having a laxative effect. There are still doubts about whether tannins actually make their way into hydrosols, but this subject is being researched. Saint John's wort is wonderfully healing on the skin and softens and clarifies the complexion, giving a dewy glow after a week or two of daily use. It is also effective as a toner and can be combined with numerous other hydrosols for skin care. I recommend it in combination with immortelle as a compress for scar treatments, since herbal preparations of *Hypericum* are extremely healing and regenerative.

The infused oil of Saint John's wort (in a base of extra-virgin olive oil) has been shown to plump up the intervertebral discs of the spine, helping relieve some back problems. In holistic health, back problems are emotionally linked to issues of support, and Saint John's wort is extremely comforting and supportive in all its forms, including the hydrosol. Internal consumption of the hydrosol has also shown some effect in reducing back pain or at least in improving the overall well-being of those with back-pain issues.

The macerated oil has also shown profound benefit in cases of multiple sclerosis, especially the early stages. Daily ingestion of one-fourth to one-half teaspoon of the infused oil and topical applications to any areas of pain or weakness bring great relief and reduction of symptoms. One client took it daily for three months and thought it had "some effect"; then she ran out and within three days could barely get out of bed. Within forty-eight hours of resuming the macerated-oil routine, her symptoms had faded to almost nothing. We are now trying the hydrosol both alone and in combination with the macerated oil to test its synergistic and solo effects on MS.

The hydrosol does not seem to cause any photosensitivity either from internal or external use.

Inula graveolens/Elecampane
pH 4.7–4.9

Aroma and Taste Minty, cool, slightly spicy fragrance with a hint of cherry floral on the edge. Taste is minty and decidedly medicinal, like a cough syrup.

Stability and Shelf Life Unstable. *Inula* has a maximum shelf life of one year but frequently lasts for only six to eight months. Very careful monitoring is necessary to protect against degradation and bloom, but it's worth it. *Inula* water is very hard to source because it is harvested from the wild and has exhibited quite dramatic differences in odor, taste, and stability from year to year. For this reason it is very hard to acquire reliably.

Properties and Applications The number-one choice for any condition affecting the respiratory system. Elecampane stops coughing "fast," even the spasmodic whooping cough; take fifteen milliliters undiluted every two hours or whenever a coughing fit seems to be coming on. Its mucolytic effects make it useful for chest congestion and phlegm, particularly bronchitis, for which it is also the best choice. You can try it for everything from laryngitis to sinusitis; it is altogether a remarkable respiratory-system tonic. Make a cough syrup with this hydrosol and keep it on hand throughout the winter: Add one tablespoon of honey and ten drops of essential oil to one hundred milliliters of hydrosol; shake *really* well before use. Take one teaspoon at a time as necessary. A three-week treatment can help re-

balance the terrain of the lungs and can be of great help to anyone suffering from chronic respiratory complaints.

Elecampane also makes a valuable cardiovascular tonic, calming, regulating, strengthening, and helping to reduce hypertension. Perhaps it just "lightens the load," as all things as rare and ethereal as *Inula* seem able to do. Its exceptional mucolytic properties make it appropriate in a douche for thrush, vaginitis, or leukorrea; this can easily be combined with other treatments, such as a tampon rolled in live yogurt and one to three drops of tea tree oil. It is experimental for leukemia and problems in the bone marrow. In Chinese medicine it is used for breast cancer and conditions of the lungs and liver. Applied one drop at a time to acupuncture points, it has astounding and instantaneous effects.

In skin care, use elecampane in combination with green myrtle to clear up infected wounds, or apply it on its own as a toner for very oily or congested skin and acne. A facial steam with this hydrolate and two teaspoons of the Swiss Kriss brand herb mixture will clean pores deeper than anything else I know and is perfect for all skin types, even delicate and sensitive. I use this combination whenever I do a liver detox with Greenland moss, as the detox always causes pimples along the liver meridians in my face within twenty-four hours of starting the cleanse, and the facial steams draw out even more toxins.

Jasminum sambac/Jasmine
pH 5.6

Aroma and Taste All my initial samples of the "real" thing were produced in India during hydro-distillation of jasmine attar, and so it retained an element of the sandalwood oil that forms the attar base. It was distinctly jasmine flowers but not like the potent and concentrated absolute. This is jasmine after a cool rain, when the blossom is still wet and its fragrance slightly retiring. The taste is most interesting, partly owing to the distillation process, so there is the edge of dry warm sandalwood as an aftertaste of the floral component. However, a recent sample from Hawaii was *Jasmine sambac* hydro-distilled only for the hydrosol. The few drops of oil it contained were heavier than the water, sinking to the bottom of the bottle, and the smell and taste were totally exquisite, very close to the absolute and better by miles than anything I've seen before. (Refer to the section Fakes and Adulteration in chapter 1 for more on jasmine hydrosol.)

Stability and Shelf Life Unknown.

Properties and Applications Unknown. The fakes, mostly from India and Egypt, are quite artificial, and I have had only one delivery of the real, *real* thing, so I have no idea what it will do, other than smell glorious. But isn't that enough with jasmine?

Juniperus communis/Juniper Berry
pH 3.3–3.6

Aroma and Taste Extremely dry, almost musty, and bittersweet in aroma. The flavor is almost woody and the astringency causes contraction of the tissue in the mouth. Diluted, it is still very dry but not uncomfortably astringent—in fact, it's a lot like really dry gin!

Stability and Shelf Life Relatively unstable. Often less than twelve months, and rarely up to fourteen months. Despite its fairly low pH, juniper berry is very prone to bloom and must be carefully monitored.

Properties and Applications   A powerful diuretic, whether used topically or internally. It contracts tissue, pushing out intracellular fluid, and promotes kidney functions. It is also a circulatory stimulant but does not seem to affect blood pressure. This is the hydrosol to use for gout, edema, rheumatic and arthritic conditions, and any water-retention-related issues. Try combining it with cypress or goldenrod. However, because of its powerful diuretic qualities, it should not be used by people with serious kidney problems or an overactive bladder. The body will not be able to excrete the fluid volumes being processed.

This is a good choice for a cleanse or as part of a weight-loss program; use alone or in a blend both internally and topically. Juniper is cleansing and detoxifying to both the physical and the etheric body. For cellulite, try a three-week protocol internally and combine it with topical compresses of juniper, cypress, and immortelle hydrosols undiluted. A daily sea-salt scrub or dry brushing will also help. If weight loss is the aim, blend juniper, cypress, peppermint, and sage. This mix will improve circulation, cleanse, aid digestion and elimination, and help control the appetite. *Note:* Daily consumption of juniper hydrosol alone gets boring because the flavor is so musty. Blending it, or adding one drop of lemon oil to the water, reduces flavor fatigue.

In skin care, juniper berry is useful for oily or acneic conditions. Use undiluted as a toner after washing with a mild cleanser. Mix it with red clay for a mask and add two drops of sweet orange *(Citrus sinensis)* or lemon essential oil. If the face is very puffy, combine juniper and yarrow or German chamomile hydrosols with green or blue clay and two or three drops of the essential oil of any one of the three (see the recipes in chapter 6 for more skin treatments).

Highly energetic, juniper berry is one of the best for vibrational work. Keep a bottle in your treatment room and mist a few sprays into the air and on the treatment table after each client to transmute any residual "vibes." Apply one drop to the palm of each hand, rub them together, and wipe them through the auric field to cleanse yourself. Very protective; use it with intention to create an effective "light shield" that blocks both the outward and the inward movement of inappropriate energies.

Delicious in cooking, in marinades, sauces, and gravies.

AVOID in the first trimester of pregnancy and in cases of kidney disease.

Larix laricina/Larch/Tamarack
pH 3.5

Aroma and Taste   One of the nicest smelling of the tree hydrosols. Fresh, resinous, a high top-note kind of odor without any of the wet mustiness one finds in so many of the conifer waters. The taste is also fresh and light but not insignificant, with only a hint of minty resin flavor in the background. Diluted, it is very mild.

Stability and Shelf Life   Stable. Lasts eighteen months to two years.

Properties and Applications   Experimental. Seems to be very effective as a circulatory stimulant, although it does not alter blood pressure in any way. On its own topically and internally larch can be used to cleanse and stimulate the lymphatic system and is wonderful in the bath or as an after-bath body splash, combined with bay laurel in synergy. Moderately diuretic, larch seems to have a positive effect on the renal system and should be considered to replace juniper berry and cypress when something equally effective but less astringent and fast acting is desired. Rudolphe Balz recommends larch hydrosol as an eyewash for infections, and the water certainly has had no ill effects, so far, when used in the eye, although I don't recommend it for this purpose. Balz also quotes Rudolph Steiner as recommending larch, lavender, and pineapple juice internally for cataracts, so perhaps this may be a fifth hydrosol appropriate for the eyes.

Larch and hemlock are extraordinary from an energetic point of view. Larch surrounds the entire being with a high vibration field and facilitates out-of-body and lucid states. Hemlock reconnects the lower and higher fields of vibration. When dowsed, the field of this hydrosol is huge. It has a particular affinity for crystals and energy clearing and healing.

Laurus nobilis/Bay Laurel/Bay Leaf
pH 4.9–5.2

Aroma and Taste   Warm, spicy, and mouthwatering when it's good; wet and musty when it's not. This is one hydrosol that smells very much like the fresh plant material or very high-quality dried leaves. The flavor is intense undiluted and remains potent in dilution. The taste is more spice than herb but has a green edge. Perhaps the most delicious of the nonfloral waters and incredible for health as well. Extremely variable in quality; I have had really, really good bay and really, really awful bay, so buyer beware; always ask for samples.

Stability and Shelf Life   Very unstable. Maximum shelf life with any certainty is eight months, although occasionally longer—and I don't care what others say! In fact, one distiller sent me a sample of his bay, claiming that all his hydrosols lasted three to five years, including bay. The bay sample arrived with furry white mold in the bottle. Bay just doesn't last. Bay must be monitored regularly and filtered promptly as soon as the slightest change in pH is noticed or it will rapidly bloom. Fortunately it can be made from dried leaves and so is available most of the year.

Properties and Applications   First choice for cleansing and toning the lymphatic system. Bay laurel should be taken in a three-week internal protocol at the first sign of swelling or conges-tion in lymph nodes anywhere in the body. The effect is dramatic and rapid, with symptoms usually disappearing in less than a week. Also very valuable for lymphatic drainage and circulation, particularly in combination with massage or hydrotherapy treatments and exercise. I have well over thirty cases of complete disappearance of lymph node swelling after treatment with bay hydrosol alone or in combination with the oil; some cases were even slated for surgery and bay was still able to clear them up. However, do not treat lymphatic congestion too casually, and do consult with your health-care professional.

In cases of cancer, replace with sweet fern combined with sweet gale, Greenland moss, or one of the hydrosols more specific to the cancer and the organs involved. Another option is to use the bay vibrationally, applying just one drop to the tumors or affected areas, rather than using the standard internal treatment.

A fairly broad-acting antiseptic, antibacterial, general tonic, and immune booster, it is good as part of a treatment for systemic infections or as a prophylactic for fast-spreading viral infections like influenza. Take bay laurel on its own or in combination with eucalyptus, tea tree, or green myrtle hydrosols internally and use an essential-oil blend topically and aerially to prevent infection. Its use in cooking tells us the herb has long been revered for its digestive properties, which the hydrolate clearly exhibits, toning the intestines and aiding peristalsis. It is a good after-dinner digestive, particularly after rich or fatty foods, and will relieve gas or bloat associated with excess. Laurel makes a delicious mouthwash and gargle for infections and general dental hygiene or bad breath and can be combined with immortelle for more serious gum problems.

Indispensable in the kitchen, bay can be added to every savory dish. Sprinkle it on cooked pasta, and add it to sauces or soups with fish or meat, salad dressings, and juices. One of the tastiest hydrosols of all. I personally find it emotionally comforting, although this is biased by a deep love for the tree and its spirit.

AVOID internally in cases of diagnosed cancer.

Lavandula angustifolia/Lavender
pH 5.6–5.9 (high mountain varieties as low as 4.6 pH)

Aroma and Taste A floral, sweet scent; instantly recognizable, although it has an added strong honey overtone and is deeper, more base-note-like, than the oil. If an azure summer sky at four P.M. had a smell, this would be it. The taste is very soapy-sweet, like eating dried lavender, and I find many people do not like the flavor unless it is sweetened or blended.

Stability and Shelf Life Quite stable. Usually lasts at least two years, frequently longer, although this may vary with growing conditions. The odor, if nothing else, may start to degrade after eighteen to twenty months.

Properties and Applications I generally recommend lavender for external application only. It is not harmful if taken internally but does not

taste very good. There are many other, better-tasting hydrosols with similar properties that can be used internally. The pH is normally close to that of most "balanced" cosmetic products, making it ideal for every skin type on a regular basis. Added to ready-made skin-care products, it will not alter their intended properties and adds a delightful fragrance and its own beneficial cooling and healing therapeutics. Lavender is rightly famed for its regenerative effects on damaged or fragile skin. Add it to masks with oatmeal for a nondrying deep cleanse; use it daily as a makeup remover and cleanser, applied with a cotton ball. Mist the face and neck throughout the day to combat excessively dry atmospheres.

Spray skin both before and after shaving or hair removal to reduce inflammation, get a closer shave, and prevent ingrown hairs. Indispensable for skin care when traveling. Use it on the plane, all over the body, including feet and legs; carry to warmer climes for calming sunburn, heat rash, sunstroke, rashes, bug bites, and itching. Mist skin with a 60:40 mixture of lavender and witch hazel, before moisturizer or sunscreen applications, when skiing or sailing, to prevent wind and temperature damage.

Its sweet and happy aroma makes lavender a natural for children. Use it to cleanse cuts and scrapes (for adults, too); a lavender kiss really "makes it better." Use it to calm cranky moods and bring an end to tearful tantrums, and add it to bathwater or spray it directly on the bed for a restful night's sleep. Little girls love to have their own perfume, and this one won't cause allergies or skin reactions. Lavender is fabulous for use with babies from birth and can be added to the bath, used to clean the baby's bottom, or combined with chamomile for diaper rash. A mist in the air in baby's room or a spritz on parents' clothing before tucking in will help make naps and bedtime easier to achieve. Combine with Roman chamomile for the ultimate baby blend.

Calming and cooling to body, mind, and spirit, lavender makes a refreshing room spray for home or office or in the car to calm, cleanse, and refresh in traffic: Good-bye, road rage. Combine it with geranium, rose, or clary sage and use it hot or cold on the abdomen and back for cramps and PMS. Combine it with a little peppermint and sage and spray it all over for hot flashes, and try a sip of this combo before your next big meeting to "pull yourself together." Use it in colonics to soothe irritated bowel. Use it undiluted in a compress on the neck, shoulders, and forehead for headaches, tension, and stress.

Lavender smells better than it tastes, but it is traditional in desserts, cookies, and ices.

Ledum groenlandicum/Greenland Moss/Labrador Tea
pH 3.8–4.0

Aroma and Taste   Highly complex scent and unusual odor. Very potent but feminine, or yin, without being floral. Wet and wild, herbaceous but not green, sour-sweet, like new-mown hay. Its intensely bitter, astringent flavor has an analgesic effect and aftertaste reminiscent of eucalyptus but fading into hay.

Stability and Shelf Life   Very stable. Lasts two years or more with little or no degradation, although after this point it may start to develop a very slight gray color.

Properties and Applications   The most powerfully therapeutic of all hydrosols. So strong that its recommended dosage is one tablespoon per one and one-half liters of water, which is less than half the normal recommended dose. Higher doses may result in "proving" of the properties; in other words, you may develop the symptoms that are normally improved or cleared up by *Ledum.* If you don't like the flavor, add a slice of fresh lemon or one drop of organic lemon essential oil.

A liver regenerator and cleanser, it detoxifies the organ and seems to improve liver functions generally. Excellent for recovering from surgery or after a serious illness or infection, as it cleans foreign substances from the system. Start with very low doses and slowly work up to one tablespoon per day over three weeks. Its bitter nature and affinity for the liver make it useful in treating digestive disorders, diarrhea, indigestion, gas, bloating, and the effects of overindulgence. Combine it with yarrow to ease withdrawal from addictive substances like alcohol or tobacco and for cleansing as part of a weight-loss program.

A general restorative, Greenland moss seems to assist the immune system and support the adrenals. It is a tonic for allergies when it is combined with topical applications of black spruce hydrosol or essential oil over the adrenal gland area. Mildly diuretic and cleansing to kidneys, it can be used with dandelion tincture to great effect. Used in a three-week protocol, it stimulates lymphatic circulation and has good synergy with bay laurel. An autonomic nervous system balancer, it is strongly sedative and works well on insomnia; try one-half teaspoon in warm water with honey just before bed.

On inflammatory skin conditions, the results are either spectacular or nonexistent, which seems to be a function of the individual constitution. Its internal anti-inflammatory properties are far more reliable, and applications for colitis and inflammatory bowel conditions are worth future study. Greenland moss is experimental for tumor reduction and treatment of liver cancers, hepatitis, cirrhosis, and ascites. May also reduce prostate inflammation when used in combination with herbal treatments. Rare and expensive.

AVOID: Because of its exceptional power, do not use on children under six, during the first six months of pregnancy, or if epileptic.

Lippia citriodora/Lemon Verbena
pH 5.2–5.5

Aroma and Taste   Distinctly lemon but not citrusy. A delicate and gently sweet fresh lemon scent, close to that of the oil but much less potent. The flavor is often not up to people's expectations owing to its mild nature, but it remains very fresh and lemony even when diluted.

Stability and Shelf Life Stable. Should last at least eighteen months or more.

Properties and Applications A powerful mental relaxant and stress buster. Verbena is used as a tea for stress and anxiety in all countries where it is grown. It has distinctly sedative properties and affects the autonomic nervous system. Good for pre-exam jitters, stage fright, and fear that creates a knot in the stomach; it can help boost self-esteem and confidence. If mental focus is required, combine verbena with a less sedative relaxant such as neroli or rock rose.

A general body tonic, it stimulates the endocrine system, particularly the thyroid and pancreas. Taken internally in a warm beverage, it relieves PMS symptoms and can reduce cramps. The essential oil is famed for its antiviral effects, and verbena hydrosol has some use as a prophylactic when taken daily during flu season. It is a digestive aid and has some effect on appetite stimulation; the results are most marked if the indigestion or appetite loss is stress related. Blend with yarrow for a gentle but effective cleanse without the weight loss that yarrow alone may produce.

A strong anti-inflammatory, it seems to have an affinity for the mucus membranes of the mouth and nose. Use verbena in a compress or mouthwash after dental surgery. Combine with *Cistus* if there is bleeding and with immortelle if there is much swelling or a tooth has been extracted. It can be used as a daily mouthwash for good oral hygiene. In cold season try snuffing a few drops up each nostril every day. It is also helpful in very dry climates or when the central heating is turned on.

Verbena's pH is very close to that of the acid mantle of the skin, and it is a clarifier for normal and combination skin. Combined with rock rose, frankincense, or cornflower, it refines skin texture and may reduce pore size. On its own or blended with lavender, peppermint, sandalwood, or calamus, it makes a wonderful conditioning aftershave and suits men both physically and mentally, being neither floral nor fruity.

Lemon verbena is one of the rarest and most costly of essential oils. The plant is highly aromatic but produces very little oil, requiring huge volumes for production. Like all the hydrosols from low-yielding plants (Greenland moss, yarrow, the chamomiles, melissa, etc.), it is highly energetic. It appears that much of the plant's life force remains in the water-soluble components like a hologram, and if the water is combined with vibrational healing techniques, the effects can be extraordinary.

Delicious in desserts, beverages, and sweets. Try it also in seafoods.

Matricaria recutita/German or Blue Chamomile
pH 4.0–4.1

Aroma and Taste   A slightly sharp, very green top note followed by a chamomile-tea middle aroma and a cool, wet bottom note. A complex and somewhat vertical aroma. Undiluted, a green-tea, bittersweet taste with a very gentle floral edge, but most of the bitterness disappears in dilution, leaving a wildflower honey aftertaste. Totally different from Roman chamomile.

Stability and Shelf Life   Quite stable; at least fourteen months, but owing to the difficulty in acquiring this hydrosol, this is based on minimal data.

Properties and Applications   A major anti-inflammatory both internally and externally and on all types of tissue. Use this alone or with lavender for bad burns or if blisters have already formed on a burn. Very serious burns requiring medical attention will often be bandaged, but try to get some *Matricaria* water on the wounds before wrapping and at each change of bandages to speed healing and reduce inflammation. All skin conditions with redness benefit: rashes, burns, sunburns, itching, even some eczema and psoriasis. Also compress on inflamed or swollen veins, hemorrhoids, varicosities, and thread and spider veins. Use alone or in a 50:50 mixture with witch hazel or rock rose hydrosol.

Reasonably antibacterial and antiseptic, it's an excellent cleanser for sensitive, inflamed, or problem skin. Use as a compress or wash for topical fungal infections, followed by essential-oil treatments if needed. Used neat in a spray two or three times a week, it will clean up sweaty foot odors. Use internally both as a beverage and as a douche for candida, thrush, and urinary tract and vaginal infections; combine it with oregano, savory, thyme, or bee balm hydrosols and essential oils or herbs if the problem is systemic. A good digestive, it calms spasms in the intestinal tract, has some effect on ulcerative conditions in the bowel, and may be used in colonics.

German chamomile is instantly anxiolytic; drink it or mist it on when stressed before exams, presentations, or major events to calm and center and get rid of a nervous stomach. Because it is balancing to the autonomic nervous system, it is particularly beneficial to the type A personality, whether male or female. It works for me every time. Men often love the aroma, and it makes a wonderful aftershave on its own and can be combined with many other hydrolates for men's body care, as it is both astringent and softening.

Roman chamomile is usually a better choice for children, although difficult skin conditions, atopic dermatitis, childhood eczema, and the like may require the extra strength of German chamomile. As it is even more sedative than Roman chamomile, just a few drops in a child's bath will slow him or her down. It can be combined with neroli for hyperactivity and added in tiny amounts to juice or drinking water.

Extremely energetic, powerfully calming, and emotionally comforting, German chamomile soothes the beast within and allows a clear approach to issues of the heart and head. It is rare because of cohobation of distillation waters.

---

*Melaleuca alternifolia/*Tea tree
pH 3.9–4.1

Aroma and Taste Smells like a disinfectant. Medicinal, sharp, acrid in smell and taste, although the flavor improves a lot in dilution, which isn't saying much really. However, as its uses are purely health oriented, you may find it easier to take it undiluted rather than sip it all day long.

Stability and Shelf Life Fairly stable; fourteen to sixteen months or better. Although one would expect that this hydrosol would never go off, it will occasionally bloom.

Properties and Applications Antiseptic, antifungal, antibacterial, antiviral: tea tree does it all. Internally it is used in many ways for many conditions, including as a gargle or mouthwash for sore throat, coughs, and gingivitis or as a cough syrup when combined with honey and essential oils. Mildly mucolytic and expectorant, it is best combined with *Inula* and eucalyptus or rosemary for chest infections. You can snuff a few drops up the nose for allergies and sinus congestion. Dilute in a douche for thrush, candidiasis, and reproductive or urinary tract infections. Internally take one-half tablespoon four times a day during a parasite cleanse or combine with pepper-

mint for bad breath resulting from poor digestion. Like the oil, tea tree hydrolol's benefits are myriad.

Topically tea tree hydrosol can be used undiluted to cleanse cuts, scrapes, and wounds of all kinds. For children, combine it with lavender and keep it on hand for all the boo-boos. Skin infections of all kinds react positively to tea tree; use as strong as you can and use clean cotton balls to wash the areas. Fungal infections under the nails should be soaked in or compressed with the hydrosol, then use one drop of clove oil directly on the nail itself. Psoriasis, which can be associated with streptococcus, may also benefit. Use the hydrosol internally for a three-week protocol and topically, combined with yarrow, directly on the affected areas.

Despite its unpleasant taste and odor, tea tree is one of the most useful hydrosols. Unfortunately, many Australian distillers do not like to ship the waters, so it tends to come from other countries. I recently received some from a distiller in Florida, where the tree was introduced to help clear swamps and is now considered a pest. Huge quantities of the tree are now being disposed of . . . perfect for distilling.

Melissa officinalis/Lemon Balm/Melissa
pH 4.8–5.0

Aroma and Taste Not at all like the herb, which is remarkably stronger. The water is a lighter, more floral version of the oil. It has an unusual edge to its scent, like both the plant and oil. The taste is mildly bitter undiluted and quite lemony but not citrusy, more the idea of lemon in a flavor. Becomes very soft, quite sweet, and delicious in dilution. A great favorite for a daily beverage.

Stability and Shelf Life Very stable; easily lasts two years or more. Melissa, thankfully, is unlikely to go off or grow a mold, and the aroma and taste remain fine for a very long time.

Properties and Applications Owing to the extremely low yield and temperamental nature of melissa essential-oil production, distillers will often cohobate the waters to improve yield. However, many distill melissa specifically for the hydrosol and consider any oil a bonus. Be sure you know what you are getting.

Melissa is calming to the body more than the mind but without being overly sedative. Use it for stress, anxiety, and childhood hysterics. Combine with rosemary while studying and with neroli to drink during exams. Has shown some positive results for attention deficit hyperactivity disorder (ADHD) and is certainly worth trying instead of drugs like Ritalin for people of all ages. For children with ADHD, use thirty milliliters in one liter of water; consume throughout the day. For adults, double the quantity of hydrosol: sixty milliliters in one liter of water. (For more on attention deficit disorder [ADD] see Scotch pine *[Pinus silvestris]*.)

During pregnancy lemon balm can be used to treat morning sickness, digestive upsets, and water retention and as a system tonic for general well-being. You can also add a small percentage of cinnamon bark and peppermint hydrosols for morning sickness to great effect. Melissa is gentle enough for use on babies; try adding a teaspoon to a nighttime bath or blend with German chamomile or yarrow for cradle cap and diaper rash (it greatly improves the aroma of yarrow). The essential oil of melissa is frequently recommended for use during pregnancy, but the real thing is very expensive and hard to find, so use the hydrosol.

Taken internally in the three-week protocol, lemon balm makes a good prophylactic in flu and allergy season and has both immune-stimulating and some infection-fighting properties. It has some effect on lowering blood pressure, although this may be due primarily to its anxiolytic properties. People who are very hypotensive should avoid the three-week protocol, as it has further lowered already low blood pressure in some clients. Lemon balm is a gentle cholagogue and has been used in digestive drinks for centuries; the hydrosol certainly aids digestion and reduces the intestinal spasms and cramps associated with colitis and Crohn's disease. In some people, however, it has shown a laxative effect, so test it on the individual before using in cases of bowel disorders. It is experimental for kidney and gallstones and, so far, works best combined with reflexology treatments.

A good antioxidant and anti-inflammatory, melissa can be used on its own or in blends as a skin clarifier and to calm rash, irritations, and eczema. Use undiluted as soon as possible after contact with poison oak or ivy. Add to propri-etary lotions and creams for antiaging and after-sun body care. The aldehydes in the essential oil are considered responsible for the pronounced antiviral properties, and the hydrosol seems to contain at least some quantity of these components owing to the large amounts of oil in solution in uncohobated waters. Apply undiluted topically to herpes sores six to ten times a day, ideally as soon as you feel them coming on, and take one-half tablespoon internally at each application. It works almost as fast as the oil.

A yummy beverage, either hot or cold. Excellent in all recipes, whether sweet or savory. Try it for steaming vegetables or fish: delicious.

Mentha citrata/Orange Mint
pH 5.9–6.0

Aroma and Taste   Light, refreshing, delicately minty but not overpowering. The taste is lightly citrus, very fresh, and you can see why the French call it bergamot mint; it has overtones of Earl Grey tea, which is flavored with bergamot. The citrus note greatly quenches the mint notes and makes this a good option for those not overly keen on peppermint- or spearmint-type flavors.

Stability and Shelf Life   Moderately stable; fourteen to sixteen months, depending on source. Slightly more stable than peppermint hydrosol.

Properties and Applications   Great for stress states, it balances and calms while focusing the mind. Take it to the office on those bad days and your colleagues will wonder what your trick is. A general system tonic, it has little effect on the digestion, although it seems to allay hunger somewhat.

In skin care it is cooling, brightening, and clarifying, with a very neutral pH. Can be used to revitalize all skin types and is particularly good for tired or stressed skin conditions.

Mentha piperita/Peppermint
pH 6.1–6.3

Aroma and Taste The aroma of freshly crushed peppermint leaves. Pungent, cool, and refreshing but significantly less intense than the essential oil. Undiluted, the flavor is very strong, but diluted it becomes softer, like a good herbal tea.

Stability and Shelf Life Unstable. Peppermint has a shelf life of around twelve months, even under perfect conditions. Although it will occasionally last longer, it is quite fragile, and I always get rid of the old crop when the new distillation comes into stock. It is one of those oddities that peppermint is considered an antioxidant, yet the hydrosol oxidizes quite rapidly. Indications are that this is a function of the high pH and the high rH_2 (electro-conductivity) factors in combination.

Properties and Applications Peppermint is most famous for its digestive, anti-inflammatory, and mind-stimulating properties. Although the essential oil must be used in low doses only, the hydrosol is problem-free, although I still consider it contraindicated for children under three years of age.

A digestive par excellence, peppermint is useful for treating colic, bloat, heartburn or reflux, and indigestion of all kinds. Try it also if you suffer from Crohn's disease, colitis, or irritable bowel syndrome, as it has provided significant relief to a number of people suffering from these conditions. It can be combined with basil hydrosol for increased antispasmodic effects and for ending the alternating diarrhea/constipation cycle. Peppermint is an effective digestive tract cleanser, having mild antibacterial and antifermentative properties, and is the hydrosol to drink, combined with Roman chamomile, during a parasite cleanse. Take sixty milliliters of peppermint combined with Roman chamomile diluted in one liter of water per day when treating parasites. Take small sips of a 50:50 dilution to combat motion sickness and nausea.

A three-week treatment of plain peppermint will do wonders for bad breath or acneic skin by detoxifying both the liver and the colon. Acne that is very red and irritated can be compressed topically with neat hydrosol; use twice daily while doing the internal treatment. Topically it combats itching and burning, providing fast relief for allergic reactions, bites, and stings, and makes a good douche or wash for genital irritation or itching in men and women.

Anti-inflammatory both topically and internally, peppermint can be used in hydrotherapy treatments for stiff muscles, aches and pains, shin splints, sprains, and strains. Added to hot water it will have a cooling effect; added to cold water it will have a heating effect. Alternating the two types of compresses is a most dramatic and profound treatment. It is recommended in France to spritz it on the décolleté as a toner for the bustline, and it is even more effective combined with black spruce hydrosol; the effect is uplifting, to say the least!

Mentally stimulating, peppermint is the wake-up water. Drink it in the morning to get your whole body going, including to the bathroom. Combine it with rosemary CT cineole to replace coffee. Spritz it on the face to revive during hot weather or when tired, or use it to soothe hot flashes. Students and businesspeople will find this an effective aid for concentration when studying or writing, as it calms and cools the nerves while stimulating the brain.

I have had a few reports of very odd effects when peppermint hydrosol was combined with alcohol or recreational drugs. It seems to markedly heighten the effects of these other stimulants, and caution should be exercised if you are inclined to experiments of this nature.

Slightly sweet, the hydrosol can be used as a sugar replacement. Try it in cooking, in ice cubes, or as a delicious beverage hot or cold. Spearmint *(Mentha spicata)* can be used in similar ways and has a 5.8 pH.

AVOID with children less than three years old.

Monarda fistulosa/Purple Bee Balm/Canadian Bergamot
Monarda didyma/Scarlet Bee Balm/Canadian Bergamot
pH purple 4.1–4.3   pH scarlet 4.2–4.5

Aroma and Taste *Monarda fistulosa* has a slightly citrus, acidy start, a green herbaceous middle, and a floral, deep-geranium finish owing to its geraniol content: an intriguing aroma that could be a lovely perfume on its own. The taste is dramatically different from the odor: sharp and spicy, mildly analgesic when undiluted. It retains an element of the floral, which comes out more when diluted. *M. didyma* is much more analgesic on the tongue than *M. fistulosa,* causing a distinct tingling sensation with a slight heat. Otherwise, there is the same slight floral edge to the taste but no geranium qualities.

Stability and Shelf Life Quite stable. Easily lasts up to two years and is usually not prone to bloom.

Properties and Applications The monardas are traditional healing plants of the Native Americans, and chemical analysis reveals that they are almost identical to two of the thyme chemotypes, *M. fistulosa* resembling thyme CT geraniol and *M. didyma* resembling thyme CT thymol. U. K. research into *M. citriodora* shows that it is a thymol-carvacrol type. As the thymes are not native to the geographic regions where bee balm grows, it is easy to see why these plants were popular and useful. As early as 1569 Spanish botanists recognized *Monarda* as a medicinal plant of the New World, and by the 1700s it was quite common throughout Europe and valued as a source of thymol. The smell of the fresh leaves is close to that of the expressed oil from the Italian bergamot orange, hence one of its common names.

Use exactly as you would the corresponding thyme hydrosols, although I tend to choose *M. didyma* for analgesic effects as well as antiseptic properties, for instance in mouth and dental care. *M. fistulosa* is more diuretic and useful for treating fungal infections.

Myrica gale/Sweet Gale/Bog Myrtle
pH 3.7–3.8

Aroma and Taste   A relative of bayberry, sweet gale has a subtler, less distinct fragrance, more on the untamed side. It is complex, bittersweet, herbaceous, and wet, with only an undertone of the bayberry spice so popular in potpourris and candles. The flavor is much sweeter than the fragrance, bordering on floral, very refreshing and light, with a slight green edge and a tiny bit of spice that is felt more than tasted at the back of the throat when consumed undiluted. The spiciness disappears completely in dilution and the flavor is sublime.

Stability and Shelf Life   Quite stable. Although this is a relatively new hydrosol, to date shelf life seems to be in the two-years-plus range.

Properties and Applications   This is one of the most powerfully energetic of the waters. I have dubbed it the WWW (World Wide Web) of

hydrosols owing to its ability to connect so many different levels, people, places, and things at one time. Sweet gale grows in clean, flowing water, and its red-and-yellow roots form a dense complex mass, allowing the plants to communicate directly with each other both chemically and by contact. Native Americans used it as a tea for communal dreaming, and the hydrosol has shown itself very powerful for lucid dreaming, meditation, group and distance healing, working with crystals, and all forms of energy work.

On the physical level it is a respiratory antiseptic, helping to loosen phlegm in the lungs, a boon for both dry and wet cough. Astringent to the digestive system, it promotes peristalsis in the bowel while calming gastric spasms and helps alleviate noninfectious diarrhea. A variety of sweet gale was a replacement for hops in old Swedish and British beer recipes, and the hydrosol makes a refreshing and thirst-quenching beverage. Interestingly, this is one of the least diuretic hydrosols despite its pH value, and it is a good choice for those wishing to flavor their waters daily.

The essential oil has been used in experimental treatments for cancer and tumor reduction and is showing great promise. Franchomme and Penoel recommend it for this purpose in *L'Aromathérapie exactemente*. We are now trying the water in a few cases, and I would consider this an important phytotherapy adjunct to any cancer treatments, whether allopathic or "alternative."

A daily intake of fifty milliliters diluted in water during mosquito and blackfly season is said to work wonders as a bug repellent; I have found it somewhat effective for this purpose when applied topically in synergy with fleabane *(Erigeron canadensis)*. It is wonderful in cooking, particularly with wild food: fiddleheads, mushrooms, game, and venison.

AVOID during pregnancy and lactation and in children less than two years old.

Myrtus communis/Green Myrtle/Myrtle
pH 5.7–6.0

Aroma and Taste   A mild aroma. Minty and dry smelling with just a hint of sugar sweetness. Very "green," really quite complex and unusual. Although a cineole chemotype, it lacks the dramatic and rather unpleasant taste of the eucalyptus, tea tree, and niaouli (another *Melaleuca* related to tea tree) waters. Undiluted, it has a bitter edge and just a hint of the mintiness of the aroma. It is most palatable diluted, as it loses its bitterness, and I find it similar to *Inula* in flavor.

Stability and Shelf Life   Moderately unstable. Shelf life is usually fourteen to sixteen months, rarely longer. All the cineole chemotype hydrosols have a level of instability, and just over a year is a safe guess for life expectancy of these waters.

Properties and Applications   *Green myrtle* refers to the high-mountain-grown myrtle that is sometimes designated chemotype 1,8 cineole. It is one of only four hydrosols recommended as an eyewash (the other three are Roman and German chamomile and cornflower). Only the green myrtle chemotype is suggested for the eyes, and this is usually what is available as a hydrosol.

Mucolytic and expectorant, it calms chesty coughs and congested sinuses and is great in synergy with *Inula* for respiratory congestion, ailments, and allergies. Myrtle may be used as a prophylactic for seasonal recurring bronchitis and chest infections. Start taking it internally two or three times a week when the "danger season" approaches, and increase daily consumption if any symptoms appear. I have several clients who have broken the cycle in this manner. Myrtle may be useful for asthmatics as part of daily care and will give best results in cases where the asthma is triggered by allergens, or pollutants, rather than stress and nerves. In the latter case, combine myrtle with melissa and/or neroli to work on the physical, mental, and emotional levels synergistically.

The mucolytic properties extend to the digestive tract, and this can be most useful in treating candidiasis. Colon health can be improved by using myrtle water in colonics, and there is extra benefit from the anti-inflammatory properties for problems like diverticulitis.

Green myrtle is a good general health tonic. Combine with other hydrosols to achieve a range of health effects for all the body systems.

Ocimum basilicum/Basil
pH 4.5–4.7

Aroma and Taste   The scent is strongly licorice in the methyl chavicol chemotype and more green in the CT linalol, although the second chemotype is extremely hard to find in a hydrosol. Neither smells quite like fresh basil or even pesto. The flavor undiluted is extremely intense and almost unpleasant, it is so strong, and again, CT methyl chavicol has a pronounced anise taste. In dilution, the real basil flavor comes out, with all the minty greenness one associates with the fresh leaves and only a hint of licorice in the background.

Stability and Shelf Life   Unknown. Although I have never had a problem with contamination, supplies have always been limited and erratic, so long-term storage has never been tracked.

Properties and Applications   This has become very difficult to find, especially the linalol chemotype, as the production of basil in Europe has decreased dramatically in the past few years owing to falling market prices. New sources in Egypt are starting to produce high-quality organic and biodynamic basil hydrosol CT linalol, and I hope it will return to the market in consistent quality and amounts soon.

An extremely effective digestive aid, it stimulates peristalsis and reduces spasm in the gastrointestinal tract. I had very good initial results for both colitis and Crohn's disease, although inaccessibility has interrupted long-term and follow-up treatments. Basil is a fast-acting carminative; add two teaspoons to a small glass of water and sip slowly for relief of gas and bloating. It can also relieve occasional constipation caused by stress or poor diet, although a teaspoon of olive oil with one drop of basil essential oil taken every thirty minutes will also clear the problem.

Basil is considered balancing to the autonomic nervous system, and the hydrosol certainly bears out this finding. Its effects on stress states are rapid and efficient, bringing a sense of calm, reducing physical tension in the body, including headaches, and calming spasms or tension in the diaphragm and digestive tract. Combine with melissa or lemon verbena to make a nervous stomach vanish almost immediately.

Other initial trials undertaken with basil include treatment of problems associated with the ileo-cecal valve and the pyloric valve. The first indications were some fairly significant relief for those with hiatal hernias, reflux, and aerophagia, although these findings are completely experimental at this stage.

Add to savory dishes, your pesto sauce, salad dressings, and soups.

Origanum vulgare/Oregano
pH 4.2–4.4

Aroma and Taste   Smells like a jar of good-quality dried oregano herb: a little sharp, slightly medicinal and pungent, strongly savory, with just a hint of sweetness. The taste is, again, very like the herb, not at all hot like the oil; it is still pungent and warm undiluted but becomes surprisingly sweet in dilution.

Stability and Shelf Life   Quite stable. Lasts two years or more and is rare to bloom.

Properties and Applications   The hydrosol is safer than the essential oil, as there is no risk of dermocausticity or damage to mucus membranes. Commercial oregano oils can cost as much as $75 for a bottle containing less than 5 percent essential oil . . . a $20 value. Despite the hype, oregano oil must be treated with real care and caution; it burns like hell both topically and internally. One drop on the tongue is like kissing a barbecue—this is no joke. Although the hydrosol has shown significant antiseptic and antifungal properties in practice, analysis of it by Dr. H. C. Baser in Turkey has shown that it contains little of the chemical functional group (phenols) associated with the effective "killing power" of the essential oil. A difference of in vitro versus in vivo, perhaps?

Specific for the digestive and intestinal tract,

oregano has traditional use in Turkey, Lebanon, Greece, and other countries where the herb proliferates as a daily beverage for overall digestive health. You can go to a café and order a glass of oregano hydrosol as easily as a coffee in some of these places. Try an aperitif of oregano before your main meal of the day or before particularly rich foods. Internally combine it with juniper berry for urinary and renal-system infections and as a blood purifier. Combine it with bay laurel in treating lymphatic infections or immune-system weakness or to bolster the system in allergy season. A general health tonic, it supports weak or delicate systems too fragile to handle essential-oil treatments.

Oregano is very healing as a mouthwash or gargle for cankers, mouth sores, gum and tooth infections, and sore throats; use one tablespoon two or three times daily until symptoms clear up. Use in a sitz bath or douche for vaginitis, candidiasis, pruritus, and similar conditions; combine it with other appropriate hydrosols like lavender, rock rose, immortelle, or one of the chamomiles. It is useful in colonics, particularly as part of an antiparasite treatment; combine it with internal oral use daily for three weeks.

Oregano is indispensable in the kitchen for sauces, pasta, chicken, meat, even fish. It is a delicious daily beverage as part of an overall health-care program.

Note: Do not confuse oregano with *Corydothymus capitatum,* or Spanish oregano, and never use the essential oil in the manner described for the hydrosol.

Pelargonium x *asperum/P. roseat/P. graveolens*/Geranium/ Rose Geranium
pH 4.9–5.2

Aroma and Taste A rich, luscious, floral, sweet fragrance with that wonderful roselike afternote. Smells remarkably similar to the essential oil. Undiluted, the flavor is overpoweringly floral, like drinking Chanel No. 5! Very cooling to the touch and in the mouth no matter what temperature the hydrosol. The flower power recedes dramatically when the hydrosol is diluted, making this a most palatable, sweet, and unusual beverage.

Stability and Shelf Life Moderately stable. African varieties usually last fourteen to sixteen months, and European varieties less. Geranium hydrosols will rapidly develop a very curious white, ball-like bloom shortly after contamination, so constant monitoring is very important to catch the signs and filter the hydrosol before the growth can take place.

Properties and Applications The favorite all-around skin-care water for everyone from the very young to the very old. Balancing and adaptogenic for oily, dry, acneic, and sensitive skin. On its own or in combination with other hydrosols it makes a magnificent addition to every kind of aesthetic product and treatment for face and body: lotions, potions, face masks, toners, moisturizers, cleansers—the works. Used daily as a compress over several weeks, it will combat rough and dry skin on elbows and knees and even calluses on hands or feet. Use it neat as a makeup remover. To repair the effects of the city environment, spray geranium directly on top of makeup throughout the day to refresh and rehydrate. Geranium hydrosol is a humectant, attracting moisture to and holding it in the skin, and may have microcluster properties similar to those of rock rose. Combine it with raw honey and use as a treatment for wind-damaged and overly dry skin or after a clay mask to give youthful dew to the face.

Anti-inflammatory and very cooling, geranium calms sunburns, rash, insect bites, and any topical conditions where heat is present. It is also effective on skin conditions with redness, such as broken capillaries, couperose skin, and rosacea, for which it can be combined with German chamomile, cornflower, or rock rose for dramatic results. Hemostatic, it slows or stops bleeding rapidly and can be used to clean wounds and cuts. Children like the smell, and it works wonders on things like scabby knees, stopping the itch and promoting healing of the new skin underneath.

Internally it combats heat and is commonly suggested as both a spritz and a beverage for menopausal hot flashes. It is adaptogenic and balancing to the emotions and the endocrine system. Geranium eases PMS, menopausal conditions, and hormone-related moodiness, especially when combined with omega-3 and -6 essential fatty acids or with internal use of the essential oil of *Vitex agnus-castus* or fleabane hydrosol.

Emotionally this is a feel-good hydrolate, balancing the twin spirits of male and female energy. On its own it makes a beautiful perfume or body spray and can be misted all over; try it directly through your stockings on tired legs! Combined with wild ginger, rock rose, yarrow, or German chamomile, it is an effective and astringent aftershave that appeals to men without being too floral.

It is delicious in sweets, with fruit, or in sauces, and it makes a marvelous martini.

Picea mariana/Black Spruce
pH 4.2–4.4

Aroma and Taste The head note is air in a winter forest: cool, dry, and redolent with complex evergreen odors and frost. This is quickly taken over by a wet, slightly musty resin aroma both akin to and quite different from the remarkable odor of the oil or tree. The taste, like that of all conifer waters, has a dry, sawdust edge to it, like chewing on a branch or twig, although it is not unpleasant. It also has the distinctly minty resin taste unique to the boreal conifers of the spruce, pine, and fir families.

Stability and Shelf Life Very stable. Easily lasts two years, although after that point some particulate matter or a faint gray color may develop. Tests have shown this is not necessarily related to any contamination and is just a phenomenon related to the tree waters.

Properties and Applications The number-one choice for the adrenal glands; use in combination with the essential oil at the change of each season for a three-week protocol. Consume thirty milliliters of hydrosol in one and one-half liters of water daily and apply fifteen drops of the undiluted essential oil to the adrenal/kidney areas on the back during your morning shower, then rinse off with cool to cold water. You will be amazed at how good you feel. The hydrosol, used one drop at a time on acupuncture points

for the adrenals, has an extraordinary effect. My TCM (traditional Chinese medicine) therapist says it feels like electricity running through her fingers as she touches the points. In high-stress periods both the hydrolate and the oil can be used as an aromatic pick-me-up that can replace afternoon or evening coffee breaks. It has been suggested that in addition to regenerating the adrenals, black spruce is supportive to thymus activity, although perhaps the thymus is responding to the immune-system boost from the revived adrenals, or perhaps both organs are supported; we just don't know for sure.

Used in a cold double compress (cold hydrosol cloth followed by warm, dry wool wrap) or bath with Scotch pine, it is highly effective for relief of pain and inflammation. It is, as yet, unproven whether the waters have the same cortisone-like effects as the corresponding oils, but indications based on results are promising. Try it for carpal tunnel, repetitive strain injury (RSI), joint complaints, back pain, muscle aches and swelling, and so on. An odd side effect of both the oil and the water is that it spruces up the bustline, adding visibly and not insignificantly to both the size and the tone of the breast tissue. Combine black spruce with peppermint hydrosol for a daily décolleté mist, but remember that the effect is not permanent and will disappear a few weeks after cessation of daily applications.

A stimulating and restorative body spray and a good aftershave, black spruce connects us with nature and the ancient wisdom of the trees. Combine it with cedarwood for use on pets in general: care of the coat, bath preparations, or as a spray for fleas and ticks. Animals tend to relate strongly to the odor.

This is an important hydrosol for the committed therapist.

Pinus sylvestris/Scotch Pine
pH 4.0–4.2

Aroma and Taste   Scotch pine has a slightly sweet and refreshing aroma. Undiluted, the flavor is quite resiny. Diluted, it becomes dryer in taste and smell and retains the minty edge of the resin.

Stability and Shelf Life   Stable. Usually lasts two years or more and does not develop the gray color of some other conifer waters.

Properties and Applications   One of the best general tonics and an effective immune-system stimulant. The essential oil has a mild hormone-like effect on the endocrine system, and the hydrosol has demonstrated similar, although less powerful, results. Try it for asthenia and loss of libido. In synergy with black spruce, it makes a powerful compress for muscle, joint, and tissue pain of all kinds. When applied as a body splash during periods of stress or when you feel run down, there is an immediate and palpable improvement in both physical and mental strength. Scotch pine improves stamina generally, and athletes will find it of great help during periods of heavy training.

Scotch pine is antiseptic, antibacterial, mildly antifungal, and decongestant; choose it for the respiratory, lymphatic, and reproductive systems in oral, internal, or topical applications. In synergy with *Inula*, green myrtle, and/or eucalyptus it provides relief for bronchitis, asthma, and chest tightness and helps with all allergic or pollution-triggered breathing problems. Use it in baths, showers, steam rooms, and saunas; it's great in the humidifier in winter, too.

Experimental properties of internal use include reduction of blood pressure, cholesterol, and arterial plaque. It treats attention deficit disorder (ADD) in adults in combination with cinnamon leaf hydrosol. (For ADHD see melissa hydrosol.)

Ribes nigrum/Black Currant Fruit and Leaf/Cassis
pH 3.6

Aroma and Taste   The first scent is sharp and acrid, very green, and smells like something starting to go bad. Immediately after that comes the sweet, juicy, mouthwatering aroma of black currant fruit, a stark contrast. The flavor is also twofold but not at all unpleasant; it just starts green and leafy and finishes dark and fruity. An intriguing combination that I really like, but many people find the first smell quite off-putting.

Stability and Shelf Life   Unknown; at least fourteen months.

Properties and Applications   Experimental. It certainly has some digestive properties, particularly after a large or rich meal, and it may contain some tannins, which are rare in hydrosols. The fragrance gives it possibilities for blending with other, less palatable waters and for use in perfumes, colognes, and aftershaves.

Makes a wicked martini and a wonderful sorbet.

Rosa damascena/Rose
pH 4.1–4.4

Aroma and Taste   Smells almost exactly like a fresh rose. Highly complex, sublime odor with the lemony edge particular to the true old varieties of rose used in distillation. Moist, cool, intensely floral scent and taste. Undiluted, the flavor is dramatic and overwhelming—far too strong—but in dilution, its intense floral nature becomes delicate, ethereal, and quite delicious. Once you have smelled and tasted real rose hydrosol, you will instantly recognize the many artificial rosewaters in the marketplace. Some distillers produce a hydrosol from *Rosa centifolia*, and I have seen the extraordinary *Rosa* x *alba* oil, so perhaps that hydrosol may become available soon as well.

Stability and Shelf Life   Quite stable. Shelf life is usually close to two years or more, although it is highly dependent on the quality of the product. Rose hydrosol made from dried petals starts to lose its fragrance around ten to twelve months, and the flavor is less intense from the outset.

Properties and Applications Divine. Because modern roses are so different in aroma, the smell of true rose hydrosol is often an eye-opener for the newcomer to aromatherapy. This is what rose is supposed to smell like! It is good for almost everything and is so nice to use that you don't need an excuse. Highly recommended as a hormone balancer for all ages when used internally in dilution. Experimental in many applications as an alternative to hormone replacement therapy in postmenopausal women and excellent as part of a program combining essential oils, herbs, and other naturopathic treatments. Combats PMS, cramps, and moodiness by virtue of its balancing effects on the endocrine system. Treats the autonomic nervous system and makes you "feel so good."

A humectant, rose adds and retains moisture and is suitable for normal to dry, mature, sensitive, and devitalized skin. Rose is cooling and very mildly astringent; use it in masks, steams, and compresses or add it to any beauty product for both its effects and fragrance. An antiwrinkle treatment when combined with rock rose, it dramatically improves the aroma of the latter. Try it in the bath for relaxation and rejuvenation or for a postpartum healing sitz bath, or use it in a douche or bidet for the most luxuriously effective personal hygiene.

Anyone suffering from environmental or chemical sensitivities could try this as an aromatic and hypoallergenic body, clothes, or room perfume. Its moisture-retaining nature makes it a good choice for the traveler, and its mild antiseptic and cooling properties make it useful for many first-aid applications. A good combination if you can take only one hydrosol with you is rose, lavender, and one of the chamomiles in roughly equal proportions (adjust to suit your nose), which will allow you to address most general health concerns, from stress and insomnia to sunburns and wound care.

Some people claim that rose exhibits the highest vibration of any essential oil. Rose has an affinity with the heart and the emotional spheres of the mind, body, and spirit. However it is applied or taken, it promotes balance, aids emotional processing, and supports you in decision making and the completion of projects. Rose lets you love yourself, but be aware that true emotional healing and opening of the heart make you more vulnerable and fragile in the short term. Make sure you request and have the support of those around you when seeking to heal these emotional, heart-centered parts of your being.

Try rose hydrosol in desserts, beverages, or a glass of champagne.

Rosmarinus officinalis CT1/Rosemary Camphor
pH 4.6–4.7

Aroma and Taste The first impression is almost floral, followed by a soft, noncamphor rosemary scent, very surprising. The flavor is also more floral than one expects, with a very soft rosemary aftertaste that has no hint of sharpness.

Stability and Shelf Life Stable; should last eighteen to twenty months. Although all the rosemaries are known to be powerfully antioxidant, the other hydrosol chemotypes have a tendency to oxidation and bloom. CT camphor has the longest shelf life.

Properties and Applications A mental and physical stimulant, it makes a good coffee substitute for those wishing to cut back on caffeine and can provide the same pick-me-up feeling. Use rosemary camphor to stimulate the liver and gallbladder, promoting release of bile and aiding digestion of rich and fatty foods. It is also useful during a fast or cleanse to reduce hunger and aid detoxification; try it combined with sage. Mildly diuretic, its ability to increase urine output may be partially a result of its hepato-stimulating properties.

Topically and internally, rosemary camphor is a strong antioxidant. In Japanese studies, rosemary scored higher than witch hazel for overall antioxidant behavior but has exhibited only low antiperoxidation properties (preventing other substances to which it is added from oxidizing), which may explain the short shelf life of the cineole and verbenone chemotypes. In skin treatments, all chemotypes perform very well, and the mild scent of the CT camphor makes it very useful as a toner for normal to oily skin. Rosemary camphor promotes healthy, shiny hair and is promising for conditions of mild hair loss when blended with cedar. Combine with goldenrod for dandruff or seborrhea. Add to shampoos and conditioners or use undiluted as a scalp tonic after or between shampoos.

A mild circulatory stimulant, it helps flush uric and lactic acids from muscle tissue and can be combined with goldenrod in topical compresses for arthritis, rheumatism, and gout. A three-week protocol during allergy season will help combat chest tightness and breathing difficulties, although the cineole chemotype works even better for this purpose.

Rosemary camphor makes a delicious cold drink and is indispensable in the kitchen for both savory and sweet dishes; it's worthy of experimentation in things like ice cream.

AVOID in cases of high blood pressure and in the first trimester of pregnancy.

Rosmarinus officinalis CT2/Rosemary 1,8 Cineole
pH 4.2–4.5

Rarely available. The shelf life is much shorter than that of either the camphor or verbenone chemotypes, and its flavor and scent are much sharper, camphoraceous, and pungent, closer to the fresh herb. The distillation parameters require that only the first 20 percent or less of the hydrosol be kept, as the later parts of the run will seriously dilute the overall product. All cineole-dominant hydrosols have a short shelf life and all seem to have a relatively high rH_2 factor, indicating high conductivity and reactivity, and this may explain the peculiarities of the product. Very nice and useful as a mucolytic; buy it when you see it from a good source.

Rosmarinus officinalis CT3/Rosemary Verbenone
pH 4.5–4.7

Aroma and Taste   Rosemary without the bite. The first note is a sweet, soft green, which is then followed by the classic sharp rosemary odor but with less intensity. Neat, the taste is pungent, herbaceous, and green with a minty, cool effect that quickly fills the mouth, less pungent than the other rosemary chemotypes. In dilution, the overall effect is sweet and cool, not at all sharp.

Stability and Shelf Life   Slightly unstable. Average life is fourteen to sixteen months, and this is a fairly consistent life span among the very few producers of this chemotype of hydrosol.

Properties and Applications   Verbenone is a worry-free ketone, making it highly useful and safe for all ages. Internal use of this hydrosol is excellent for treating the respiratory system and conditions of congestion and mucus. On its own or combined with *Inula*, take one to two teaspoons at a time up to ten times a day to loosen phlegm in the lungs and sinus. Snuff a few drops up the nostrils every morning in winter to keep the airways clean and moist and combat the congestion associated with central heating. Internally the three-week protocol can help clear mucus from the digestive tract, improve liver function and digestion, and clear the skin.

Use topically in a hot compress for ear infections to speed drainage of pus and to disinfect; do not put hydrosol directly in the ear canal but compress on and around the ear. Follow with one or two drops of lemon eucalyptus and lavandin or spike lavender essential oils applied at 50 percent dilution around and behind the ear and down the neck, repeated three or four times a day. Candle the ears on the first and fourth days.[3] This treatment works wonders, even on the recurrent, antibiotic-resistant ear infections so common in children. It is experimental in combined internal and topical use for decongestion of the prostate associated with aging.

The aesthetician's friend, rosemary verbenone works on the middle layers of the skin, calming irritations, bumps, pimples, and roughness from the inside out. In a steam or hot compress it helps bring impurities to the surface and decongests clogged pores, toning and refining. It clarifies and brightens all complexions and can be combined with rose geranium, melissa, the chamomiles, lemon verbena, and carrot seed hydrosols for a serious skin-regenerating protocol. All the rosemaries are known to exhibit strong antioxidant properties, and this variety is no different, possibly exhibiting stronger free-radical-scavenging traits, although the data is currently inconclusive on this.

Its antioxidant properties on the skin do not seem to help its shelf life, probably because of the high rH_2 factor.

Salvia apiana/White Sage/Desert Sage
pH 3.6

Aroma and Taste   The fragrance is overpowering. A very intense mixture of sage and rosemary, but much stronger than either. The flavor is completely the opposite: very gentle even undiluted. Sweeter than *Salvia officinalis*, neither herbaceous nor floral. Very unique and quite delicious.

Stability and Shelf Life   Unknown.

Properties and Applications   Although the flavor is very nice, I do not recommend white sage for internal use. Its sphere of activity is energetic. This is the desert sage that has been used by Native Americans for ritual, smudging, and healing as far back as traditions go. The energy field of the hydrosol is unbelievable; the pendulum is almost horizontal, its swing is so strong. Use as a smudge or mist for the auric field, use to cleanse and program crystals and other healing tools, apply by anointing to the chakras and energy points of the body, and mist through the air to disperse negative energies in healing rooms or your home. Avoid applying directly to polished metal objects, as it can affect the finish. Really most extraordinary and powerful.

Salvia officinalis/Sage
pH 3.9 – 4.2

Aroma and Taste   One of my all-time favorites for both smell and taste. Strongly herbal but not harsh, and instantly recognizable as sage. The flavor undiluted is extremely potent, with a rough edge and rather overpowering sage flavor, like a high dose of the dried herb. Diluted, all the harshness disappears and you are left with a savory, herbal taste that is extremely delicious and very satisfying to consume.

Stability and Shelf Life   Very stable; lasts two years or more. Rarely problematic, rare to bloom, and maintains its aroma and fragrance right to the end.

Properties and Applications   Sage is one of the most maligned of essential oils, often labeled as highly toxic owing to the ketone thujone, which can be present in concentrations of over 60 percent in some varieties. There is a small-leaf variety of sage, sold either as *S. officinalis* or as *S. angustifolia,* that contains less than 12 percent thujone, usually somewhere around 7 percent, which should be better known and more widely available; both varieties have exceptional healing properties if judiciously used. The properties of both hydrosols are the same, although the small-leaf variety is less hypertensive than the regular variety and tastes slightly sweeter; it is the one I tend to use.

An exceptional circulatory stimulant, sage tones the venous system, improving circulation both in topical and in internal use. A mild diuretic, it is useful as part of a detoxification or fast. It improves digestion as well as suppressing the appetite or allaying hunger, so it helps in a weight-loss program, especially when combined with diet, exercise, and lifestyle changes. Quite stimulating both mentally and physically, it can be used as a pick-me-up beverage as needed or to restore vitality and energy levels with a three-week protocol. Cases of chronic fatigue can benefit both from the immediate energizing effects and over the long term from the antibacterial, antifungal, antiviral, and regenerative nature of sage.

Balancing to the autonomic nervous system, it works to reduce sweating, especially sweating of the armpits and feet triggered by an imbalance between the sympathetic and parasympathetic nervous systems. A renowned hormone balancer, it regulates the menstrual cycle, reducing symptoms of PMS, cramps, bloating, and water retention, even when misted topically on the lower abdomen. It is equally suitable for menopausal symptoms used internally and combined with topical essential-oil use. For issues of infertility, take sage internally for three weeks combined with topical aromatherapy treatments using a carrier oil infused with plantain *(Plantago major)*. Sage's effectiveness may, again, be a combination of the balancing of the autonomic nervous system and the directly physical effects on the hormones. Sage hydrolate has never shown itself to be emmenagogic, even after weeks of continuous use. After bay laurel, sage is the best lymphatic stimulant and cleanser and can be used at the first signs of swollen glands in the neck, which often precede a cold or infection.

In a compress or bath it aids removal of fluid and acids in the joints and gives exceptional results combined with goldenrod for topical use and with cypress or juniper berry used internally. A very powerful antioxidant, sage is excellent in antiwrinkle and antiaging treatments and can be sprayed on skin prior to and during exposure to sun, wind, and the elements. Mildly astringent, it works as a toner for normal or combination skin and with variable to good results on oily skin. Combine with cedar hydrosol as a leave-in rinse for stimulating hair growth or use on its own to give shine and luster to dark or red hair. Herbal traditions promote sage to reduce gum inflammation, and it can be combined with immortelle as a mouthwash for oral health or used on its own for toothache.

Wonderful in the kitchen, its savory-sweet flavor improves most sauces, pastas, marinades, and dishes with heavy meats or fatty fish.

AVOID in cases of hypertension and in the first trimester of pregnancy. Sage hydrosol will raise blood pressure significantly more than the essential oil; the lower the dose, the stronger the effect. This is the most distinct contraindication for any hydrosol; *ignore it at your own risk.*

Salvia sclarea/Clary Sage
pH 5.5–5.7

Aroma and Taste Smells like a really good cup o' tea—Earl Grey tea, to be precise, because there is a distinct bergamot edge to the aroma. The water is distinctly clary sage, although less potent and much, much softer than the oil. The flavor is also remarkably Earl Grey–like, with the bergamot citrus quality stronger even than in the odor. In dilution it is sublime either hot or cold, any time.

Stability and Shelf Life Slightly unstable. Clary sage has a quite variable shelf life; some batches last less than twelve months, others last well for two years or more. The plant is a biennial or perennial, and this may have something to do with it, since at least two years' worth of weather and environment affect the plant and therefore the hydrosol. Generally I would give sixteen to eighteen months as a safe range.

Properties and Applications Clary sage essential oil should not be used in combination with alcohol owing to the adverse interreactions between the two. Clary sage hydrosol is safe to use if alcohol will be consumed and, in fact, is a traditional addition to the May wine in Germany.

This is the "woman's choice" water, and it makes a great life-affirming beverage at any time. Use for hormone-related cramps, bloating and water retention, moodiness, and other symptoms of PMS. A three-week protocol can help regulate the menstrual cycle, reducing excessive bleeding and helping reestablish the cycle after cessation of birth-control medication. Menopausal symptoms also respond well, particularly in synergy with sage hydrosol. Try a three-week treatment with a 50:50 combination of the two hydrosols or alternate clary one day, sage the next, to reduce hot flashes. Do not use sage hydrosol if you are hypertensive. During the birth process make a hot compress with two hundred and fifty milliliters of undiluted clary hydrosol, three drops of clary oil, and three drops of blue tansy oil; apply it to the lower abdomen and back during contractions for really amazing pain relief. If the birth is taking place in water, skip the essential oils; add the hydrosol directly to the tub and put some in the mother's drinking water.

Clary is lovely misted on the face or combined with peppermint, rose, and/or rose geranium, all of which will give a moist dewy glow to the skin. On its own it is astringent and toning for oily skin and can be used in combination with Roman chamomile as a makeup remover. A mild antispasmodic and anti-inflammatory in both topical and internal use, it has at least some effect on many of the body systems—circulatory, endocrine, digestive, muscular, and nervous—and can be taken in synergy with yarrow for overall health benefits and to improve the flavor.

Clary sage is a euphoriant and antidepressant; some find it an aphrodisiac. Either way it provides emotional support and a feeling of well-being. It makes a good beverage for those giving up the alcohol habit and can calm some symptoms of withdrawal. Profoundly energetic; use it with any form of vibrational work, particularly for emotional traumas and heartache.

Clary sage makes a delicious martini or white-wine punch and is wonderful on fresh fruit and in sorbets and ices.

Sambucus nigra/Elder Flower
pH 4.0–4.2

Aroma and Taste   Sublime. It is floral but not sweet, delicate but with a wonderful and firm presence both aromatically and in the flavor. In dilution it is exceptionally delicious.

Stability and Shelf Life   Stable. Should last for eighteen months without problems.

Properties and Applications   Experimental. Unlike the extracts or berries, which contain high levels of vitamin C, there is no confirmed evidence that this vitamin is present in the hydrosol, as vitamin C is both water-soluble and destroyed by heat. However, it works synergistically when taken with vitamin C and does seem to have fairly distinct immune-boosting properties. Take one teaspoon every hour at the first sign of a cold and you will probably never succumb to the infection. A gentle circulatory stimulant, elder flower can be compressed on muscle aches or sports injuries, or you can drink it as a beverage to tone the venous system. Mildly diuretic and a specific for the kidneys, it detoxifies and restores and is experimental to reduce the pain associated with arthritis, rheumatism, swollen joints, and acid deposits in tissue.

Elder is renowned for its effects on the nervous system; it reduces physical and mental stress and promotes a sense of calm. A delicious cold beverage; sweeten it with honey for children. Use it in ice cubes, punch, or alcoholic drinks; add it to desserts, jams, jellies, and fresh fruit.

Santalum album/Sandalwood
pH 5.9–6.0

Aroma and Taste   A soft, dry, unmistakable sandalwood odor that is highly aromatic despite its extreme delicacy. Must be at room temperature to give off an odor at all. The flavor is more pronounced than the smell, as is the case with all the wood waters; it is dry and pleasant and holds up well in dilution.

Stability and Shelf Life   Stable. Should be in the range of eighteen to twenty-four months.

Properties and Applications Experimental and rare. Certainly some of the sandalwood hydrosol in the market is the oil, or synthetic oil, added to water; the real thing is as rare as the real oil, so buy carefully. Government-controlled forests in India have been the only reliable source for many years, as poaching of the wood led to its eradication from the wild in most of the world, including India. However, in recent times Australia has started producing a beautiful sandalwood oil, but it is an absolute extraction, not a distillation. There is also the West Indian sandalwood *(Amyris balsamifera)*, which is quite nice but completely unrelated to the true Indian sandalwood of the Santalaceae family. You will find all of these products on the market at some time or other.

Sandalwood shares many properties with cornflower, and they can be used interchangeably in topical applications, although men, and many women, prefer to use sandalwood, if only because it sounds more exotic than cornflower.

Do not put sandalwood in the eyes.

Topically it is exceptional in skin care. It is only slightly drying and astringent; use it as a compress on delicate and mature skin, in the eye area for crepey lids, and with variable results for acne, rosacea, couperose skin, eczema, and psoriasis. For these last conditions try combining it with other suitable hydrosols; synergies nearly always work better. Add sandalwood to your shampoo, or use it combined with cedarwood and/or goldenrod as a rinse on oily hair and for seborrhea.

Mildly anti-inflammatory, it is a great aftershave, balancing and calming the skin and the mind, preparing you for the day ahead. Combine it with immortelle as a mouthwash for gingivitis or post–dental surgery. Ayurvedic uses include possible applications as a douche for vaginitis and candida. A three-week internal protocol has proved effective in recurring bladder infections and cystitis.

Satureja montana/Winter Savory
pH 4.1–4.2

Aroma and Taste Smells medicinal and powerful, like a strong cough syrup or mouthwash. The taste, undiluted, is very potent, sharp, slightly hot, tingling, and analgesic in the mouth and distinctly "therapeutic." Diluted, the warmth disappears, but the analgesic and me-dicinal flavor remain. Not delicious, but you can feel it working.

Stability and Shelf Life Quite stable. Should last two years without problems. I have had California savory, distilled in a copper still, that was quite salmon pink in color and much hotter on the tongue, and some distilled in stainless steel that also had a pinkish color but was more in the normal flavor and heat range. The European variety usually has little color. Shelf life of all the varieties is very good.

Properties and Applications Safer than the essential oil, which is not much used except internally in the world of medical aromatherapy, its value being its high phenol content and exceptional anti-infectious properties. Topically, savory oil is dermocaustic, causing burning sensations, redness, and skin irritations. Happily, the hydrosol will not cause any of these problems, although it is still on the hot side. Do a patch test to check for sensitivity before using on broken skin.

A very powerful antiseptic, antibacterial, and antifungal, savory can be used undiluted or at high strength topically as a wash for skin infections, diluted in a douche or sitz bath for vaginal or urinary tract infections, and in combination with allopathic medicine for sexually transmitted diseases. Try it in combination with thyme CT linalol and rosemary CT verbenone or *Inula* hydrosols for candidiasis. Use it in colonics, where it will help kill infections and get rid of parasites without damaging the healthy intestinal flora. Combine it with yarrow or German chamomile for inflammatory bowel conditions that may be of an infectious nature. In a gargle or mouthwash it is effective against sore throat, tonsillitis, gum infections, abscesses, cankers, and bad breath. As a steam inhalation combine it with essential oils for infections of the respiratory tract and sinuses. If you use winter savory oil for an inhalation, use only one or two drops and keep your eyes closed throughout, as it can irritate the eyes, even in a steam. Along with oregano, the thymes, and the monardas, this water is the first choice for any serious infection in any part of the body. However, *never* put it into the eyes or ears.

Regular use boosts immune functions, particularly of weakened systems or those too sensitive to handle essential-oil treatments. Use fifteen milliliters in one liter of water for fragile systems. Use it diluted 50 percent with water as a body splash during flu season for protection from infection; it's an amazing feeling. It enhances body functions without overstimulating. As a digestive aid, savory is a mild hepatostimulant, promotes secretion of bile, dispels colic and bloat, and rapidly eases the effects of overindulgence. It is experimental for the adrenal glands, particularly the adrenal cortex, which may partly explain its immune-boosting effects. Stimulating and energizing, it is useful for states of asthenia, along with cinnamon and oregano hydrolates, and may enhance libido.

A great morning drink. Good in cooking in small amounts, as flavor may be pervasive.

Solidago canadensis/Goldenrod
pH 4.1–4.3

Aroma and Taste   The odor is very green, slightly weedy like wet hay. The taste is the same, although it leaves a dry feeling in the mouth, indicating its diuretic nature. Diluted, it loses its musty-hay taste and becomes slightly nondescript. Not particularly interesting but worth using for its properties.

Stability and Shelf Life   Very stable. Very few problems, and normally lasts two years without much degradation, although the taste is slightly better in the first year.

Properties and Applications   One of the "sleepers" of aromatherapy, since many people who are allergic to the highly reactive ragweed confuse the two plants. Goldenrod rarely causes allergies.

Goldenrod is a strong diuretic, and taken internally it may aid the treatment and prevention of kidney stones and is cleansing to the entire hepatorenal system without having the "squeezing" effects of juniper berry or cypress. Although not a digestive per se, it can stem diarrhea, depending on the cause, and is very useful for treating stress- or diet-associated "runs" in both people and animals. Topically, use it as a compress for fluid retention and uric acid in joints and tissue or add it to the bath for soothing rheumatic and arthritic pain. This hydrosol is a strong anti-inflammatory and moderate antispasmodic for sore muscles, stiff neck, tendonitis, and repetitive strain injuries. It can also prevent inflammation if used as a friction rub before or after a workout or physical labor.

The oil is known for its cardiotonic properties, which seem to be present to a slightly lesser degree in the water. Goldenrod hydrosol lowers blood pressure in both the hypertensive and the hypotensive. Those with extremely low blood pressure should avoid internal use. The effects on the heart seem to be a result of the anti-inflammatory properties, and this should be explored further for conditions like endocarditis and pericarditis, as suggested by Rudolphe Balz. Applied topically, goldenrod reduces swelling in thread varicose veins and broken capillaries.

Remarkably energetic for such a "common weed," goldenrod carries the intense vibrations of heat and sun; it opens the solar plexus and diaphragm, bringing calm. It is wonderful in energetic healing for the emotions and the heart and for helping to release old anger.

AVOID internal use in cases of hypotension and consult with your health practitioner before internal use if you suffer from liver, kidney, or heart disease.

Thymus vulgaris CT1/Thyme Geraniol
pH 5.0–5.2

Aroma and Taste   The distinct smell of geranium is the overriding scent here. The flavor is also very floral and sweet, undiluted, although you can also taste the thyme. In dilution it loses much of the sweetness but retains the floral element, and the thyme flavor begins to dominate.

Stability and Shelf Life   Stable. Usually lasts two years.

Properties and Applications   This hydrosol is hard to obtain, but it shows up from time to time. I tend to use *Monarda fistulosa* to replace this chemotype, as I have a more regular supply.

This is a good choice for fungal infections of all types. Use it undiluted as a wash or douche for the skin and genital areas; it is very mild but effective. Foot fungus will benefit from regular washes or soaks in thyme CT geraniol, followed by applications of undiluted essential oil of palmarosa and/or tea tree or niaouli. Apply this hydrosol in a compress to herpes blisters as soon as they threaten to appear; it can prevent the outbreak.

Thyme geraniol is a good choice for use on children, as the odor is sweet, the hydrosol is mild, and the effects are significant. Use on infected cuts, scrapes, and wounds, either undiluted or at 70 percent dilution. Teenage acne can be reduced with daily applications, undiluted, with a cotton ball; wipe the whole face, not just the acneic areas, and consider taking some internally as well: drink two teaspoons in a glass of juice or water at breakfast every day. Makes a good mouthwash for children prone to cavities: dilute one-half tablespoon in a small glass of water and rinse with it after brushing twice daily. It can also be made into tea for treating childhood infections of all types, as it boosts the immune system and helps kill germs, and kids don't mind the taste.

Thymus vulgaris CT2/Thyme Linalol
pH 5.5–5.7

Aroma and Taste   A sweet, somewhat fruity, floral aroma, with just the tiniest hint of herb as an after-smell. Interesting. Undiluted, the flavor of thyme is detectable and the aftertaste is slightly cool and analgesic, but again, the fruity-floral taste dominates. Diluted, it is simply delicious and difficult to recognize as thyme.

Stability and Shelf Life   Stable. Normally good for two years.

Properties and Applications   A mildly antiseptic, antiviral, and effective antifungal hydrosol. Use it to clean wounds, prevent and clear up infections, and soothe insect bites. As a steam or undiluted as a wash it treats acne, impetigo, and dermal infections. Its antiinfectious and healing properties make it a specific for bedsores, and it is gentle enough for even the very ill. Topically, apply on normal to oily skin for a balanced deep cleanse; its pH is very close to that of the natural acid balance of the skin. Combine with neroli and rock rose to compress enlarged pores. Internally thyme CT linalol is a digestive and intestinal cleanser; it is very effective in colonics. Balancing to mind and body, it makes a healthy daily tonic and could be thought of as a supplement, like vitamins.

When infants and children require some stronger healing power, this chemotype makes a safe and effective choice. Add it to baby's bath for diaper rash that won't respond to chamomile or lavender; apply one or two drops to the feet for chesty coughs and colds, or add one drop to one hundred milliliters of fluid in the baby's bottle. It can also be added to the washing machine's rinse water for baby's bedding, clothes, diapers, and so on. I add it to my dish soap. In the treatment of animals, add it to the drinking water for bad breath or as part of a natural feeding program.

The sweetest of the thymes, CT linalol makes a good drink hot or cold and is an unusual addition in soups, stews, and the like. Thyme CT thymol has a more traditional thyme flavor for cooking.

Thymus vulgaris CT5/Thyme Thuyanol
pH 4.6–4.8

Aroma and Taste   Distinctly thyme in scent, it's very close to the fresh herb straight from the garden. The taste is also strongly thyme, but with no element of heat. A soft, sweet thyme flavor that borders on the flowery. In dilution, the flavor becomes very mild indeed.

Stability and Shelf Life   Very stable. I have never had this hydrosol go off, even after three years or more.

Properties and Applications   This is a most unusual and rare type of thyme that must be propagated by cuttings or clones to grow true to chemotype. This unfortunately means that there are very few producers, but at least you know the hydrosol will be the real thing when you find it for sale. Incredibly useful, this chemotype is as strong as the thymol chemotype in its ability to combat infections, bacteria, even a virus, but it is as gentle and mild as the linalol and geraniol types. What more could you want?

Choose CT thuyanol for serious conditions, especially those of a chronic nature when treatment is likely to be long-term. Recurring infections like bronchitis and other respiratory complaints, systemic candidiasis, and tropical infections of undiagnosed types have all responded wonderfully to internal use of this hydrosol. Treatment can be continued in three-week cycles for several months if necessary, and the immune system will be greatly revived, as chronic infections are particularly hard on the immunity. If parasites are suspected, CT thuyanol is a good hydrosol choice. Always start treatments on the new moon, as the parasites are more active while the moon waxes, less active and harder to get rid of when the moon wanes. Animals can also be treated for parasites with this hydrosol in combination with oils or conventional medicines.

Allergies and allergy-induced asthma also respond well to this water, although the mechanism is unclear. Perhaps it is the immune-stimulating effects, or perhaps it is the ability to reduce the likelihood of secondary or opportunistic infections taking hold when the respiratory system is full of mucus. Try snuffing a few drops up each nostril two or three times a day during allergy season; it can really help.

At the first sign of a cold or flu, take one tablespoon undiluted every two hours and then add thirty milliliters to a liter of water and drink it over the day; this is often enough to stop the cold. Combined with "living embalming," with oil of palmarosa, even the worst of colds is short-lived. When children (not infants) get caught by the flu bug, give them a bath with fifty milliliters of thyme CT thuyanol hydrosol added to the tub or rub them down after the bath with a small amount of undiluted hydrosol, then put them to bed.

Thymus vulgaris CT6/Thyme Thymol
pH 4.5–4.6

Aroma and Taste Here be thyme! No question in the aroma or taste of this one. Strong thyme smell and very close to the fresh plant picked at the height of summer under the Mediterranean sun. The flavor is intense, quite hot, and almost burning to the mouth undiluted. When it is diluted it becomes quite palatable, although it is still distinctly thyme and slightly warm.

Stability and Shelf Life Very stable. Even after nearly three years this hydrosol remains in perfect condition

Properties and Applications Antibacterial, mildly antiviral, antifungal, and antiseptic, this is the big gun of the thyme family. Like the oil, the hydrosol is hot, literally causing a burning sensation on the tongue if undiluted, although it is not dermocaustic like the oil. Choose CT thymol when you need a killer.

This hydrosol makes a great gargle or mouthwash for sore throat, tonsillitis, laryngitis, or any throat infection. Use it as strong as you can bear, given the taste and heat, two or three times a day; it usually takes only a couple of days and is rather like the old commercial suggesting that Listerine tastes lousy but it works. In fact, Listerine contains thymol. For colds, flus, and respiratory and gastrointestinal infections, take 1 tablespoon of a 60:40 hydrosol-to-water blend, sweetened with honey if you want, every hour up to 6 P.M. during the acute phase. This is dramatic but it works, and for those who refuse to rest even when they're ill, you have the added benefit that CT thymol is quite stimulating—which is why you stop at 6 P.M.

As a prophylactic to prevent infections and boost the immune system, blend CT thymol with melissa, sweet fern, and/or *Echinacea* and drink it at normal dilution (thirty milliliters to one liter of water) three or four days a week. A good digestive in low dilution or in blends, it cleanses the colon and is recommended for use in colonics when treating antibiotic-resistant gastric infections.

For severe acne, impetigo, or dermal infections, blend CT thymol with one of the other thymes and use it as a steam or wash daily; do not use it undiluted on broken skin, as it will sting. Animal skin conditions also benefit from this hydrosol. Wash cuts, bites, hot spots, and sores with a 70 percent solution and add two tablespoons to the rinse water after shampooing your dog. Avoid using it on cats, as it is too strong; use CT thuyanol or bee balm instead. Add one teaspoon to your pet's dinner for bad breath or gas, and rinse all animal feeding dishes with the pure hydrosol to disinfect them.

This hydrosol makes a delicious drink and is great for cooking in soups, stews, and vegetarian meals.

Tilea europaea/Linden/Lime Flower
pH 4.3–4.6

Aroma and Taste Very difficult to describe this aroma: slightly floral but with a wheat-beer freshness and overtone that makes it almost herbal. The flavor is superb—more flowery, less beer, but refreshing and light, unlike the floral intensity of rose or neroli. Diluted, it is very mild but distinct and makes a delightful beverage in hot weather and a lovely tea if served hot. Particularly good with linden blossom honey.

Stability and Shelf Life Slightly unstable. Linden starts to fade in flavor after twelve to fourteen months but generally remains free of bloom a little longer.

Properties and Applications A word for herb teas in Europe is *tilleuil,* which is also a name for linden, from the Latin *tilia.* Linden herb tea can easily go bad, and it is recommended that it be used fresh, as older products have been known to cause psychotropic effects, perhaps resulting from specific molds that can grow in the tea bags. The hydrosol is a wonderful and safe substitute for the tea. In North America it is often called basswood.

Linden is distinctly sedative and a true stress buster; use it for insomnia, anxiety states, and nervous exhaustion. Very useful when the body wants to stop but the mind keeps whirring. The "Mom" of hydrosols, it provides emotional comfort, making it a good choice for babies and animals. Its synergy with Roman chamomile is extraordinary. It has a calming effect on the nerves both internally and externally and can be used either way for shingles. Try blending it with rosemary essential oil and linden-infused oil or absolute and applying it in a compress at the first signs of the shingles rash or itching.

In skin treatments, it works well on dry eczema and itchy eruptions and can be combined with yarrow, witch hazel, or both for psoriasis and eczematous conditions. Use it undiluted in a compress on the forehead and scalp for headaches and migraine or combined with lavender or German chamomile for sunstroke. It is mildly anti-inflammatory and works well in masks and treatments for puffy or devitalized skin. In hot weather linden cools the body and soul. Add it to a cold bath or mist it over the sheets, pillows, and skin in hot, humid weather for a good night's sleep. Energetically very alive, the linden has been considered a magic tree by many cultures for centuries. It promotes lucid dream work, especially when combined with sweet gale, and fifteen milliliters (one tablespoon) of undiluted linden can help in achieving deep meditative states.

Linden makes a really lovely beverage hot or cold, and it's great combined with other hydrosols or teas. In cooking it lends itself to both sweet and savory dishes of a delicate flavor.

Some New Hydrosols

Finally, I just can't help adding a few notes about some of the newest goodies in my cupboard. What I know about many of these would fit on the head of a pin, but it is worth knowing that they are out there. These are all real, bona fide hydrosols, produced either by steam- or hydro-distillation specifically for their therapeutic effects . . . whatever they may turn out to be. They have provided quite a lot of fun and diversion while writing this book.

Aniseed	*Pimpinella anisum*
Black Austrian pine	*Pinus laricio*
Black butt eucalyptus	*Eucalyptus pilularis*
Caraway seed	*Carum carvi*
Katrafay	*Cedrelopsis grevei*
Champa	*Michelia alba*
Clove	*Eugenia caryophyllata*
Dandelion	*Taraxacum officinale*
Dill seed	*Anethum graveolens*
Fenugreek (leaf)	*Trigonella foenum-graecum*
Feverfew	*Chrysanthemum parthenium*
Frangipani	*Plumeria apocynaceae*
Ginger	*Zingiber officinale*
Gingergrass	*Cymbopogon martinii* var. *sofia*
Greek sage	*Salvia triloba*
Hyssop	*Hyssopus officinalis*
Lotus, pink, white, and blue	*Nelumbo nucifera*
Lovage	*Levisticum officinale*
Mastic	*Pistacia lentiscus*
Mushroom	*Boletus* spp.

Myrrh	*Commiphora molmol*
Nettle	*Urtica urens*
Nerolina	*Melaleuca quinquinervia CT nerolidol* and *linalol*
Niaouli CT 2	*Melaleuca quinquinervia CT cineole*
Nutmeg	*Myristica fragrans*
Orange peel	*Citrus aurantium* (z)
Patchouli	*Pogostemon cablin*
Plantain	*Plantago major*
Spike lavender	*Lavandula spicata*
Tuberose	*Polianthes tuberosa*
Valerian	*Valeriana officinalis*
Vetiver	*Vetiveria zizanioides*
White ginger lily	*Hedychium coronarium*
Zdravetz geranium	*Geranium macrorrhizum*

FOUR

⁓

The Hard pHacts

Science is strong on description; we know so little that scientists make discoveries everywhere they look. But each discovery merely reveals the magnitude of our ignorance.
David Suzuki, *The Sacred Balance*

ydrosols, unlike most essential oils, have a finite shelf life. Although it is true that some oils, notably the conifer and expressed citrus oils, do have a shelf life of around two years, most of the oils will, if stored correctly, last indefinitely. Some, like patchouli, vetiver, sandalwood, and the resin extracts like myrrh and frankincense, can actually improve with age, like fine wine. However, hydrosols are a different kettle of fish, and we must develop a new way of thinking to fully understand their needs.

Establishing and monitoring the shelf life of hydrosols has, until now, been largely a matter of experience combined with guesswork. The result has been that if a distiller or seller of hydrosols actually gives them a best-before date, it seems to be regardless of bottling standards, storage conditions, or plant-material source. Some

people say one year on everything, others say three years on everything—they can't both be right, and they're not. Each hydrosol is totally unique, just like the oil and plant from which it is derived. The shelf life of each hydrosol is also unique and is affected considerably by storage conditions, packaging, and a few chemistry factors.

When I started working with hydrosols, I wasn't much concerned with the issue of shelf life of hydrosols or contamination. I bought only from reliable sources, and as hydrosols were even harder to find then than they are now, these were just about the only sources for most of the varieties that were of interest. I also kept them in the fridge, bottled mostly to order, and sterilized my packaging. I figured that if any contamination was present, I would surely see it in the water. And see it I did, although not very often. But it was bay laurel hydrosol that made me start to think about the issue of shelf life—that and the frequent questions of colleagues who wondered if I didn't have contamination problems.

At first I put down the concerns of colleagues to the fact that one of the great fictions of aromatherapy is that hydrosols are really unstable and nearly always full of contaminants like mold. This really is a fiction. Of course hydrolates, like any natural substance without preservatives, can develop bacteria, and they do go off. But—and here is the important thing—they are not that unstable for the most part. Take Roman chamomile, for instance. Early on I started buying chamomile by the gallon. It is so lovely and sweet and has so many uses that I figured I could sell it quickly enough to justify buying what was then large bulk to me. Of course, I was wrong. That first gallon of chamomile did go fast, but the second took over eighteen months to sell, and it never changed one iota during the whole time: The taste, smell, look, or pH was not altered in any way. So what was the problem with this contamination malarkey, I thought to myself. Then came bay leaf.

Whenever I get a new variety of hydrosol I always do a three-week protocol myself to see what happens and to gauge the physiological, emotional, and vibrational response within the body. Over three weeks one consumes 630 milliliters of hydrosol: 30 milliliters a day for twenty-one days. So I always buy at least a couple of liters to allow for experimentation. But with bay the results seemed so good and the health benefits so palpable that I went for the gallon and then watched in amazement as it started to bloom after only five months in the fridge. I called the

supplier and checked the distillation date, which was around ten months previous. What was going on, I wondered. Why did chamomile last and bay degrade?

I had to rethink everything, and soon I realized that I had lumped all hydrosols together as far as stability was concerned, just as we tend to lump most essential oils together in the same regard. I realized that every hydrolate was unique and probably had a specific shelf life. Eventually I realized that the individual pH was the key to understanding the whole problem.

Because of this, the easiest, most effective method to determine and monitor shelf life is to measure the pH value of the waters. Each hydrosol has a unique pH or a pH range into which it will fall. This may vary from year to year and is affected by all the same conditions that affect the essential oils: weather, altitude, harvest times, and so on. They have chemotypes; different countries of origin; and variability in yield, chemistry, taste, and aroma, just as the oils do, and this is important to remember. However, the pH is a reliable indicator of the potential life span of a hydrosol—it is not the only relevant parameter, but it is the easiest to measure for the home user or small distributor, and except for a few anomalies, it is a very reliable standard.

In the future I hope that distillers will start testing the pH of the waters during the distillation process so an absolute value or range can be assigned to each and every hydrosol produced, year after year. This will be an extremely valuable sales tool for producers, distributors, and practitioners, as you will see by the end of this chapter. It will also be fascinating to see the differences in pH and therefore effects, aroma, taste, and so on of hydrosols produced in different years by the same distiller and in the same year by different distillers in different areas or countries. Until then, you can use the pH table supplied in chapter 2 as a starting point. The data are based on my own tests conducted over the last three and one-half years and are an accurate reference for good-quality organic and wild-crafted therapeutic products.

Note: If you know about pH, you will know that each tenth of a point on the scale represents a factor of ten; thus some of the pH ranges presented for hydrosols actually represent quite high variables in actual pH. Chemists out there may find these ranges too wide, and in a way, so do I, but as the ratings are based on averages of hydrosols received over a four-year period, from many sources and of many species, this is as accurate as I can be at the moment. Also, as these are natural compounds, their values change from season to season, from country to country, and of course, because of distillation methods. It is better to have a normal range to work from then a finite value that may not be applicable to your next batch.

The Key, or More Correctly, the pH

When I started testing the pH of the waters, I had no idea why I was doing it. I was given a meter by my brother, *L'Aromathérapie exactemente* listed the pH values for a few hydrosols, and I was curious. Also, it was the only "scientific" test I could conduct in my kitchen.

I knew that distilled water has a 7.0 pH, and I already knew that hydrosols were not "just water," as some would have it. They have aroma and flavor, unlike distilled water, so at the very least these were substances comparable to herbal teas. What the tests showed is that hydrosols are nothing like water or even herbal teas. And although the waters are distilled, not one has a 7.0 pH—far from it. I was excited!

If we look at the pH of a few other common substances, we can see that the acid nature of hydrosols, while not immediately apparent, is very important. Compare the pH values of various hydrosols (pages 69–72) to the substances listed in the table on the next page. Lemon juice is highly acidic, as is vinegar, and we can taste and feel this acidity in the mouth and in the way our body reacts. Rock rose hydrosol is as acidic as some vinegars, but we do not taste or feel the acidity in the same way at all. Tomato juice is too acidic for some people's taste, and sugar is often added to tomato sauces and juice to reduce the acid effects. Elder flower, German chamomile, neroli, fennel, and several other hydrosols have a pH value equivalent to that of tomato juice—4.0—but we find no acidity in their flavors; on the contrary, they seem quite sweet. This does not, however, change the fact that they are acid by nature, and this is an important consideration in how, why, and when we use them. Only peppermint and linden blossom hydrosols have a pH close to that of our own saliva, which is very near neutral.

pH Table of a Few Comparative Substances

Substance	pH
Saliva	6.5
Tomato juce	4.0
Vinegar	2.5–2.9
Lemon juice	2.0
Human tears	7.2
Ethyl alcohol	6.9

I compared my first hydrosol pH tests with those of Franchomme and Penoel, and the measurements didn't all jibe. Some were spot-on, but for others there was a huge difference between their figures and mine. Too much difference to be right, I thought. So I started testing every batch soon after it arrived but without developing any clear picture of what the data meant. Really, I just wondered why my numbers were so different from the only reference numbers I could find. Interestingly, my tests were usually pretty close to each other; that is, geranium was always in the 4.7 to 4.9 pH range, different from the 3.3 pH in Franchomme and Penoel but relatively stable within my own tests. Other glaring differences were green myrtle, 3.95 pH versus my reading of 5.8; rosemary cineole, 3.7 versus 4.2 pH; and oregano, 5.2 versus 4.2 pH.

However, some hydrosols, specifically neroli, or orange blossom, were quite variable in my own tests, ranging from as low as 4.0 pH to as high as 5.5 pH. The hydrosols came from several different countries and sources, and at the time, I put the differences down to those variables. I now believe that some of the neroli waters contained preservatives, probably alcohol. Ethanol, or 95 percent ethyl alcohol, has a 6.9 to 7.0 pH; distilled water also has a pH of 7.0 and is considered neutral. No hydrosol has a pH in the alkaline range above 7.0; they are all acid—either slightly, like lavender (*Lavandula angustifolia*, 5.7 pH), or very, like rock rose (*Cistus ladaniferus*, 2.9 pH). According to data, the pH range of authentic essential oils is around 5.0 pH, with a maximum of 5.8 pH.[1] I have never tested individual oils but must assume that there are distinct ranges for each oil, as there are for each hydrosol. Balz and others go on to say that the acidic nature of oils contributes to their antibacterial properties, as an acid environment inhibits the growth of bacteria and can even kill some bacteria. When we are dealing with the huge range of pH values in hydrosols, we can see the importance of using this knowledge in judging appropriate therapeutic applications. We can also see that they must work.

For the most part I tested each bottle of hydrosol only once, usually on or shortly after receipt. Then I decided to test the bay that had bloomed—bingo! The pH was way off, infinitely more alkaline than the original reading. I ran the hydrosol through a paper filter, and although the pH dropped by 0.15, the reading was still nowhere near where it should be. It was clear that a change in pH can be triggered by the appearance of bacteria. (Okay, so maybe this would have been obvious to a chemistry student, but to me it was . . . Eureka!). After numerous tests of this kind, I would suggest that as soon as a change in pH is noticed, one should suspect that the hydrosol has become contaminated in some way. I now test each bottle of hydrosol every three to four weeks.

Hydrosols are really remarkably stable for natural, preservative-free products. As was discussed in chapter 2, many products, including beer (Budweiser's shelf life is 110 days), have a much shorter shelf life than hydrosols. Regardless of our former thinking, if we want to embrace this new aromatherapy, that is the first bite of the cookie to digest. They don't last forever, but they are not totally unstable! Contamination can happen in many ways, from nonsterile bottles, shipping and transport conditions, formation of condensation inside the bottles, plant matter or residue from the distillation stage, heat and light damage, just smelling the bottle directly under your nose, and so forth. Even aerial contamination during the bottling stage could undo all the precautions and sterilizing techniques you may employ; it's not common, but it's certainly possible. One distiller I know puts a small piece of the plant material into the finished hydrosol and leaves it there for two to three months to "revive" the hydrosol. While energetically this is a nice idea, it raises serious issues concerning contamination.

Say a hydrosol blooms. You will see some evidence of residue in the bottle. It may be tiny bits of particulate matter, a furry algae-type growth, spirals that look like frog's eggs, wispy ghostlike bits—each one seems to develop its own unique pattern of growth. But you can *see* it. Even if the smell and taste have not changed, you can see this stuff floating around in the bottles. It's a pretty simple and unmistakable clue. But what if the hydrosol is contaminated and just hasn't had time to actually grow a bloom? It doesn't make it any less contaminated; you just don't have any way to know about it . . . until now.

A change of more than 0.5 pH from the initial reading on any given batch is positive indication of bacteria. Testing should be undertaken at least every two months (sixty days), and more frequently if you resell the products. At present I have only my own benchmarks to work with, but within five years I believe hydrosols could come labeled with their pH at the time of distillation, giving everyone involved in their handling a perfect reference point for both contamination testing and therapeutic action.

Now, does it matter? Are they still safe to use if we can't see a bloom? Difficult questions. I have drunk hydrosols with bloom, just filtered through a paper coffee filter, to see what would happen. Nothing so far. I am fairly sure that friends, colleagues, and maybe even some clients have consumed hydrosols that were contaminated but not blooming. I would certainly *never* knowingly give anyone a "contaminated" water, but without a bloom, how would we have known, before the pH test? I am pretty sure that *anyone* who has worked with hydrosols has consumed "contaminated" but nonblooming waters, probably many times. But what comes out of your tap could be almost as bad, depending on where you live. All I know is that I am alive and well and have never been made sick by a hydrosol. However, there can be some unpleasant organisms contaminating hydrosols, and it is obviously much, much better never to drink or use contaminated products.

What matters most is that we now have a simple method for monitoring hydrosols, checking for contamination, and choosing what to do about the knowledge that we have. We also have a way to filter them, as I've mentioned. Testing the pH of hydrosols will monitor more than bacterial contamination; it can also reveal the addition of preservatives like alcohol. Ethyl alcohol is 6.9 pH; as you'll see in the table below, if alcohol is added to a hydrosol to prevent bacterial growth, it will change the pH of the water.

Let's use rock rose as an example, since it has such a low pH to start with and is so important in therapeutic care.

If you were to conduct a test and find the pH to be 3.6 instead of the normal 2.9 to 3.1, you could assume one of two things: either bacteria are present or alcohol has been added.

To determine which is the problem, you could smell or taste a small amount to see if alcohol was detectable. Although at less then 5 percent it's hard to detect alcohol from the odor, if you are sensitive you will usually notice the slight "rush" of alcohol entering the bloodstream if you drink the hydrosol undiluted; whereas, if the problem is bacteria, you will not feel the same alcohol effect. But do you want to taste a potentially bacteria-carrying hydrosol? Probably not. You can also spray the hydrosol on your skin; if alcohol is present, it will be quite drying, usually leaving a light or white patch on the skin if the alcohol content is over 5 to 7 percent, but at lower concentrations there may be no immediately visible effects. In any case, you will know that something is wrong with the hydrosol, and you should either filter it, return it to your retailer, or use it to wash the floor.

The pH will also give us scientific information as to the potential therapeutic applications of the waters. Rock rose, as discussed, is the most acid of all, with a 2.9 to 3.1 pH, so it is highly astringent. It will constrict cells and reduce blood flow, which is why it is used as part of an aromatherapy protocol for fibroids. That is also part of the reason why it reduces wrinkles, since it tightens and tones the pores, reducing visible fine lines. Rock rose will also slow or stop bleed-

	STANDARD pH	5% ETHANOL ADDED	10% ETHANOL	15% ETHANOL
Rock rose (*Cistus ladaniferus*)	2.9 to 3.1	3.2 to 3.3	3.4 to 3.5	3.5 to 3.6

ing by the same astringent action; it can be used on cuts that bleed profusely, like those on the fingers or on animals pads, and it makes a wonderful addition to men's aftershaves. Of course, if the cut is deep, it may require medical attention, but this is what to use first, before you panic. The essential oil does the same thing, only more powerfully, but at forty dollars or more for 5 milliliters, compared with fifteen dollars for 120 milliliters of hydrosol, it's more likely that you'll have the water on hand. Rock rose has other unique properties that you will find described in chapter 3.

ESTABLISHING SHELF LIFE AND STABILITY

The pH

Generally hydrosols with a pH of 5.0 or less last longer than hydrosols with a pH over 5.0. As a very broad rule of thumb, I rate those under 5.0 pH at two years and over 5.0 pH at twelve to eighteen months. There are some exceptions, of course. I rate bay laurel *(Laurus nobilis)* at eight to ten months only. Although it is 4.9 to 5.2 pH, bay is quite unstable and will easily go off, even when kept sealed and under refrigeration. I would like to get my hands on some bay with a 3.9 pH, as listed by Franchomme and Penoel, to see if it lasts any longer. Perhaps it is the nature of the plant material, perhaps it is the distillation, but it is fragile. It is also very difficult to get a good one. I have had bay from four different sources and two were downright awful:

musty, tasting more like branch or weed, no spice, no complexity, no relation to the plant I so love. The other two were both good, but only one of them was excellent. I always try to buy laurel from this distiller now, and this is the one that has achieved the brilliant and remarkable results in dealing with swollen lymph nodes. This hydrosol is very close to the oil in smell and tastes just like the fresh leaf picked from the tree. I used to have an ancient bay growing near my house in England, and we would wander up the hill whenever supplies were low and pick what we needed for the kitchen. The tree was magical, full of faeries I'm sure, and although I already had a strong love for the herb in cooking, I developed a special resonance and love for this tree and its gifts of flavor and smell. If you are lucky enough to live in a climate that allows you to grow bay trees, do it! You will never regret it, and although they grow slowly, they live long—much longer than you will.

Another fragile hydrosol is juniper berry. Again this is odd, because juniper's pH is usually 3.3 to 3.6, so one would assume that the shelf life should be long, but that's not always the case. Juniper berry water tends to grow a gray, frog's-eggs-like spiraling mold if you let it bloom; this bloom is very distinctly different from any of the blooms in other hydrosols. It always fascinates me to see what form a bloom will take, but the grayness and spiral of the juniper is most unique. Somehow I feel that it is energetically quite different, taking the form of a spiral. Spirals are a powerful geometry and exist in many forms in nature, from how leaves appear on branches to the convolutions of seashells to water turbulence. Bearing in mind the vibrational properties of juniper, it is perhaps not surprising that the bloom assumes this DNA-like spiral, and I don't mind terribly if I miss the cues in pH change and lose some juniper to bloom; it's intriguing.

My two suppliers of juniper hydrosol both sell essential oils of juniper branch with berry and pure juniper berry but offer hydrosols only of the berry, so I assume that they are telling the truth and that there is no branch or green material in the distillation that produces the hydrosol. The chemistry of the branch oil differs greatly from that of the berry oil, as does the cost. The berry oil is much lower in monoterpenes and in therapeutic applications would be a better choice if you had concerns about kidney health; however, the berry oil costs about twice what the branch or branch-and-berry oil costs, so most people don't use it. The fragrance of the pure berry oil is much more rarefied, as well, and is my personal preference. I have never seen a hydrosol offered of the branch or branch-and-berry distillation; I don't know why except to assume that the extremely high terpene constituents of the oil, which are non–water-soluble, make this hydrolate rather uninteresting from a therapeutic viewpoint. Whatever the reason may be, this is one of the "fragile" hydrosols, and I normally give it only a twelve-month shelf life.

Anomalies

On the other hand, some waters with a pH over 5.0 do have long lives. *Myrtus communis*, specifically the high-altitude green myrtle, is quite stable, even though it is 5.7 to 6.0 pH (*L'Aromathérapie exactement* lists myrtle at 3.95 pH). Is this because of its chemistry? Unlikely, since the high-altitude myrtle is a cineole-rich plant and the cineole-rich hydrosols tend to have shorter life spans. Is it because of the growing conditions at this higher altitude? Perhaps, as high-mountain lavender has a much lower pH than midaltitude lavender. But there are no confirmed answers yet, I'm afraid, just lots of ideas, and this is the kind of thing that I hope will be answered by research in the next couple of years. Good thing, too, that green myrtle lasts so well, since this is one of only four waters that is recommended for use in the eyes. Shock, horror?! Yes, some people actually put hydrosols in their eyes, just like a saline solution or eyedrops, and they are lovely to use in this manner. Look in the monograph section for more information on this subject.

Lavender, our precious stalwart, has a pH of 5.6 to 5.9, and as low as 4.5 from the wild highland varieties, yet it will sit on the shelf for two years without a problem—that is, if your supply lasts that long. As interest in hydrosols grows, more and more people are experimenting, but nearly everyone starts with lavender, since they know it so well. I can barely keep enough in stock to get me from season to season these days, and although I still think the French true lavender water is the best, my Canadian distiller produces a lovely product, and I may need to add California production to my inventory if demand keeps growing. (Until now the U.S.–Canadian exchange rate has rendered this product rather expensive by comparison.) But here we enter the sticky world of botanical specificity and chemical analysis.

My French hydrosol and oil both come from the same producer. It is true organic French *Lavandula angustifolia*, and I've seen where it grows and where and by whom it is distilled. I have had the oil analyzed, and as the oil and water batch numbers agree, I can be sure that the therapeutic parameters are within the desired range. My Canadian distiller also provides analysis of the oil that comes with the hydrosol, and although it doesn't grow at one thousand meters above sea level, it, too, fits within the desired parameters when chemically analyzed. This is really what you want when you buy a hydrosol. It is a coproduct of essential-oil production, and you want to know that truly therapeutic oil was produced so you can feel certain that the properties of the hydrosol are also therapeutic. It's not just a smell thing. And I still believe that you get a better hydrosol if the distillation produces oil rather than just water, assuming the plant produces oil.

It has been mentioned several times that botanical specificity is absolutely necessary for essential-oil plant production, or for any plant being grown for therapeutic applications. Even

then, the chemistry of the plant changes and your active ingredients will be quite variable from year to year and from producer to producer. That is the argument for standardized extracts, at least on the surface. Until the day comes when labs can assess hydrosols by GCMS (gas chromatography, mass spectrometry) as easily as oils, we must rely on this cross-referencing system when we buy our waters. For the moment no one is offering analysis of hydrosols, but a project is under way that I hope will soon change this situation.

However, I have digressed wildly. Back to the stability issue: As I said, 5.0 pH seems to be the point at which the shelf life of a hydrosol starts to change; more acid than that and you have a longer life, more alkaline and you have a shorter life. Why is this?

Other Factors

Perusing the medical aromatherapy literature didn't yield many answers and even less any suggestion as to why my little "rule" didn't always hold true—except that that's the way of rules. Then I found a few paragraphs in the famous text *The Practice of Aromatherapy* by Dr. Jean Valnet, and I knew I suddenly had more than a clue. He talked about the importance of acid and alkaline substances as bacteriostatic agents, things that stopped or killed bacterial growth. He says, "Vitamins have an acid reaction less than 6 or 5—fruit and fruit juices of low pH value are sources of vitamin. Wine ferments in an acid medium, as does milk when it turns into yogurt, a powerful intestinal disinfectant. On the other hand, rotten eggs and bad meat produce an alkaline reaction. This is why we keep gherkins in vinegar, which is acid, rather than in, say, Vichy water, which is an alkaline."[2]

What Valnet was saying is that the more acid the substance—hydrosols in our case—the better a preservative and the more potential therapeutic benefits. Why, then, are we so often told to eat alkaline foods and to make our digestive tract more alkaline? Well, the funny thing is, many acid substances, like lemon juice, create more alkalinity in the digestive tract, thus fitting both requirements. This also explains why more-acid hydrosols last longer; they are more naturally preservative, even to themselves. However, this was not all. Valnet then went on to discuss the rH_2 factor, which defines the charge in electrons of a given pH value; "for the pH value there will be an infinite number of rH_2 values."[3] Eh, voila! The answer was becoming clearer.

Without getting into this too heavily, the rH_2 factor, which measures the conductivity of a substance, relates to the "potential of oxido-reduction," the activation or reduction of oxidation.[4] In other words, antioxidants or "reductive agents" have a low rH_2 value; that's part of how they work. They also tend to be on the acid side of 5.0 pH or less. We know that oxidation of essential oils and hydrosols causes their degradation, so perhaps part of the reason that the anomalies exist in the pH rule is because of the rH_2 rating. I am positive this is what is going on with bay laurel and juniper berry: they have a high rH_2 value and a low pH and are therefore oxidizing in the bottle; whereas lavender and green myrtle have a low rH_2 value, even though their pH is above 5.0, and therefore they last longer.

Then there is the subject of resistance, which creates an environment hostile to infection. Valnet states, "Generally speaking, natural essences have an acid pH value and, which is important, high resistance. For instance the resistance of cloves is measured at 4000 (20 times that of human blood), thyme at 3,300, lavender at 2,800 and mint at 3,000. A mixture of essences, which, as we have seen, has strong bacteriacidal properties through nebulisation in the atmosphere, has a resistance of 17,000—thus the resistance of the mixture is much greater than its component essences. Its pH is very acid at 4.6. Alkalinity favours the rapid multiplication of microbes whereas acidity opposes it, hence the bacteriacidal properties of the essences. The high resistance also encourages the diffusion of infections and toxins."[5] Do we know what the resistance values of hydrosols are? Not yet, but we're working on it.

On one page, which I'm sure I had read at least half a dozen times, I had suddenly found a significant clue to the anomalies in the pH–shelf-life rule. Research currently under way will take a close look at these ideas, and by the time you read this book, we will probably have answers to some of the questions still unresolved on this subject. But let's look at one more little anomaly.

Natural Antioxidants

Extract of rosemary is used as a natural preservative and is considered an active antioxidant compound. However, rosemary hydrosol, depending on the chemotype, has only a short to medium shelf life and is definitely on the unstable side. Japanese research testing the antioxidant properties of plant extracts found that although rosemary inhibited peroxidation and exhibited strong antioxidant properties, it "had a lower activity than *dl-x*-tocopherol, a positive standard." The reaearchers go on to say, "Rosmarinus officinalis and Salvia officinalis are reported to have antioxidative activity, however, Rosmarinus officinalis was found to exhibit a low activity against both active oxygen species and peroxidation under our experimental conditions."[6] None of the test parameters included looking at the pH or rH_2 values of the plant extracts, and it is quite possible that this is the reason that rosemary was such a poor show on the antioxidant front. One must then wonder where rosemary actually got its great reputation. However, the same study found that rosemary had the highest "superoxide anion scavenging activity," so there you go! In real terms, witch hazel, sage, and even *Eucalyptus globulus* hydrosols can outperform rosemary hydrosol as antioxidants, although the verbenone chemotype ranks with sage in practice.

There are also lots of confusing signs with hydrosols, and only working with them will teach you what they mean. Earlier I suggested that you use a wine glass to decant new batches of hydrosol. The shape of the glass is designed to augment the aromatic elements of wine, and it works equally well for hydrolates. It also allows you to look at the color and clarity of the water, both of which contain important information. Some hydrolates have a slight color; others, like the pink, copper-distilled savory, are intensely hued. By using a wine glass, with its broad surface area, you will also notice if there is a visible oil slick or drops of oil on the surface of the water. Sage frequently contains a visible slick, as do melissa and rose if the waters are not cohobated.

Sometimes these signs can be disconcerting and confusing. Recently, while desperately awaiting a large shipment of neroli water, I received a call from the supplier, who thought there might be a problem with the hydrosol: It might have become contaminated and was being tested. It appeared that some "matter" had formed on the sides and surface of the jug and hydrosol that was suspect, but on analysis this turned out to be the oil residue floating to the surface and oxidizing as the hydrosol matured after distillation. It was a very good batch, but I'm grateful the supplier was aware enough to notice the anomaly and give it attention.

I also consider the viscosity and surface tension. Just as wine is said to have legs, which are the rivulets returning to the liquid after it has been swirled in the glass, so some hydrosols exhibit a similar if less dramatic tendency. The surface tension may be visible in the shape of the meniscus, that is, the upper surface of the water where it touches the glass. You can also look at surface tension by pouring a little hydrosol onto the back of your hand in the dip by the thumb. Some waters have such a high surface tension that they sit in an almost spherical drop; others have so little surface tension that they are difficult to keep on the hand at all, tending to dribble onto the floor. I don't yet understand all of what the surface tension means, but I believe it is higher when a higher portion of oil is in the solution, as it tends to appear in hydrosols that are more difficult to separate. It is also higher in hydrosols that are more stable, regardless of pH.

There is still so much to learn about why, how, and under what conditions hydrosols degrade, but we are getting there.

FILTRATION

Two years ago some hydrosols I bought arrived with filtration information on the label. I was impressed. The date of filtration was noted and the size of the filter—0.3 microns—given. The shipping date was on the bill, and it was the day after filtering, so for the first time I had a product that I knew was clean at the time of dispatch to my door. Since I received the goods just four days after they had been shipped, this gave me the best benchmark I had to date.

The filtration process used was reverse osmosis. Although very few distillers use any method of filtration for hydrosols, reverse osmosis is perhaps the most common process currently used when they do. There are other options, however, so let's look at the parameters of the filtration process.

- ✧ Temperature of hydrosol before, during, and after filtering

- ✧ Availability and ease of handling of filter system

- ✧ Efficiency of filter

- ✧ Speed of filtration

- ✧ Sterilization of vessels

- ✧ Cost

Temperature of Hydrosol

As was mentioned earlier, a constant temperature is as important as the actual temperature for storage and handling. If the storage temperature is thirteen degrees centigrade (fifty-five degrees Fahrenheit), then, in an ideal world, the filtration process should take place at approximately the same temperature. Therefore it would be nice if the filtration device were actually in the same cold-storage area as the hydrosols are kept. If the filtration is done in a different location, it would be most desirable if the area were similar in temperature to the storage room, and if it were not the same, then the filtration should be completed fast enough that the temperature of the hydrosol does not have time to come up to the new ambient temperature, only to drop after being returned to the cold store afterward. It is not that a short period at a higher temperature will be the death of the hydrosol but rather that putting a warm, clean, filtered water into a cold environment may prompt the formation of condensation inside the bottle, and condensation can cause problems.

Condensation causes pure water molecules to be drawn out of the hydrosol and to form into drops on the upper regions of the container. As the condensate "evaporates," these pure water molecules go back into the hydrolate. The hydrosol reacts as though the condensate water molecules were fresh water coming from an outside source. As I have mentioned, diluting hydrosols with water shortens their shelf life, and condensation will shorten their shelf life in the same manner. My current estimates are that diluted hydrosols, regardless of type, have a reliable shelf life of no more than four months, and in some cases less.

So cold-storage facilities could be designed to include a filtration system as part of the setup. The cold store could be a clean room of sorts; dust-free; doors always closed; with work benches for sterilization, filtering, and bottling; and with storage for both bulk and bottled quantities and a temperature- and humidity-controlled environment. Of course, it would be like working in a fridge, but oh, how I have dreamed of such a room.

Availability and Ease of Handling of Filter System

It's no use talking about filter systems that we can't get access to or that are too complex and expensive for all but laboratory conditions. Perversely, the unfortunate state of municipal water supplies has made the business of water filtration a lucrative and innovative one. Water companies abound, both those that supply bottled water and those that supply systems to do the filtering. Everything from tabletop distillers to carbon and charcoal filters is out there. UV light can be used and makes a neat substitute for chlorine in purifying swimming pool water but is of no use for hydrosols. Some filters spin the water to affect an electrostatic charge; other devices such as the Brita remove chlorine, lead, and some organisms and improve the flavor but require basically clean municipal water to start with. One of the best filter systems involves a huge tank of coconut-shell charcoal and is attached to the water source where it enters the house. Because the water is filtered at the point of entry, it is filtered before it gets to the hot-water tank, thus eliminating the problems most filtration systems have in dealing with hot water from the tap.

But what are the options for our specific purpose? The filter should be compact, possibly transportable. It should be easily set up and maintained to prevent contaminants from building up in the filter and being introduced into, rather than removed from, the hydrosol. The filter itself and all necessary parts for maintenance, repair, and use should be available locally. If it takes four weeks to get a replacement filter, you had better order early or you'll be out of business for a while. The filter should also be easy to use. Part of the success of the Brita brand filter jug is its ease of handling. It requires no installation—even a child can do it. It is reasonably quick, and Brita has dealt with the problems of maintenance by introducing filter monitors. Now when your filter needs replacing, a little arrow on the filter tells you. Idiot proof! But hydrosols are not water, and we want something that works for us.

Efficiency of Filter

Sometimes it works to equate hydrosols with drinking water. I drink them a lot and so do many others; it is one of the nicest ways to benefit from their therapeutic properties. Hydrosols must also be able to conform to any laws that may exist regarding the sale of cosmetic, aesthetic, supplement, and therapeutic products or food products. Not all countries have applied their laws to hydrosols specifically, but some have, and any filter system must be sufficient to render the filtered product in accordance with the legal requirements, should they ever be introduced.

The particulate matter is easy to filter and it can be done with coffee or paper filters. But what about the stuff you can't see? Bacteria are usually 0.1 to 0.8 microns in size. Viruses can be smaller then 0.03 microns, but they usually bind to other material that tends to be larger. So we

want a system that will remove everything down to at least 0.2 to 0.4 microns, which is almost the same as the 0.1-micron EPA standard for bottled water in the United States. The efficiency can be determined with lab tests; however, the home test will be that the pH of the hydrosol will have returned to the benchmark point after filtering. As was said, an increase in pH is the indication mark for the presence of bacteria, visible or not. After filtering, if the contaminants have been removed, it stands to reason that the pH will return to its original point.

With hydrosols, unlike drinking water, the filtration is not to improve the flavor of the water or to get rid of odors. In fact, it is critical that the system not alter the flavor or aroma of the hydrosols; it should remove only undesirable, not desirable, elements. If the smell or flavor of the hydrosol has degraded or gone off, I do not bother trying to filter—I just dump the stuff. When in doubt, throw it out. The loss factor is part of the reality of dealing in natural products, and I'm just glad I don't sell strawberries.

Speed of Filtration

The system should be relatively quick. Time is money, and if you are working with hydrosols, you are probably dealing with many liters at a time. Most of my containers are twenty-liter carboys, with the occasional five-liter jug. If the system filters at one liter per hour, it will take twenty hours to filter a carboy, and if you stock forty or fifty waters, as I do, you will be filtering constantly. The other problem with slow systems is that they need to be closed to the environment or you risk recontaminating the filtered water in the receiving vessel during the filtration process. Twenty hours is a long time to leave the lid off a bottle while it fills, and only the most ultra-pristine and controlled conditions would allow this kind of process to occur without your being guaranteed that aerial contamination occurs with it. And who has this kind of time?

Sterilization of Vessels

It's a big help for the vessels that receive hydrosols at the still to be sterilized before use. Hydrosols come off relatively slowly, two to four liters per hour, depending on the plant material being processed, so the same problem exists as with slow filtration: Your vessel and your product can be contaminated during filling. But the risks would be tremendously minimized by the use of sterile containers and some minimal dust filter to keep out particulate matter. The Canadian distiller with whom I work extensively sterilizes everything before filling and uses a paper filter to seal the mouth of the receiving vessel. We have noticed the difference these little changes make.

Every vessel at every stage of a hydrosol's life should be sterile, as should lids, sprayers, drippers, and any packaging component with which they come in contact. It is an easily achieved control that makes a huge difference in storage capability, but as of this writing I can

assure you such is not the case. Some simple methods of sterilizing were discussed in chapter 2, and I would urge the distillers, exporters, and distributors in particular to make this effort part of their normal routine. At the very least, bottles for packaging hydrosols should be washed in a dishwasher or boiled; it would be better yet to sterilize them with alcohol or food-grade hydrogen peroxide. All components of the packaging must be sterilized, not just the bottles, and gloves should be worn so that bare fingers, however clean, do not come into contact with either the clean components or the hydrosols.

I want access to hydrosols uncontrolled by government agencies. If contaminated products continue to be put on the market, regardless of their intended use, we run the risk of the imposition of laws and regulations that will undoubtedly affect our access to these and many other natural products. We must self-regulate; we must take care. The European Union has already demanded the addition of 13 percent alcohol to any hydrosol being sold for "cosmetic" use. In Europe, as in the United States and Canada, *medicines* enter a sticky world of regulations, so health products are often marketed as cosmetics, perfumes, flavorings, and foodstuffs. I don't want to put alcohol on my skin, and I much prefer single-malt scotch to ethyl, thank you, so I won't be drinking commercially available hydrosols off the shelf in Europe any more. Sterilization of all packaging material at all stages should be a minimum standard in the handling of hydrosols.

Cost

At their source, most hydrosols are still relatively inexpensive, even cheap in some cases. Unfortunately, that source may be Bulgaria, Morocco, Turkey, or islands like Madagascar. By the time a hydrosol is shipped by air to its final destination, the cost per liter will have doubled, tripled, frequently quadrupled. Loss owing to contamination, whatever the cause, also increases price, and those companies responsible enough to filter, sterilize, and do all the extras have every right to charge more for their products. When choosing a filtration system, you must factor the cost of the system into the final price at which the hydrosols will sell. Until the day when consumers are willing to pay extra for their hydrosols to be preservative-free and retailers follow the model of juice companies by installing fridges, we will unfortunately continue to find adulterated, preserved, contaminated, and poor products in the market.

Water filters can cost between ten and ten thousand dollars, and your final choice will depend on the scale of your business, the volume processed, the end use of product, and the range of your products. If I carried only five different waters, I would probably use a glorified up-market version of the Brita system. Same idea, more efficient filter. If I were Primavera Life in Germany and sold two tons of rosewater a year plus twelve other hydrosols as well, I'd be looking for something mechanical that required less manpower to operate while still meeting all parameters.

What follows is an examination of a variety of filter systems currently on the market with possible applications in the filtering of hydrosols.

TYPES OF FILTERS

Paper Filters

Clean, unbleached paper coffee filters can be used to give a just-for-safety's-sake filtration to waters from unknown sources that seem to be clear but—you never know. They can also be used to remove particulate matter either before further filtering or as the sole means of filtering for noninternal use, at the consumer's discretion. A paper filter is an effective device used at the distillation moment. A filter in a funnel reduces the orifice of the receiving vessel, and anything entering the vessel would have passed through the paper. This makes the time the container takes to fill less important, since it would be exposed to less contamination. Lab-supply companies have sterile disposable filters, which are available by mail order, and even the dairy filters used in the milking process are wonderful for hydrosols. Paper coffee filters can be sterilized in a microwave oven, but be careful—you don't want to start a fire; just use several very short blasts.

Distillers

Home water distillers are common and highly effective, resulting in a pure, neutral 7.0 pH drinking water. However, distilled water is so clean that the beneficial minerals and micronutrients in the water are removed along with the contaminants, and it is recommended that you add colloidal minerals or special water supplements back to the distilled water if you drink it on a daily basis. Otherwise distilled water can, over time, leach these nutrients out of your body instead of supplying them, as water should. Home distillation is also slow and will usually produce no more than five liters in six to ten hours, depending on your distillation unit.

Redistillation of hydrosols is not a good option. The resulting product is more like plain water than the original plant water: The pH tends to be close to the 7.0 mark, and although some smell and taste remain, they are significantly reduced. I also believe that reboiling the hydrosol damages both the water-soluble components and the essential oil in suspension.

Reverse Osmosis

Reverse osmosis (RO) was invented for the desalination of seawater for ship-bound naval and military personnel. This system pushes water through a semipermeable membrane that traps impurities, dissolved material, and contaminants, allowing only pure water to pass through. There are few better filtration systems than reverse osmosis, and the technology is now quite developed and complex.

The problem with RO is the speed—or lack of it. Although there are many different membranes available, depending on the nature of the contaminants and the end purpose of the water product, it is still an extremely slow process. It takes several hours to filter five liters (approxi-mately one gallon), easily as long as distillation, in some cases longer. The water passes through the membrane literally one drop at a time. Now, this is satisfactory for a home unit if you have a sufficiently large storage tank to hold the filtered water and the system runs all the time. But when your undercounter tank runs out, the wait until it fills again can seem interminable, and you better not be thirsty.

Most RO systems are also closed systems, meaning that there are no open, or exposed, elements between the point of entry and the point of exit in the system. The water main attaches directly to the filter unit, which drips directly into the sealed storage tank, which pumps straight to the tap. It doesn't really matter, from the point of view of contamination, if the system drips the water or pours it in a stream. The lid of the storage tank is sealed shut and drop by drop the water remains clean.

Filtering hydrosols by reverse osmosis is a different matter. A closed system is not really viable, since it would have to be opened and cleaned every time you changed hydrosol type. Also, the membranes themselves would be more likely to develop or hold flavors, and they are much more difficult to clean than the receiving vessel. RO systems are available that back-flush the membranes, and this can deal with the flavor issue, but you will still have either an open system, meaning that the hydrosols are dripping into your jugs in the open, or a labor-intensive closed system.

Then there is the issue of maintenance. If you do not keep the membranes clean, replacing them as often as or more often than manufacturers recommend, and also maintain the rest of the system, you will have a product loaded with toxins, far, far worse than anything you may have had in your hydrosol to start with. Don't forget that the membrane is holding all the "bad stuff" that you are removing from your water; eventually it will become full and all these contaminants will start entering the finished product. It's too disgusting to think about!

Where reverse osmosis is showing the greatest potential is in removing some of the water content of the hydrolates, concentrating the soluble therapeutic properties. Developed for use in the food and fragrance industries, these concentrated hydrosols are easier to analyze chemically and are being promoted as easier to store, since they are less bulky, being reduced four- or fivefold in volume, and seem to have a slightly improved shelf life. There are obvious benefits and drawbacks to this concept. First, a concentrated product is stronger. It will be critical from a therapeutic point of view to know just how strong it is, so appropriate dilution rates can be established before therapeutic protocols are developed. This will be difficult, as every system may produce a different level of concentration, and standards will be very difficult to establish.

Second, if thyme CT thymol hydrosol, for example, is hot to the taste in its standard form, how much hotter will the concentrate be, and will this alter its application potentials? If the shelf life is improved, that's a plus, but how much is it improved? Do we know? Can we extrapolate from the concentration, or do we need three to five years to make actual tests?

The biggest single advantage to the concentration is that shipping costs are reduced, since you ship smaller amounts. However, a concentrated product will be more expensive, as the cost of the processing must be factored into the price, so my guess is that the final savings to the buyer will be negligible.

One distiller who is using this method told me that there was "no problem" with this concept. If the hydrosol was concentrated by the removal of four liters of water, you just add four liters of water back to the product when it arrives. Unfortunately, adding water to a hydrosol immediately reduces its shelf life, so the only efficient way of using the concentrate would be to dilute it just before use. Of course it's possible to concentrate hydrosols, we do it with oils, but you wouldn't spray a concentrated hydrosol on your face, and diluted hydrosol is much less viable than the unconcentrated hydrosol you started with. I also question whether the "energetic" and healing properties of a reconstituted hydrosol can be the same as the original product. My gut feeling is no, although I have not had the time to test these products properly.

Although the process of creating a concentrated hydrosol is still experimental and rare, it's being explored and at the very least gives us a better way to analyze the chemical profiles of the waters.

Charcoal

In addition to the Brita system, which is discussed next, many tap and shower filters use charcoal as the filtering medium. Charcoal is very porous, which gives it a large surface area. Water passes over all these surfaces, leaving behind residue and contaminants. Charcoal filters come in a multitude of sizes and price ranges, from the top-of-tap model for thirty dollars at the hardware store to the two-thousand-dollar scuba-tank, coconut-charcoal, point-of-entry system. The overall effectiveness of any charcoal system depends on correct maintenance and design.

Charcoal filters have a finite life, depending on use. The surfaces of the charcoal become saturated with the pollutants; when these surfaces become clogged or full, they can start releasing them back into the water being filtered. Shower filters, which filter hot water, are rated for twelve to eighteen months but frequently last less than a year, as hot water tends to contain trihalomethanes (THMs), and they clog the filter fairly rapidly. However, charcoal is effective for filtering hydrosols only up to a point, and with larger systems you must deal with other technical issues. Do you pump the hydrosol through the filter? Then you must find a pump made from stainless steel or inert plastic and must make sure no lubricants come into contact with the water. If you use gravity to force the hydrosol through the filter, what happens if you have only one liter? The wastage is quite high. If you have fifty liters, to what height can you elevate the container to give you enough clearance and gravitational force to get the pressure just right? How do you clean the filter between different types of hydrosols? Do you use water, knowing that water added to a hydrosol shortens its shelf life

and that it would be virtually impossible to eliminate all the water inside the filter after a water flush? I have yet to find a charcoal system that fits the desired parameters, although they do have some hydrosol applications.

Brita

Invented by a Canadian, the Brita filter is one of the success stories of the 1990s. Now sold in over a dozen countries, Brita is the quick fix for already-potable but unpalatable tap water. Brita uses a charcoal filter that lasts from four to six weeks, depending on the quantity and quality of water filtered. Brita removes some heavy metals and nearly all chlorine and THMs, as well as bacteria like giardia and cryptosporidium.

If a hydrosol's pH has changed only slightly (0.2 to 0.3) and there is no particulate matter or growth in it, a Brita filter can sometimes restore the pH and therefore the product. If you want to use a Brita, you must have a fresh filter for every hydrosol or run several rinses of clean water through the filter between hydrosols. Before filtering, you must also first soak the filter in a quantity of the hydrosol to be filtered. Brita is not a viable option for the distributor or reseller of hydrosols but may be used by the consumer who wants to be on the safe side or who is buying from unknown sources.

Ceramic

There are a number of ceramic filters on the market, and they are both effective and cost-efficient options. Ceramic may filter down to 0.2 microns, and the filters come in a variety of sizes, from palm to industrial volume. They have been used in hospitals and manufacturing and are commonly part of multisystem filtration protocols in technology.

Some ceramic filters are impregnated with silver nitrate, a sort of colloidal silver, to boost their effectiveness. Colloidal silver burst onto the health scene a few years ago as an alternative to antibiotics and is useful for treating antibiotic-resistant infections. Many books have been written about colloidal silver's effectiveness, and testimonials are excellent. Silver enhances ceramic's filtering capability because it acts even on germs that are smaller than the size to which the ceramic alone is effective. Impregnating the filter with silver also prevents the growth of bacteria within the ceramic matrix of the filter itself, an important benefit that makes maintenance much simpler. The Katadyn filter, for example, is impregnated with silver nitrate, which works to help kill anything smaller than 0.2 microns, such as viruses, while keeping the filter itself free of contaminants, removing the need for water flushing.

Katadyn Filters

The hand-held Katadyn is rated to pump five liters per minute, although in practice it is more like one-quarter to one-half liter per minute for hydrosols, and even this will bring beads of perspiration to your brow. This is still astonishingly quick for an effective filter when compared with the systems described above. This also refers to the smallest model, which is designed for travelling; the larger commercial systems are faster and either work by gravity or are mechanically powered.

The unit is easily disassembled for cleaning; it just unscrews and separates into its components, which can be individually washed and dried. The ceramic-and-silver filter will pump up to approximately fifty thousand liters before needing replacement, depending on the level of contaminants in the water and the cleaning required after each use. The only difficult thing is drying the inside of the uptake hose.

The filter comes with a three-foot-long hose that has a conical screen at the end that is placed into the water supply. This screen prevents big chunks and fish or other water creatures from entering the unit if you happen to be in the Amazon rain forest. It is nigh impossible to remove this tip. The other end is attached to the base of the filter system where the water enters the unit; it is also nearly impossible to undo this end, and if you do you'll have a devil of a time getting it back on. So the hose portion needs to be dried intact—and it's three feet long! In the beginning I found that not even twelve hours in the oven would dry up all the water drops, and I'm a bit paranoid about condensation. I finally started blowing down the hose to remove water droplets because I realized that any germs I was introducing would be filtered out, but it was an unsanitary method, and I now force canned pressurized air through it. When storing the unit for more than a couple of weeks, I leave it—filter, hose, and all—in a gas oven with only the pilot light on for four to eight hours, until it is bone dry.

I had to keep reminding myself as I learned to use this filter that if I were trekking in the Himalayas I probably would not even have the opportunity to properly clean, much less dry, the unit for the duration of my trip. But that's the kind of treatment and conditions the unit is designed to deal with, after all. It is considered the top-of-the-line filter for just these situations, so anything I throw at it in the way of hydrosols has to be a piece of cake. I would also say that I bought my Katadyn amid a series of the most serendipitous events you can imagine and even got an impromptu phone consultation with a water-filtration expert during the transactions, so I knew I was on the right track.

If you have a cold store for your products, filtering can easily be done in situ, or it can be set up wherever and whenever needed. The Katadyn changed a lot for me, as I can now be absolutely certain that I am not selling contaminated products. I have my pH parameters and my filter to back me up and am glad that I will be pouring less hydrosol into my compost heap this year than in years past.

Testing

Of course the Katadyn required testing. The pH test was the first to be conducted, and it showed that the Katadyn works like a charm. More than 85 percent of the time, even hydrosols full of particulate matter will filter out crystal clear, and the pH will usually be spot-on, back to its original point. Interestingly, even though I have what I consider to be great suppliers who know and care about hydrosols, most of them still don't even sterilize their containers. I received some geranium water last year that measured 5.6 pH and was starting to develop little balls of fluff. It was less than six months old at the time. We filtered the water through paper to remove the particulates, then pumped it through the Katadyn into sterilized bottles. The resulting crystal-clear liquid had a 4.8 pH and tasted and smelled just wonderful.

I sent samples of the filtered and unfiltered geranium to be analyzed. Here are the results. Sample 1 is the bloomed, unfiltered hydrosol; sample 2 is the filtered hydrosol; sample 3 is a clean geranium hydrosol from another batch.

PARAMETER	UNITS	SAMPLE 1	SAMPLE 2	SAMPLE 3
Heterotrophic plate count	CFU/ml	›57,000	0	0
Yeast	CFU/100 ml	‹2	‹2	‹2
Mold	CFU/100 ml	›400	2	‹2

CFU=colony-forming units

A count of less than two (<2) for each of the parameters is normal for a plant extract, as it is in part a measure of the water-soluble components thought to be plant carbohydrates. I am assured by the lab that hydrosols with counts of less than two are acceptable for consumption.

Of course, there are times when a hydrosol is too far gone to be saved by any filtration method. I received some *Inula* last year that was only two months old but arrived milky and full of "clouds," little white chunks of floating gunk. I was shocked that the stuff had even been bottled, much less shipped. The pH was 6.3; *Inula* should be 4.6 to 4.8 pH or even less. *Inula* is exceedingly hard to get and very powerful. Since we were at the beginning of a terrible flu season, I was more than a little frustrated. I needed this hydrosol; my clients needed this hydrosol. This particular flu virus settles in the lungs and *Inula* is your lad for that specific problem. In this case, not even the Katadyn was able to restore the pH, although it did filter out quite clear. I resorted to using eucalyptus, bee balm, and savory in the end.

If a hydrosol's odor has changed, filtration will not bring it back. If the contaminants are smaller than 0.2 microns, they can't be filtered out with this method, although the silver will probably kill the bacteria. If the hydrosol is really getting old, there is only so much that a filter will do, and there comes a point where it is just not worth it to try to save the water. But as hydrosols are relatively inexpensive, it seems a small price to pay if the occasional bottle goes to floor cleaning or plant feeding or into the compost pile.

AFTERCARE AND PACKAGING

Although I talked about bottling and storage in chapter 2, I think it worthwhile to look at this in a little more depth. Packaging of hydrosols and their care is a major contributing factor to their shelf life. Since I am a proponent of internal use, it is also something in which I place a fair amount of importance.

When a distillation takes place, the hydrosol and essential oil are normally separated during the process by a Florentine flask. The hydrolate flows out into a collecting vessel or is allowed to flow back into the fields, while the more precious oil remains in the flask, floating on the surface of the hydrosol that remains. There is a variety of views among distillers on the importance of this separation, but it is generally agreed among those for whom the oil is the primary product that it is quite important to separate the oil and water components fairly soon, ideally immediately, after distillation is complete. When the run is finished, the oil—and only a small amount of hydrosol—is collected in another vessel. This vessel is usually some type of laboratory glass that will allow the oil to float on the surface and the hydrosol to remain underneath, where it can be drawn off by a spigot or tap. The oil is left to sit in this container for anywhere from six to thirty-six hours, depending on the plant species, and during this time the microdrops of water suspended in the oil will have time to sink to the bottom and be removed. Once completely separated from the water, the oil may be allowed to sit open to the air for an additional period of time to allow it to "dry" further and for the aroma and chemistry to rebalance after the shock of distillation. This is a key practice in aromatherapeutic distillation that is often not practiced by the unskilled distiller. I once bought a kilo of patchouli oil from which the lid literally blew off in my hands owing to the fermentation taking place in the oil. The smell was quite awful. It was very obvious by the cloudy, not to mention bubbling, nature of this oil that it still contained a fair amount of moisture and had certainly not been left to dry after distillation.

I have been told that some oils require two weeks or more of unlidded rest before they are considered dry enough to bottle. Who but a skilled distiller would leave a bottle of fresh oil unstoppered for that length of time? Everything we are taught says that bottles should remain tightly lidded at all times, but I frequently leave large containers of oil unstoppered if their odor tells me they are not fully dry. My apprentices complained about a new batch of basil recently, but upon smelling it the problem seemed clear. After being left open for twenty-four hours, the basil smelled terrific—and we all had learned something new.

When Wet Is Dry

But oils are not hydrosols, so does the same hold true for the waters? Most definitely, although we allow them to "mature" with lids on. Very fresh hydrosol has a very wet odor. You might say they all have a wet odor, but this is really wet, a damp-dog kind of wet. It takes time for the components to come into full resonance with each other, to get to know each other, as it were: "Oh, hello, so you're from Madagascar are you, cinnamon bark you say, well howdy, my name's H_2O and I come from that little spring round the back, how're you doing?" Or something like that. Hydrosols require at least a week before the odor and taste start to stabilize, and they reach their full flavor after about two months. They do actually "dry" in much the same way as the oils, and although they are always wet, they lose that musty damp scent that they have when fresh. You can use them before this time, but they taste and smell better if you wait.

Now comes the revolution. As distillation of plant material just for hydrosols has become more common, on both a home and a commercial level, a divergent theory has appeared. This theory proposes that the distillation run be stopped when the maximum quality of hydrolate has been collected but before all the oil is distilled, as the hydrosol is the primary product. (Or all the hydrosol and all the oil are both collected and saved.) Any oil that is collected during the run is allowed to stay floating on the surface of the hydrosol, which is stored in glass containers with a spigot on the bottom. The belief is that the oil on the surface prevents oxygen from coming into contact with the hydrosol, slowing or preventing oxidation. The hydrosol is decanted from the bottom, not disturbing the oil on top.

Some distillers say they are able to store hydrosols for several years without any degradation using this method, but I have my doubts. Just as the neroli oil coalescing out of the hydrosol made my supplier suspicious of bacteria, so many distillers report that improperly dried oils will not only ferment, as we have seen, but also oxidize more quickly if not dried or if left in contact with the hydrosol. What I do know is that oils floating on the top of hydrosols in the bottle do not extend their shelf life in the least. It is an interesting idea, however, and I'm sure that as more distillers experiment along these lines we'll have more concrete proof one way or the other.

Plastic versus Glass

Then there is the issue of storage containers. Most shipping containers are plastic for bulks of one liter or more. It's just not feasible to ship gallons in glass; it's too heavy and it's breakable. But there are conflicting views on plastic, and in some ways it's a matter of making an educated choice. Glass is actually a liquid flowing at a very slow speed. For this reason most glass bottles would actually hold more liquid than they say. They are designed so that, when filled, an air space remains at the top so the liquid expanding and contracting inside the glass will not cause it to explode. Essential oils, like most liquids, expand and contract a lot, and overfilled bottles can explode just from changes in barometric pressure. The same is true for hydrosols. The batch that froze on its way to Alberta would have

blown a glass bottle to smithereens. Fortunately a phenol-resistant, rigid plastic bottle with sufficient air space and a responsive air-pocket lid allowed the hydrosol to expand in freezing without breaking and ruining the entire shipment.

If you wish to store hydrosols with a layer of oil on top, you must use glass, as most plastics, even those that are phenol resistant, will break down from contact with the oils. But if you are storing hydrosols that have been carefully separated, then these phenol-resistant rigid plastics seem to offer no hazard of any kind to the waters. Very few suppliers, whether large or small, sell their hydrosols in glass. Most don't sell even small quantities of one hundred to two hundred milliliters in glass, choosing instead these resistant plastics. They come in all sizes, shapes, and colors; I have seen several shades of blue, purple, red, green, orange, and even amber plastic bottles for hydrosols. But what do the hydrosols think?

Again we enter territory full of divergent opinions. Many very good distillers and practitioners who have worked extensively with hydrosols claim that plastic is just fine as a storage container. Assuming that we are using sterilized containers, plastic does not seem to shorten a hydrosol's shelf life, at least not in my tests. Dark plastic provides very little more protection than clear plastic; ultraviolet (UV) protection is more a function of the type of plastic than the color of the container, whereas in glass the color creates the protection. What makes the difference is the type of plastic itself, and any supplier will provide you with data about the UV protection, oxygen permeability, reactivity, and chemical resistance of all the various plastics available. For one- to five-liter jugs, I buy a high-grade, phenol- and alcohol-resistant, rigid plastic with a low oxygen permeability and good UV protection. It is not quite opaque, and the lids contain a bladder that can expand and contract, which seems to help reduce condensation.

There is another choice in plastic, and that is Nalgene. Developed by NASA for astronauts, this is a totally inert plastic that will withstand the most extreme conditions . . . like space. Nalgene is resistant to most chemicals and solvents and poses no danger at all to hydrosols. It is usually tinted somewhat and has good UV-protection capabilities as well as extremely low permeability to oxygen. Nalgene is manufactured in a variety of densities, from very rigid to squeezably soft, and its nonreactivity has made it a new standard in many science and hospital laboratories for all kinds of chemical substances.If you can find them at a reasonable cost, Nalgene containers would be the ultimate nonglass storage vessel for natural products.

In the next few years a number of other containers will be tested. One, designed for liquid foodstuffs, consists of a very rigid plastic outer shell with a complex polycarbonate soft liner bag. The idea is that the liquid is inside a vacuum in the inner bag, which is protected by the hard shell. As the liquid is removed from the inner bag, it collapses to prevent air from getting in contact with the food, reducing the likelihood of degradation. Another innovation is the new range of airless sprayers introduced by the cosmetics packaging companies. Because shelf life and product degradation are big issues for cosmetics as they begin to incorporate more natural ingredients, airless sprayers were designed to prevent the oxidation process that can happen inside standard spray bottles whether you take the lid off or not. Most of these airless sprayers are plastic or rubber, so reactivity may be an issue, but some are glass, and some of the plastics are very high quality, so we shall see what options these components provide to aromatherapists and hydrosol users.

Black Amethyst Glass

But I ask again, what do the hydrosols think? Ultimately they prefer glass, and of all the colors of glass, they prefer the blue-to-violet spectrum best. Amber glass is fine, but just as humans respond more favorably to water that is blue than water that is brown, I think the hydrosols, too, have a color preference. They want us to like them—and too bad if that's not scientific. Most blue glass is no longer made with cobalt—it's just colored blue—although true cobalt is still available, at twice the price. Real cobalt glass seems to affect the vibrational health of a hydrosol, and in tests where samples from just one hydrosol was put in a number of different vessels, when dowsed, the true cobalt was found to increase the energetic field by a significant amount. Interestingly, the plastic did not diminish the vibration any more than amber glass, and neither seemed to affect shelf life to any certain degree.

But that's not all there is to glass. A couple of years ago I received an e-mail that claimed that the life span of my hydrosols could be extended dramatically simply by using violet glass. Sure, sure, more hype. Well, not completely. Black amethyst glass, or violet glass, as it's now known, was developed in the early 1800s in Germany for a specific line of products. These products were "cured" in the blazing Mediterranean sun for weeks or even months, then stored in these special glass bottles that would allow only certain frequencies of light to pass through. It is believed that these frequencies enhance the bioenergetic nature of the plant remedy and the sun energy they have absorbed. The glass is so dark that it looks opaque and black, and the deep violet hue is obtained by the addition of a host of ingredients, including ground amethyst, hence its original name.

But what of the claims? Having put a number of hydrosols in Miron violet glass, I can say that there seems to be no more than a 10-to-15-percent increase in shelf life; I will run the tests again this year for a longer duration to check yet again. What I can say, however, is that the hydrosols love the violet glass. An increase in the energy field is visible by dowsing within ten minutes of decanting hydrosols into these bottles and seems to increase for about eighteen to twenty-four hours, when it reaches its peak and stays there. The difference is significant, far greater than with cobalt, and if you are using hydrosols primarily for vibrational work, you would do well to invest in some of these bottles to store your energetic waters and blends.

Even a 10 to 15 percent increase in shelf life is nothing to sneeze at, particularly with the more fragile waters such as bay leaf. One company in Germany sells all its hydrosols in violet glass, having found that it helped slightly with shelf life. The biggest drawback to these bottles is their price and weight. Just as real cobalt is more expensive than plain blue glass, violet glass is costlier than standard glass, and it is also thicker, thus increasing the shipping cost. But the significant effects on the energetic field make it worth using for this reason alone.

So the learning curve seems endless, as it always does. For every discovery in the areas of preservation, storage, monitoring, and shelf life, there are a host of new questions that arise. But today the issue of contamination and degradation worry me no more than they did in the early days of blissful ignorance. Yes, hydrosols require some care. Yes, hydrosols can go off. But also, yes, hydrosols can be monitored. Yes, hydrosols can be tested easily at home. Yes, hydrosols are safe, fun, and effective to use. And finally, yes, hydrosols are totally delicious and worthy of exploration for the sheer pleasure they can add to our lives. Those, in the end, are the hard facts.

FIVE

Now What Do I Do with Them?

The system of life on this planet is so astoundingly complex that it was a long time before man even realised that it was a system at all and that it wasn't something that was just there.

Douglas Adams, *Last Chance to See*

In the monographs you will find specific information on the properties and applications of individual hydrosols. However, there are some general rules, a variety of dosages, and many different ways to design protocols for their use. There are also areas of special interest that require exploration, particularly applications for babies and children, aesthetic uses, detoxification programs, and use by those with immune concerns.

It is interesting that when one starts looking for scientific research into oils and, specifically, hydrosols, all sorts of odd data come up. The exploration of potentially marketable properties of plant material and botanical extracts is a huge business, and millions of dollars can ride on the findings. Fortunately for us, we can use and build on this information as we dis-

cover the real power in this new aromatherapy.

Let's look at some of this research, shall we?

"Many reports on the relationship between skin aging induced by UV-irradiation and the active oxygen suggest that the prevention of 'skin-aging' can be achieved by active-oxygen scavengers." In this study the researchers not only looked at the antioxidative, free-radical-scavenging properties of sixty-five plant extracts but also tested their ability to prevent and/or repair damage to the collagen- and elastin-forming fibroblast cells in the skin. The most active plants were rosemary, horse chestnut, and witch hazel, followed by common burnet, red oak, bistort, sage, *Eucalyptus globulus*, thyme, and coltsfoot. The first seven herbs were tested for a variety of scavenging activities as well as for their ability to protect cells from matrix damage caused by ultraviolet exposure. Both horse chestnut and witch hazel achieved top marks in virtually every test and were considered by the researchers "to be effective anti-aging or anti-wrinkle agents for the skin." Rosemary, which received the highest overall score in "superoxide anion scavenging activity," had a widely variable effect in the other tests, although rosemary extract is widely recognized as an effective antioxidant substance. Sage had really interesting dose-dependent effects in protecting skin cells, with maximum effectiveness achieved at a comparatively low concentration.[1] Interesting when one considers the hydrosols.

A study on the ability of essential oils to scavenge free radicals found that several chemotypes of thyme and eugenol-containing herbs like basil and clove were most effective. It was the phenolic compounds that inhibited the energy metabolism catalyzed by isolated cell membranes. Compare these findings to the Japanese research cited previously.[2]

Hamamelis virginiana shows up in a pile of documents that look at the antiviral, antiherpetic, anti-inflammatory, and protective properties of aqueous and alcohol extracts prepared from witch hazel bark and branch with leaves. In one, witch hazel outperformed the control substance ascorbic acid dramatically.[3]

Another study showed that it is not just the tannins in witch hazel that contribute to its potential antiviral and proven antiherpetic properties. Since few if any tannins show up in hydrosols, might these "other" compounds make

witch hazel hydrosol a possibility for inhibiting herpes and HIV? The same study showed that *Hamamelis* extract also helped diminish the damage created by polymorphonucleotides (PMN) influx in herpes-induced lesions on the skin and mucus membranes.[4]

Then there is my favorite, the paper reporting that although it is not quite as effective as topical hydrocortisone treatments, *Hamamelis* distillate (hydrosol) is very close. The authors discuss the many adverse effects inherent in the use of glucocorticoids such as hydrocortisone, which are "varying from mild to life threatening," and state, "Fearing adverse effects, physicians as well as patients try to avoid glucocorticoid therapy as far as possible. This holds true especially for atopic dermatitis, because its chronic course and frequent relapses require long-term treatment." In fact, *Hamamelis* was so effective in two randomized, double-blind studies, far more effective even than German chamomile, that the authors suggest it should be considered as a non-damaging treatment option for inflammatory skin disease, in particular atopic dermatitis.[5] In my own work I've found that both German chamomile and witch hazel hydrosols can clear up atopic dermatitis, even in very young infants.

Then there's yarrow. Crude aqueous extracts and lipophilic extracts (teas, hydrosols, and oils) of five species of *Achillea* were examined for their antiedematous activity in the croton-oil ear test, and common yarrow, *A. millefolium*, scored highest. The authors state, "All sesquiterpene lactones showed topical edema inhibition. . . .

As all substances are transferred into herbal teas they must be accepted as part of the antiphlogistic properties in millefoil."[6] Is this why yarrow hydrosol has such dramatic results applied topically to eczema and psoriasis? Is this why it is so good as part of a detoxification program, helping the body rid itself of excess fluid, cleaning the bowels, and balancing the endocrine system? Surely there is a connection here.

TOPICAL USE

Health Applications

Hydrosols are mild but effective. They can be used undiluted without problems for most topical applications. In some ways you can treat them like water, for instance, to wash a cut or scrape, but it must be remembered that they differ from water in many ways. Hydrosols do contain some essential oils, so whichever one you use will contain some but not all of the properties of the oil, and you will receive some of the benefits that you would get if you used the respective oil. Hydrosols have a very different pH than water; they are always either slightly acid, like lavender (5.6 to 5.9 pH), or very acid, like rock rose (2.9 to 3.1 pH). The pH of hydrosol greatly influences its effects as a healing substance. Rock rose, because of its extreme acidity, is highly astringent and will constrict cells where it is applied. This means it is useful to stanch bleeding; it is also great for tightening pores and reducing wrinkles. Lavender, with an almost neutral pH, may be a better choice if a wound contains dirt or pus, since it can wash the debris out of the cut more easily, as the cells remain open and bleeding will help clean the wound.

A spray makes it easy to apply undiluted hydrosols; it allows a small amount of the water to be directed at the desired area quite precisely. Sprays are efficient, do not waste the hydrosol, and allow the container to remain closed, reducing the risk of contamination. (For more on storage and issues of contamination, see chapter 2.)

Undiluted hydrosol can also be sprayed all over the body as a quick refresher, to stimulate circulation or cool the body temperature, as a subtle perfume scent, to reduce the impact and damage of sun exposure, and even as a deodorant. Neat hydrosol can be used to make your own wet wipes, for both adult and infant personal hygiene; as a hand spray to prevent the spread of germs in cold season; and for whatever other applications you can imagine.

Undiluted hydrosol is the best choice for treating skin conditions. Dermatitis, eczema, psoriasis, poison ivy, and cuts and wounds respond very well to topical applications of neat hydrosol. If you are treating a skin condition such as these, several small applications per day are more effective than only one or two large applications. The general rule would be no less than three and as many as a dozen small localized applications per day, every day, until the symptoms resolve. In cases of eczema, for instance, the hydrosols can greatly ameliorate the itching, pain, and redness of the skin. They can slow down the flaking process and speed the healing of the bottom layers, meaning that when skin does flake off, the exposed tissue is less fresh, less sensitive, and less painful. With poison ivy, a combination of hydrosols and oils can slow or even stop the spread of the rash, which frequently will travel throughout the body, affecting far more surface area than was originally exposed to the plant toxins. Tea tree is the best choice for poison ivy and should be used topically and internally in both hydrosol and essential-oil form.

With conditions like psoriasis and eczema, I'd love to say hydrosols could be a cure, but, alas, they are not. These complex *dis*eases require healing on many levels, and in holistic health, psoriasis, eczema, and asthma are considered symptoms of a constitutional imbalance rather than conditions that should be treated directly. However, you can do much to alleviate the itchiness, pain, and peeling by applying waters of yarrow and witch hazel liberally and undiluted.

Certain very astringent hydrosols can be too much for sensitive skin. Neroli, another of the very acidic waters, can dry out already-dry skin. Repeated applications, once an hour every hour for ten applications, result in the test area of skin on the top of the forearm turning slightly white. One test subject was a woman of fifty-five, postmenopausal, who had extremely dry skin, crepey in texture, slightly wrinkled and damaged from years of overexposure to the sun. The same patch test was conducted a week later with rose geranium hydrosol, and at the end of the ten applications the skin was softer, more supple, and less wrinkled than before the neroli test and exhib-

ited none of the whiteness that had been created by the more astringent water.

Bearing this in mind, it is easy to see how important it is to buy preservative-free hydrosols. If pure neroli can have this effect on dry skin, what would happen if it were preserved with 14 percent alcohol or contained the synthetic preservatives that some companies use? If you buy your hydrosols in health-food stores or from retail outlets where they are not refrigerated, ask for quality assurance and inquire why, if they are indeed preservative-free, they are not cold-stored. The seller may not be able to answer you, but if every customer asks the question, the store personnel will start asking the supplier and will become better informed about these products in the future.

Topical Dilutions

Hydrosols are not expensive—I think they are cheap—but some people just don't value themselves enough to spend much on their health. Although there is nothing nicer than splashing yourself all over with undiluted hydrosol, it is not something everyone will do for themselves. However, diluting hydrosols is often as effective as using them undiluted and will save you money.

Compress

In a bowl, dilute three to five tablespoons of hydrosol in one liter of water at the desired temperature. For children dilute two to three teaspoons of hydrosol per liter of water. Soak a clean, lint-free cloth in the mix and apply it to the affected area, holding it there until the cloth changes temperature, that is, the hot cloth becomes cool or the cold cloth becomes warm. Repeat until the water in the bowl changes temperature. I say water "at the desired temperature" because you will sometimes want a hot compress, sometimes a lukewarm one, and sometimes an icy-cold one. It depends on the condition you are treating. Always heat or cool the water on its own, then mix in the hydrosol, and never use a microwave for anything to do with healing.

Compresses are fantastic treatments for all kinds of issues, from muscle aches and strains to infected wounds, scar tissue to bronchitis, varicose veins to menstrual cramps and ear infections. When you really think about it, most conditions will benefit from a compress application, if only by virtue of the temperature issue; add therapeutic botanicals and you create a healing synergy. As a general rule use cold for inflammation, cool or lukewarm temperatures in cases where there is great heat (especially fevers), and heat when there is tightness and lack of flexibility, but be sure to ask the client what feels best.

Sitz Bath

Dilute one hundred milliliters of hydrosol in the appropriate-temperature water in a small basin or a specially designed sitz bath; in a pinch fill the bathtub with three to four inches of water and sit in that for fifteen minutes. This seems like a lot of hydrosol, and it is, but sitz baths are often used to treat specific and somewhat severe conditions like hemorrhoids, postpartum damage, severe cystitis, and thrush and vaginal infections, and you don't want to mess around.

Most frequently it is recommended that you prepare two sitz baths simultaneously, one hot, one cold, and that you alternate between them, two minutes in each bath, with at least four or five sits in each one. This creates a dramatic increase in circulation to the area and is the tried-and-true healing method. If you undertake the two-bath method, split the hydrosol between the two baths—fifty milliliters in each. Start with warm water in one and cool in the other; every time you switch baths, make the warm water a little hotter and the cool a little colder until the two temperatures are as opposite as you can comfortably bear.

Bath

For babies up to six months old add one teaspoon of hydrosol to an infant-size tub of water or two teaspoons to an adult tub filled to baby depth. For children up to twelve years, add to the tub one teaspoon of hydrosol per year of age, up to a maximum of eight teaspoons. Adults can use from 30 to 250 milliliters per tub; the amount is dependent on personal taste, whether the bath is therapeutic or for pleasure (they are always both, really), and the size of the tub. A "normal" tub, which requires that adults bathe themselves one half at a time, needs 30 milliliters; a Jacuzzi for four needs 100 to 250 milliliters.

Note: Hydrosols, unlike some essential oils, will not harm the pumps used in whirlpool baths.

Dilution Mediums

When we think of diluting hydrosols, the first medium that comes to mind is usually water. After all, they are water, so . . . However, hydrosols can be added to almost any medium other than an oil with excellent results. Some products have such a high oil content that you will find it impossible to incorporate hydrosols into them; this also holds true for products that have a mineral oil or petroleum jelly base (such as many zinc ointments). If in doubt, try putting a little of the proposed dilution medium on the base of your hand, then flick a few drops of hydrosol on top. Using your fingers, try to combine them. If it works, try a batch; if the water just slides around on top, you are out of luck. You can often tell from the way the hydrosol reacts upon contact with the base if mixing will work, since the distinctive beading of the droplets usually indicates a heavy oil content in the base product.

Here are a few suggestions for usable dilution mediums:

Aloe vera gel or juice. Aloe vera is used topically for burns, rash, and dermal conditions to reduce itching and to coat wounds. Internally aloe cleans and heals the digestive tract and is an effective laxative. Choose the appropriate hydrosol for the condition that you are treating and use it to dilute the aloe vera by 20 to 50 percent. Use as you would pure aloe.

Rescue Remedy cream. This Bach flower remedy ointment can be squeezed into a clean container; hydrosol can be added by the drop and stirred in with a small spatula or spoon. You will be able to add only up to about 10 percent hydrosol effectively before the mixture either becomes too liquid or separates. I have used this as a topical ointment for very raw skin when I wanted a less viscous cream that could be spread without pulling at the delicate tissue and with the added benefits of the hydrosol.

Proprietary lotions and creams. There are many products in the marketplace—some natural, some less so—that can be used as a base for hydrosols. One client I have insists on using Lubriderm for her excessively dry body skin but found that the addition of 30 percent hydrosol did not lessen the effect of the Lubriderm; in fact, it enhanced her skin's ability to retain moisture. In this case a blend of rose geranium and rose hydrosols was used. You can add up to 50 percent hydrosol to a standard cream or lotion but may find that 30 to 40 percent is the best range of dilution. Even 5 percent will have an effect and will add a distinct note of luxury.

Calamine lotion. The classic treatment for sunburn, itchy skin, chicken pox, poison ivy, and a variety of dermal problems, calamine is a soothing, cool, pink liquid that dries on the skin, leaving a powdery residue behind. Hydrosols can be added to calamine in dilutions of up to 25 percent, and the appropriate hydrosol should be chosen based on the application.

Hydrogen peroxide. Usually sold at 3 percent strength for topical use in cleaning and disinfecting wounds, killing germs, and healing septic conditions, hydrogen peroxide can be diluted with 10 to 15 percent hydrosol to or up to 25 percent when using it on children or pets. The hydrosol will reduce some of the sting of the peroxide and at these dilutions will not inhibit its effects. I have also used 20- and 30-volume hydrogen peroxide, such as that sold in beauty supply shops for bleaching and dying hair. In the case of 20-volume peroxide (note this is 20 volume, not 20 percent) I add just 2 percent peroxide to 98 percent hydrosol or hydrosol and water. *Never* use stronger than 3 percent hydrogen peroxide on the skin undiluted; it is unnecessary and will bleach and burn the tissue. You may also find a food-grade 11 percent peroxide for sale in health food stores. This is used for oxygenating the body and treating certain infectious pathologies; it is not the same as the 3 percent topical peroxide and must not be confused with it, as it will sting and bleach the skin. Hydrosols may be added to food-grade peroxide up to 70 percent.

Unscented gels. There are a variety of unscented gels available; some European brands are even produced specifically for the addition of essential oils. These water-based gels can become a base for hydrosols, and you will have to experiment to determine the quantity of liquid that each brand will hold. It is usually safe to add at least 10 percent hydrosol, although in some cases the gels will take up to 50 percent. One client adds a blend of rose and neroli hydrosols to an aseptic gel and says it has done wonders for her sex life. No comment, really.

Milk. Even skim milk has some fat content, although full-fat milk is best for mixing with hydrosols. Milk can be particularly nice in a bath. Milk will also help disperse essential oils for those times that you may want both oil and hydrosol in the tub. At bedtime you can also flavor hot milk with sleep-inducing hydrosols.

Paper towels. Paper towels—not really a medium, but sort of—can be used to make your own towelettes or wet wipes. Choose a good-quality paper towel that holds up when wet and doesn't just turn to mush. If possible remove the cardboard tube from the center of the roll and cut the roll in half crosswise. Put the half-roll of towel upright in a suitable container to which you have added two tablespoons of pure hydrosol. Now sprinkle an additional two tablespoons of hydrosol on top of the roll so the paper absorbs from both top and bottom edges. Put the lid on and voilà . . . wet wipes. These homemade versions will not withstand being pulled out through a dispenser top, as the paper will shred. Some companies in Europe are now producing all-natural commercial towelettes containing herbal extracts and essential oils using the same fiber base as standard wet wipes.

Topical Applications

Aesthetic/Cosmetic

Many years ago, the Erno Laszlo beauty company ran an ad that described their philosophy of skin care. I was only about ten, but I remember being fascinated. The basic advice was to use *only* water on your face, exactly thirty splashes of clean fresh water, not too hot, not too cold, on the face and neck every morning and every night. For a ten-year-old this was affordable and fun, and I have done it ever since. Water is the greatest treat for your skin, which suffers seriously from dehydration, but unfortunately tap water is not pure water anymore. Chlorine, fluoride, and the residue of chemicals that modern water treatment can't remove mean that tap water is less of a boon than Laszlo may have had in mind. Of course, water filters help, and a bath or shower in filtered water will make a difference to hair and skin almost from day one. But hydrosols can also help.

Fill the sink with water and add a splash of the appropriate hydrosol. Now rinse your face with this water. Or splash the hydrolate on already-clean skin and allow it to dry naturally.

Here are some other ways that hydrosols can be used in beauty-care treatments:

Makeup remover. Roman chamomile, cornflower, and geranium are the most effective, in that order. Use as you would any makeup remover by applying the hydrosol to a cotton pad and gently wiping it over the skin, moving up the face. Chamomile will even remove some waterproof types of mascara, although not all of them. Follow with a splash—or thirty—of fresh water or water-hydrosol blend.

Toner. Neroli, rock rose, yarrow, and sage are some of the most astringent and therefore most toning choices; they also have antioxidant effects. Again, use as you would any toner by patting the hydrosol on clean skin from cotton pads or spritzing it lightly over the whole face and allowing it to air dry. Many other hydrosols can have toning qualities, so refer to the pH chart and individual profiles and make a custom blend for your particular skin.

Steams. Remember the face-steaming contraptions from the late 1960s? They were cone-shaped devices into which you placed your face, with a steam unit underneath that would allow a gentle, not-too-hot steam to open pores and cleanse skin. Perform the same treatment by boiling water, then diluting it up to 50 percent with hydrosol and pouring the hot liquid into a bowl. Now tent a towel over your head and sit with your face over the steaming vapors. This is an excellent method for deep-cleaning pores and removing stubborn impurities without damaging the tissue. Follow with a cold water-hydrosol rinse to close the pores afterward. Diluting the boiling water with room-temperature hydrosol means that the steam won't burn. Steam for a maximum of ten minutes only. Use hydrosols in the 4.5 to 6.0 pH range for steaming, and follow with a hydrosol with a pH of 4.5 or less to tighten the pores afterward.

Masks. Facial masks can be made from many different substances, although clays are some of the most common and popular. You will find green, red, blue, gray, and white clays, as well as bentonite and pascalite clays, which come from the fossilized remains of ancient seabeds. They are favored for their fine texture and high mineral content. There are mask recipes in chapter 6 for specific skin conditions. For one treatment, take a heaping tablespoon of clay and add the appropriate hydrosol or hydrosol blend drop by drop until the desired consistency is reached. The clay should be neither so stiff that it is hard to spread on the face nor so runny that it won't stay where you put it. You may also wish to add one or two drops of essential oil to your mask, choosing the oils corresponding to the hydrosols used or different oils to create a synergy. Oatmeal, mashed avocado, eggs, honey, and even banana and papaya can all form the base for a mask, and many beauty books can give you recipes for facial masks. In each case just be sure that the amount of hydrosol added balances the final texture of the mask. There is nothing worse than having egg dripping all over the place, even if your skin looks fabulous afterward.

Scrubs. Scrubs and polishes are now available for every part of the body, and they are wonderful for the circulation, remove dead and dry surface skin, promote detoxification, and leave you silky smooth. Except when the recipe also calls for sea salts, hydrosols can usually be added as a component of homemade scrubs. If you do want to use sea salt—which is especially good for the legs and in cellulite treatments—wet the skin with a hydrosol first, then use the salt or salt–essential oil combo on the already damp skin, and rinse with cool water.

Face and décolleté scrubs must be gentle and can be made from finely ground almonds, pin or ground oatmeal, coarse cornmeal, ground rice (not rice flour), and even ground adzuki beans,

although I prefer to use adzuki for foot scrubs. Add a few drops of a carrier oil like hazelnut, peach kernel, jojoba, or carrot to the dry base, then your essential oils, and finally, drop by drop, your hydrosol—only enough to moisten the mixture, not to turn it into soup. Again, look to the recipes for other ideas. My favorite scrubs are produced in Toronto by Aroma-Terrapeutics, using exotic additives like volcanic ash, moor muds, and even ground-up loofah and pumice stone, depending on the part of the body being treated. Aroma-Terrapeutics has provided a number of the recipes in chapter 6.

Compresses. Our mothers used slices of cucumber; we have hydrosols. Puffiness, redness, and swelling in any tissue, but especially in the face, can easily be reduced with a hydrosol compress. Take cotton balls or pads, saturate them with the appropriate hydrosol (but don't make them dripping wet), then lie down for ten minutes, feet up, compresses in place. This restful treatment can be used for tired eyes, computer eyes, and conjunctivitis or as a five-minute lift before applying makeup. Use rock rose, witch hazel, and German chamomile on the cheeks and nose in a compress for rosacea or spider veins and redness. Use rosemary, sage, juniper, or thyme linalol for oily skin and add a little peppermint, bee balm (geraniol type), or thyme thymol for acne and spots. Try rose or rose geranium on a bad day, just because you'll feel so much better afterward. This treatment should become a weekly habit to combat the dryness of central heating in cold winter climates.

Moisturizers. Straight hydrosol, either singly or in blends, misted on the face before applying an oil or cream will help skin stay moist longer while balancing the overall condition and texture. Depending on your activities, lifestyle, and climate, change your hydrosol from winter to summer. And since most lotions are a blend of oil and water, you can create a lotion right on your face by spritzing on a generous mist of hydrosol and then applying an appropriate carrier oil–essential oil blend to the still-wet skin. Both substances will be emulsified and rapidly absorbed in the process.

Moisture mist. Any time your face feels the ravages of the elements—dryness, humidity, stress, smoking, fatigue, climate-controlled air—a hydrosol mist can bring relief. Applied in a fine spray it will not ruin makeup, and you will feel and look better for it.

Certain hydrosols like cinnamon should not be sprayed on the face; refer to the monographs chapter to choose the best water for the conditions being treated.

Shampoos, Conditioners, and Rinses

Hydrosols can be added to any proprietary hair-care product with great results.

Shampoo. Dilute shampoo 50 to 70 percent with the hydrosol of your choice. This sounds like a lot, but most shampoos are much stronger than is needed to wash your hair and scalp. With a shampoo diluted to 70 percent you will still get a lather, if that is an issue (although lather usually signals the presence of sodium lauryl or laureth sulfates, undesirable foaming agents), and your hair will be totally clean, but you will be preserving the acid mantle of the scalp, smoothing and giving shine to the hair shaft, and feeding the condition of your scalp and the hair follicles. Choose cedar, rosemary (any chemotype), or geranium for most hair conditions; sage for oily or dark hair; chamomile for blondes; and goldenrod with cedar or rosemary for dry hair, dandruff, or flaky scalp.

Conditioners. Dilute conditioners 20 to 30 percent with hydrosol. You can choose a hydrosol for its conditioning properties or for its fragrance. Neroli, rose, and rose geranium all leave your hair with a light and beautiful fragrance and shine. Any of those mentioned for shampoos can be added to conditioners for the same effects.

Rinses. Hydrosols can be used as a leave-in rinse after washing and conditioning or as a scalp treatment used daily when styling the hair. For serious scalp problems like seborrhea, difficult dandruff, hair loss, or uneven growth, pour thirty to fifty milliliters (one to one and one-half ounces) of pure hydrosol through the hair before getting out of the shower; do not rinse out; dry and style as usual. A daily treatment can be achieved by misting the hydrosol directly on the scalp, wet or dry, or by taking a small amount in the palm and using the fingertips to massage it into the scalp. Particularly effective combinations are goldenrod or yarrow with rosemary for seborrhea, dandruff, and itchy, flaky scalp; cedar and rosemary for hair loss; German chamomile for sensitive scalp; and sage with rosemary or neroli for excessively oily scalp.

Any of the treatments described can be used on the body as well as the head. It takes very little time, and the improvement in how you feel will be as great as the improvement in your looks.

INTERNAL USE

Water can be made not only more palatable but even healthier with the addition of hydrosols. If you want to start drinking more water but don't really like it, choose three or four of the yummiest hydrosols and start by spritzing very small amounts, just enough to taste, into each glass of water you consume. Vary the hydrosols to give your taste buds something to look forward to or until you find a flavor that you like enough to drink all the time.

Oral

Beverage. Add only enough hydrosol to flavor the water as a tasty method of increasing daily water intake.

Therapeutic beverage. Add two tablespoons of hydrosol to one liter of water and consume it over the course of the day. Plain water may be alternated with the hydrosol water, as it is best if one and one-half to two liters of water can be consumed daily during a treatment. Repeat the process with the same hydrosol, or hydrosol blend, daily for three weeks, than take one week off to allow the body to assimilate the changes

of the treatment. Reassess your condition at the end of the week off.

Gargle / Mouthwash. Combine one part hydrosol with four parts water for a general-purpose mouthwash that will help maintain oral hygiene and sweet breath. For children over three years, dilute one part hydrosol in ten parts water. If you are dealing with specific mouth or gum conditions in adults, such as cankers, ulcers, gingivitis, sore throat, or infections, use neat hydrosol, twenty milliliters at a time, and hold it in your mouth around the sore spot. For a gargle, using a total of thirty milliliters of hydrosol, gargle with fifteen milliliters twice; spit out the hydrosol, don't swallow it. Repeat two or three times daily.

Tonic or "Remedy." Take one-half to one tablespoon of undiluted hydrosol three to six times a day or as required for specific purposes or conditions. An example would be tea tree or eucalyptus hydrosol for coughs and colds, basil or fennel for digestion, sage for chronic fatigue or hypotension, or German chamomile or Greenland moss for insomnia.

Non-Oral

Eyewash. Green myrtle, Roman and German chamomile, and cornflower are the only hydrosols that should ever be used in the eye. Other hydrosols can be used on the eyelid or in eye compresses, but only these four may ever be put *in* the eye. It is imperative that you make sure that any hydrosol you wish to use in this manner is absolutely fresh and uncontaminated and that it contains no preservatives, alcohols, or other dilutants. If in doubt, don't. Mucous membranes are extremely sensitive, and essential oils should never be applied directly to them, especially not the membranes of the eyes. The four hydrosols mentioned, however, can be gentle and effective substitutes for commercial eyedrops. Either mist the eye area, blinking rapidly to get the waters into the eye, or use a sterilized eyedropper to place two or three drops directly in the eye. This works equally well for serious conjunctivitis, allergy eyes, or just plain tired eyes.

Eardrops. Experimental. I am not a big fan of putting much of anything in the ear, especially because the rate of chronic ear infections in adults, children, and pets has increased so dramatically in the past three decades. However, this is an occasion where eardrops with hydrosols worked wonders: A case of chronic ear wax buildup and flaking and peeling of the skin inside the ear was cleared up by daily application of the following mix for one week: ten drops of calendula tincture in ten drops of Roman chamomile hydrosol. Put two or three drops in the ear two or three times day. Ear candling was done on the first, third, and seventh day.

Nose drops. Ayurvedic medicine suggests cleansing the nose and sinus cavities with sea-salt water daily, and you may have seen people who could put a string soaked in salt water up their nose and bring it out their mouth, almost like flossing. Fleurs de Sel is a superfine, solar-dried sea-salt product sold particularly for this purpose, as the salt dissolves totally and is easier on the nose than regular sea salt. One to two milliliters of hydrosol may be diluted at 30 percent in water or used straight and snuffed up the nose a few drops at a time, then blown out to achieve the same cleansing action. It is much healthier and far more pleasant to repeatedly snuff two or three drops than to try to snuff a larger amount at one time. Anyone who has ever had water up his or her nose knows what I mean. *Eucalyptus globulus* or *polybractea*, elecampane, or myrtle would be good nose-drop choices for treating sinus congestion or allergies. Thyme chemotypes or the bee balms are good as immune tonics in flu season, and German chamomile can help relieve inflammation of the mucosa and the effects of excessively dry environments, including airplanes. Before using undiluted hydrosol for cleansing the sinuses, try it diluted first; it's quite a "blast" snorting some of the stronger varieties neat, and it's not always necessary.

Douche. The acidic nature of hydrosols makes them a good choice for use as a vaginal douche or wash; after all, that is part of the theory behind using apple cider vinegar. Dilute one part hydrosol in four parts warm distilled water; use no more than five hundred milliliters total volume per douche, which means you add one hundred milliliters of hydrosol to four hundred milliliters of water. If you are treating a specific problem, for example, cystitis, endometriosis, or thrush, you will need to use a stronger hydrosol concentration or a smaller total volume of liquid. See the recipe section in chapter 6 for more information.

SPECIAL APPLICATIONS: BABIES AND CHILDREN

Before the eyes can focus clearly, a baby's sense of smell is its most important sense, especially in the first few days after birth while bonding with parents and food sources. During the first year, as the other senses become attuned and develop, smell slowly decreases in importance, but the olfactory sense remains highly acute and sensitive, and what may be a mild odor for an adult may be overpowering for a child.

Scientific studies into the phenomenon known as synesthesia show that this linking of the senses is the result of synapse connections in the brain; smell has sound and visuals, sound has a feel and a taste, touch has color and sound—each sense is linked to all the others and experienced simultaneously. At birth we all have synesthesia, or at least we all have the synapse connections in the brain that are observed in synesthetic adults. What happens, researchers believe, is that as speech develops (usually between two and three years of age) these synaptic connections gradually separate, until the links are broken and each individual sense stands on its own. We no longer smell sound or feel sight and taste; however, until a child can talk, we can assume that he or she is synesthetic. So what happens when the child perceives an odor? It may well be a cacophony of sound, taste, physical sensation, and sight that is quite intense, so it is important to watch an infant's reaction to sensory perception and stimulus.

A more metaphysical understanding of this phenomenon proposes that the synesthetic connections are dissolved as speech develops, since this is when the filters and views of those around us come into play. If, for instance, a child is told that smell has no visual expression, he or she will start to introduce this concept and so filter out the sights he or she may normally experience when smelling. Children are also able to see things adults may not, again owing to the lack of filters in their perception. Historically, children were often the subjects of ghostly visitations, as in the film *The Sixth Sense,* not because the spirits meant them harm but because they were the only ones who allowed themselves to see things that are unseen or imaginal. One child told me rainbows were common, the trees make them when the wind blows their leaves. Yogis spend their lives trying to regain this unfiltered vision.

Therefore, when considering any treatments or health options for babies and toddlers, we must be sure that we recognize their needs as different from our own. The treatments must be infinitely gentler, even subtle. Odors should be kept at a very low concentration, and touch must respect the fragility of their being, inside and out. Hydrosols are a much better option for babies and toddlers than essential oils, in virtually all instances. They are safer, easier to use, nonirritating and gentle, and able to speak to the vibrational state that children are easily able to perceive. It is far less likely that any accident or unpleasant experience will occur when mixing children and hydrosols than with children and oils.

When you first encounter hydrosols, you

may be surprised at the odor intensity of these waters. No, they're not as strong as essential oils, but they do have an intense aromatic component, and undiluted, their smell will fill a room just as oils' will. So undiluted hydrosols, just like essential oils, are usually too strong a fragrance for an infant. However, one drop of hydrosol diluted in a cup of water decreases in odor intensity far more than one drop of oil would. Hydrosols are not volatile like the oils, and they do not evaporate into the environment in the same manner. Thus, when they are diluted, all their elements are diluted quite dramatically, including odor.

Considering the sensitivity and interconnectedness of smell for children, the ability to reduce a hydrosol's scent to almost imperceptible levels is quite handy. And although the delicate physiological properties of the substance are also diluted, babies don't need a very strong dose to register an effect. Less is more, especially with kids. Then there is the subtle energy of hydrosols; diluting them does not seem to diminish these effects—the energy is just redistributed holographically and remains the same. Then we could take a homeopathic approach and extrapolate that the more a hydrosol is diluted, the more its energy is increased. Either way, or even if it is as diluted as the odor, the subtle energy is a definite part of how hydrosols benefit health for children and everyone.

But one major factor to remember is that children love to learn and experiment, and they also love to emulate the adults around them. If children see parents using aromatherapy, they will want to use it too, and with hydrosols they can,

safely. One client of mine made a hydrosol kit for her two-and-a-half-year-old daughter. Now she can ask for "her oils" and go off and play with her bag of aromatic goodies to her heart's content. Children can make choices based upon their personal response to the odors and will soon develop favorites for play, bath, "perfume," and bedtime. You may wish to dilute hydrosols in advance for children, and placing them in spray bottles or dropper-top bottles will give the child reasonable control over dispensing his or her own aromatherapy, thus learning the "less is more" concept right from the start. Adults can feel safe in the knowledge that these scents will not harm their child, as synthetic fragrances and perfumes can do when allergies, asthma, or other sensitivities are an issue; in fact, your child will benefit from the aromatic play in ways that may surprise you.

"Kid Scents"

To make a kit of aromatics for your child to play with and explore, use 10 percent hydrosol to 90 percent distilled or springwater, place the hydrosols in unbreakable bottles with a spray top or some kind of dispensing top, and let the child go wild. You may want to sit with your child and make up suitable names for each of the "scents." One child I know calls Roman chamomile "honey water" and loves to drink it, and lavender is "quiet time." Making up the diluted hydrosols and bright, colorful labels for the bottles can be a wonderful activity to do together, and you may be quite surprised to hear how a child perceives the fragrances that you know so well. You can also relax, since spilled hydrosols will not damage carpets, furniture, or little people, even if a child pours the whole bottle over his or her head. Appropriate choices, in addition to those mentioned, would include rose geranium, melissa, linden, angelica, sandalwood, purple bee balm, and petitgrain, depending on the child's age and sex.

The Safe List: Not all hydrosols are suitable for use on children, and they should never be administered to children under ten in the manner suggested for adults. For children less than two years of age use only lavender, Roman chamomile, and German chamomile. After that use your common sense and be guided by the child. Children's sense of what is right for them has fewer filters than our own, and if we listen to them we will learn. Check the profiles for age contraindications and . . . if in doubt, don't!

Undiluted

There are times when undiluted hydrosols may be used on babies and children, but generally it is unnecessary. Try a very diluted solution first and slowly increase the concentration of hydrosol only if and as needed. *Do not* use an undiluted hydrosol without trying it in dilution first.

If the condition requires the topical use of undiluted hydrosols, it should be for a localized application on a small area for a short period of time only, just as you would use undiluted essential oils on an adult to treat a very specific and localized area.

Undiluted topical. Apply hydrosol to a cotton ball or cotton pad and compress on the affected area for thirty seconds to one minute. Repeat with a fresh cotton pad. Use for conditions like stubborn cradle cap, eczema, teething, or diaper rash. Try German chamomile or, if it's very bad, witch hazel, but ensure that the witch hazel does not contain any alcohol, as this will aggravate skin conditions. One drop of neat hydrosol could be applied to the soles of baby's feet for a cough or cold; try purple bee balm *(Monarda fistulosa)* or myrtle in addition to the hydrosols on the safe list (see page 180).

Undiluted oral. Only to be used for teething pain and inflammation. Wash your hands or wear a disposable clean surgical glove or finger cot. Put one drop of Roman chamomile hydrosol on your finger, or use a cotton swab, then rub it very gently over the swollen gums. Repeat no more than three times a day. Try diluted hydrosol first, which can be used more frequently—up to five or six times daily.

Undiluted nontopical. As mentioned, babies, and especially newborns, are heavily dependent on smell. If a mother has help in caring for the child, the transition from one caregiver to another can be easier for the child if there is a similarity in smell between the caregivers. Using a spritz of lavender or chamomile water as a scent on the mother's skin will create a link for the child between that smell and food, protection, love. If all the caregivers of the child wear the same hydrosol, the child will immediately feel relaxed and more secure in the arms of someone other than *Mom*. One drop of hydrosol on baby's pillow will have the same effect, and all three waters suggested on the safe list will probably help sleeping patterns.

Dilutions

Diluted topical. You can dilute, dilute, dilute. Add one drop of hydrosol to one tablespoon of distilled water. Take one drop of that mixture and add it to a tablespoon of distilled water. Now add one drop of this second dilution to your baby's preparation; it is less than one five-hundredth of a drop of pure hydrosol. That is about the dilution you can start with, and if it has little effect, you can always add two or three drops of your first diluted blend until the desired response is elicited. But do give the "remedy" time to work. These are not pharmaceutical drugs and should not be expected to act in the same way; apply, wait, and observe before you use more. You could try this for babies who have trouble sleeping, using Roman chamomile in their bottle or applied to their feet, wrists, or back with a little massage.

Bum spray. Mix equal portions of lavender and Roman chamomile, dilute 50 percent with water, and put this in a sterilized bottle with a spray top. Spritz this mixture on whatever tissue you use to clean your baby's bottom. If you want to spritz it directly on the baby's bum, make sure it is not too cold and that you have a fine mist sprayer, not a jet stream, which could hurt your child. In many cultures a diaper wet only with urine is used to wipe the baby's bum, thereby preventing diaper rash by preserving the acid mantle of the skin. Hydrosols are slightly acid and can do the same thing.

Baths. Add one-quarter to one-half teaspoon of hydrosol to a baby bath of warm water. If you use the big tub, add no more than one teaspoon. Lavender and Roman chamomile are both sedative and good for the delicate skin.

Baby lotions and creams. Add one or two drops of hydrosol per ounce of lotion or cream. Shake the cream well and use it as normal. Please do not use any baby preparations that contain mineral oil, as this is a petrochemical product, as is petroleum jelly, and they are not natural products. Hydrosols will not mix into diaper rash ointments that have a petroleum jelly or mineral oil base.

Wet wipes. Not really a medium, more a carrier. Paper towels can be used to make baby's bum wipes. Choose a good-quality paper towel that holds up when wet and doesn't just turn to mush. If possible, remove the cardboard tube from the center of the roll and cut the roll in half crosswise. Put the half-roll of towel in a suitable container to which you have added two tablespoons of pure hydrosol. Now sprinkle an additional two tablespoons of hydrosol on top of the roll so the paper absorbs it from both top and bottom edges. Put the lid on and voilà . . . chemical-free wet wipes. These homemade versions will not withstand being pulled out through a dispenser top, as the paper will shred. (I am told that Bounty brand paper towels work best.)

Laundry. Add one-half cup of hydrosol to the final rinse water when you do baby's laundry. For real germ-killing power, you could use three or four drops of essential oils in the soap wash, but hydrosols in the rinse impart a beautiful fragrance when germ killing is not the main issue.

SPECIAL HEALTH CONCERNS

Today herbal "medicines" are being qualified and quantified by laboratory studies and double-blind placebo trials. Methods of validation for certain chemical components of herbs are big news, since our scientific approach is to believe that one or two chemical constituents of an herb may be all that matter in healing. If we can prove this, we can patent (and make money on) methods of extracting these substances, the substances themselves, and any preparations that can be formulated based on these chemicals or synthetic versions of these chemicals. No longer is the anecdotal validation of several hundred years of use enough to prove that an herb works and that it is safe for the public. At the turn of the millennium, money is finally being invested in phytomedicinal research on a grand scale, but it remains to be seen whether it is being done for the benefit of both nature and mankind or just for the pocketbooks of the multinational pharmaceutical companies that are financing the studies.

In most people the immune system is capable of dealing with health concerns. Colds and coughs are usually gone in a few days, cuts and wounds heal quickly and leave little or no scar-ring, and indigestion or diarrhea is short-lived and passes after a day of rest. Most herbal or non-pharmaceutical supplements and remedies are based on the premise that if you stimulate the immune system and give it a bit of help in combating whatever ails you, you'll be right as rain in no time. That is why and how we have always used phytomedicines, not as killing agents targeting bacteria and shooting them down on their own, but as stimulants to the body's natural defense mechanisms and our built-in ability to stay healthy and balanced. We must remember that for most of the history of natural medicine we didn't know what germs were, much less viruses and microorganisms. The cause of disease was, and in some places is, more likely to be attributed to the wind or rain or to evil spirits than to a pathogen or germ. We didn't use herbs because a laboratory study told us what germs they killed; we used herbs because we could see and feel their effects and our bodies responded by becoming stronger and healing more quickly with their help. We used herbs because they were all we had other than ourselves.

The discovery of the "germ" and the move to a scientific approach to health and the body changed all that. Now that we could isolate the "cause" of an illness, we could target the cause directly. The concept of healing through restoring balance to the whole organism (read human) went the way of the dodo. Those must have been heady times, and we certainly have benefited in miraculous ways from the science of health. But perhaps we have suffered, too, and the changes we see today in the mass consciousness are the result of the suffering. People need to be treated as people, not as diseases. We need to look at the cause, not the symptoms, of illness. Balance in the whole body is key to healing. Moving the pendulum of medicine all the way from one side to the other to effect a "cure" is no cure; the pendulum must be at rest, balanced in the middle, not under the strain of extremes. Advocates of natural healing understand this as one of the basic concepts in "soft medicine." Terms like *integrative medicine* are being coined to indicate that the treatments integrate the whole body, healing philosophy as well as integrating the approaches of modern medicine with natural healing. Even the hallowed halls of Stanford, Yale, and Harvard have schools of study pursuing these ideas and now host conferences and courses in everything from acupuncture to healing touch, phytomedicine, and biofeedback. The times they are a-changin', oh, yeah!

Perhaps part of what has spurred on this research, besides public opinion and spending, is studies on the effects of drugs on severely depressed immune systems. Sometimes the immune system becomes so damaged by illness or lifestyle, addictions, long-term use of medication, chronic malnutrition and/or dehydration, or the effects of age that it is no longer able to respond to stimuli that are intended to increase its effectiveness and action. The system is simply not capable of rallying if overstimulated. The net result can be a negative response or crash. It doesn't matter whether the stimulus is natural or synthetic in origin; if it is too strong for the body, it is too strong, period.

Essential oils can easily be too strong a message for a weak immune system. Highly concentrated, highly aromatic, and easily absorbed via dermal, olfactory, and oral applications, essential oils can send too much of a signal to someone in a fragile state. Do pregnant women develop an increased sense of smell by accident? Or is it to prevent them from using or eating anything that is too strong for the growing fetus? Is this a natural safety mechanism to prevent overdosing? Pregnant women are not sick, but their body and immune system are very busy, and the fetus is fragile and easily overstimulated.

Although in the British school of aromatic practice the applications are usually via inhalations or topical in fairly low dilution (1.5 percent being recommended for those seriously ill or elderly), the French and so-called aromatology approach frequently uses much higher dilutions, neat applications, and internal doses when healing a pathology or infection. Even in very low doses of 1.5 percent or less, oils are potent chemical messengers and can bind to receptor sites on cells and cross the blood-brain barrier. They are also highly complex chemical compounds. Clary sage contains about 250 different chemicals, and the one that gives it its distinctive smell has yet to be identified and seems to be present in such microamounts that it may resist detection. If something at that small a dilution in the chemistry of clary gives it such a potent aroma, how much information do all the other chemicals carry?

When I teach about essential oils I spend a lot of time trying to make the chemistry comprehensible and therefore usable. My practice changed dramatically when I could marry the scientific knowledge (having finally understood the chemistry and its implications) with the anecdotal evidence and the palpable energetic effects of real essential oils. I really "got it" when I could see and understand the whole complex relationship. Just as we must be holistic in our approach to the human body, factoring in emotions, attitudes, and belief structures with physicality and knowledge of how the body actually works, so we must be holistic in our understanding of the tools, the aromatics, understanding their various parts and moods, attitudes and predispositions, likes and dislikes. Get out the conifer oils at the autumn equinox and use them until the spring equinox. This is their season; conifers stay green when all the other trees are bare, sending us this message, "Pick me, I'm alive; when all is asleep I am here." The high monoterpene content of conifer oils makes them ideally suited to easing bronchial conditions, fighting colds, and killing germs both aerially and on contact. Just what we need when it's winter outside. Larch, on the other hand, is the only deciduous conifer (it loses its needles), and it enjoys the summer as well as the winter. Its aroma is lighter, more ethereal, than most of the needle oils, although its chemistry is similar.

Drug Interactions

Chemistry must be considered when you are dealing with anyone who is receiving other treatments or taking medications of any kind. Drug interactions do not happen just between pharmaceutical drugs. Where do you think the theories behind food combining come from? Any substances taken into the body, regardless of the method of absorption, combine in the body with each other and with the body's own chemistry. There are now many reference books available on pharmaceutical drugs, which include their side effects and information about contraindications and possible effects in combination with other drugs and chemicals. Some blood thinners given to people with high blood pressure may carry warnings that they should not be taken in combination with any coumarin-containing substances. You may find, if you wish to use an essential oil to help someone sleep, that coumarins are in the oil, as they have a sedative effect and show up even in sweet old lavender, as we saw in chapter 1. So cross-referencing essential oils with pharmaceuticals can be very important. Many phytomedicine texts and books on phytopharmacognosy will also include information on possible interactions and contraindications between various herbs and herbal preparations. The American Botanical Council offers a huge array of books on just this subject. They are valuable texts and should be part of anyone's library, particularly if your practice deals with anyone on multiple treatments, medications, and/or supplements.

Whether you choose aromatics because they can improve the mental state of the individual or the life force of the body and thus help heal, or because you feel that the properties of the oil may heal an illness or kill a pathogen, remember: If the person is in a fragile or weakened state, use the tiniest dilution you can or turn to hydrosols.

As discussed in the section on babies and children, hydrosols offer a soft, aromatic approach. They are water-soluble and therefore quickly flushed through the system; mostly terpene-free, so gentle on internal organs and unlikely to accumulate in fatty tissue like the liver and kidneys; extremely gentle in aroma, especially when diluted; and with few if any contraindications—here are the "homeopathic" versions of essential oils.

In chapters 1 and 2 you will find information and ideas on using hydrosols in the manner of homeopathy, but remember the golden rule in any special health concern: Less is more. You can always increase a dose if you need to, but once given it is much harder to dilute in vivo, or to turn back the effects caused by too high an initial dose. Hydrosols can easily be diluted infinitesimally. Just keep adding water. Hydrosols will not damage skin or mucous membranes; they require no special carrier other than simple water, so no additional ingredients need to be factored into the healing equation. They are simple, easy to use, and highly unlikely to cause any kind of interaction with any other treatment or medication being given or used.

If you work with immune-compromised clients, use hydrosols as you would essential oils in treatments, and start with the dilution rates suggested for babies and children. Always ensure that both you and the person you're treating exchange as much information as possible on the effects of the treatments, and keep lots of notes. This is not just for professionalism but because long-term treatments may result in some pretty fabulous results, and it is of benefit to everyone if this data is carefully recorded and can be shared so that many more can benefit from the experience.

Undiluted

As with babies and children, there are times when undiluted hydrosols may be used on fragile individuals, but generally it is unnecessary. Try a very diluted solution first and slowly increase the hydrosol only if and as needed. *Do not use an undiluted hydrosol without trying it in dilution first.*

If the condition requires the topical use of undiluted hydrosols, it should be for a localized application on a small area for a very short period of time only, just as you would use undiluted essential oils on an adult to treat a very specific and localized area.

Undiluted topical. Apply hydrosol to a cotton ball or a cotton pad and compress the affected area for thirty seconds to one minute. Repeat two or three times, using a fresh cotton pad each time. Use for conditions like bedsores, intravenous points, rashes, lesions, and slow-healing cuts and sores. A few drops of neat hydrosol could be applied to the soles of the feet for a cough or cold, or bee balm, *Inula,* eucalyptus, or green myrtle could be used in a footbath.

Undiluted oral. For mouth ulcers, gum infections, and cankers, take ten milliliters of hydrosol and rinse the mouth for forty-five to sixty seconds. Then spit out the water.

Undiluted nontopical. Hydrosols can be used as a linen mist to impart a gentle scent to bedding and to reduce stress and aid relaxation and sleep. Spritz a fine mist down the edges of the bed or on the pillow, but not enough to make the linen wet.

Dilutions

Diluted oral. Add one-quarter to one-half tablespoon of hydrosol to one and one-half liters of water. Sip the water throughout the day. Even if the hydrosol can barely be tasted in the water, do not increase the dilution until you have tested this dilution rate for at least three days. If there is no effect after three days, increase the hydrosol one-quarter teaspoon at a time, testing for three days each time you raise the strength, to gauge the results, until the desired effects are achieved.

Diluted topical. You can dilute extensively. Add one drop of hydrosol to one tablespoon of distilled water, then take one drop of that mixture and add it to a tablespoon of distilled water. Now add one drop of this second dilution to your base; it is less than one five-hundredth of a drop of pure hydrosol. That is the dilution you can start with, and if it has little or no effect, you can always add two or three drops of the first diluted solution until the desired response is elicited. Remember, homeopathic remedies are infinitely more dilute than this.

Skin spray. Dilute a hydrosol 50 percent with distilled or deionized water and put it in a sterilized bottle with a spray top. If you want to spritz it directly on the skin, make sure that you have a fine-mist sprayer. Research and a long historical tradition have proved that urine can be effective as a skin wash in treating eczema, psoriasis, Kaposi's sarcoma, and other lesions and serious skin conditions; it is the acidity that rebalances the acid mantle of the skin. Hydrosols are acid to varying degrees and do the same thing. Yarrow, melissa, and witch hazel have proven particularly beneficial in practice.

Baths. Add one tablespoon of hydrosol to a tub of water to begin with, and add no more than one tablespoon at a time until the desired concentration and effects are attained. Usually two to three tablespoons are ample for a bath.

Lotions and creams. Add ten drops of hydrosol per ounce of lotion or cream. Shake the cream well and use as normal. Check the ingredient list for additives or medicinal ingredients. Creams may be medicated or contain cortisone or corticosteroids, which are seriously strong drugs. Witch hazel has been proven to be a viable substitute for cortisones. If you are using a prescription topical formula for a specific skin condition, talk to your health-care practitioner or pharmacist or get some good reference books before blending in a hydrosol. Do not use any preparation that contains mineral oil, as this is a petrochemical product, as is petroleum jelly, and they are potentially carcinogenic and damaging to the immune system. Hydrosols will not mix into ointments that have a petroleum jelly or oil base.

Mouthwash. Use 15 milliliters (one tablespoon) of hydrosol in 120 milliliters (four ounces) of water. Rinse the mouth well or gargle for at least thirty to forty-five seconds at a time. Repeat two or three times. Do not swallow the hydrosol after rinsing out your mouth, especially if you are treating a condition like gingivitis or an infection.

Laundry. Add one-half cup of hydrosol to the final rinse water. For real germ-killing power in sickbed laundry, you could use five to seven drops of essential oils in the soap wash, but hydrosols in the rinse impart a beautiful fragrance when germ killing is not your primary concern.

AROMATIC TINCTURES

I woke up one morning a couple of years ago laughing at how dense I can be, at how it is always the most obvious things we tend to overlook. The idea? Combine hydrosols and tinctures and you will have remedies with numerous traceable physiological effects from both the alcohol-extracted elements in the tincture and the water-soluble and microoil particles in the hydrosol, a product that truly contains all the therapeutic properties of the plant(s) in question *and* the energetic properties of the hydrolates to boot. I called a distiller friend with whom I work on hydrosols, and we laughed because no more than two days previous she had woken up with the same thought. Not two months ago I discovered that Avicenna in England had started working on the same idea at almost exactly the same time, calling the product distilled tinctures. Serendipity indeed.

I call my hydrosol–tincture mixtures Aromatic Tinctures, and they are wonderful and amazing and seem to be extremely powerful. They are also easy to make; even off-the-shelf tinctures can be turned into aromatic tinctures by the addition of hydrosols, although in that case you are watering down the tincture a little, but you're adding the therapeutics of the hydrosol, so it should balance in the end.

Aromatic Tinctures allow you to create remedies that use both aromatic and nonaromatic plant materials, and you can create single-plant tinctures or combination tinctures according to your needs, whims, and inspiration. Milk thistle, for instance, which is extraordinary in a tincture, is not made into either an oil or a hydrosol, but it is the only substance known that can reverse liver damage and prevent death by poisoning from certain mushrooms or liver failure from overdoses of drugs like ibuprofen. Think about the synergy of this tincture combined with Greenland moss, a detoxifier so powerful that you use the hydrosol at half the normal dosage, and which also has extraordinary liver-regenerating properties. What happens when you combine the two? Magic!

Preparation

You will need 95 percent (190 proof) ethyl alcohol, sometimes called ethanol, to get the best results, although you can use a lower-percent alcohol and either add less hydrosol or have a lower alcohol-by-volume finished product.

There are two methods you can use to make aromatic tinctures. The first is to make your desired tincture using undiluted ethanol. This is most appropriate for woody plants, bark, and root material. Fill a clean sterile jar with washed and thoroughly dried plant material, cover with alcohol, and put a tight-fitting lid on the jar. Leave it to sit for two weeks, inverting the jar once a day and giving it two or three raps on the table and a gentle spin or shake after each inversion to make sure all air bubbles make their way to the surface. After two weeks filter the tincture through a muslin cloth and add enough hydrosol to dilute the finished product to 60 percent alcohol by volume. You can dilute to as low as 40 percent alcohol by volume and maintain a shelf life of approximately two years. You may wish to use a hydrosol from the same plant you've tinctured or a complementary hydrosol (or two) that will act in synergy with the tinctured plant.

The second method is to dilute your ethanol down to 60 percent (120 proof) by adding the hydrosol of choice in the beginning. Then follow the instructions above for making the tincture, omitting the last step of adding the hydrosol(s), as you have already done this.

If you start with one liter of ethanol, you must add 570 milliliters of hydrosol to get a 60 percent alcohol solution or 1,375 milliliters for a 40 percent alcohol-by-volume product.

The possibilities are endless, and of course you can simply use the hydrosol of the plant in your tincture, which is the best way to start. I began my experiments with a 60 percent by volume Greenland moss tincture to which I added Greenland moss hydrolate, diluting it to 40 percent alcohol by volume. Besides having had the

Suggested combinations:

TINCTURE PLANT	HYDROSOL
Melissa	Neroli / German chamomile
Milk thistle	Greenland moss / calamus
Echinacea	Black spruce / bay laurel
Greenland moss	Sweet gale
Arnica	Immortelle
St. John's wort	Melissa / rose / neroli
Astragalus	Angelica
Goldenseal	*Inula / Eucalyptus globulus*
Vitex agnus-castus	Clary sage / sage / rose
Dandelion	Artemesia / cypress

epiphany of making aromatic tinctures, I was also looking for a way to use Greenland moss water, which is extremely powerful. The resulting product was really exciting, and I believe that this is an important place for hydrosol use in the materia medica.

Avicenna offers the widest commercially available list of distilled tinctures, and has wholeheartedly embraced this idea. Although they are selling only single-plant products at the moment, after our conversations, combination tinctures will be coming soon. It is interesting to me that Avicenna's primary clientele have been herbalists and practitioners of traditional Chinese medicine. The products have been largely overlooked by the aromatherapy community in the United Kingdom thus far, perhaps because this is being construed as internal application and thus outside the scope of practice for aromatherapists in England. I trust that as hydrosols grow in popularity this will change.

PETS AND DOMESTIC ANIMALS

Like babies, animals have an extremely sensitive sense of smell. It is said that a dog's nose is thirty times more powerful than a human's, and a cat's nose is ten times more powerful than that. Birds may detect electromagnetic frequencies that guide them in migration and homing through sensors in their smell organs. Lions and tigers and bears . . . oh my! Smell is more closely linked to survival and communication in animals than it is in modern speech-dependent humans. We must be aware of their sensitivity in dealing with

them and aromatics, just as we must remember this in dealing with babies or fragile adults. Animals are also generally more "aware" energetically than humans. They can sense thunderstorms and earthquakes, epileptic seizures or severe anxiety, and they sense unseen presences around and among us. Hydrosols speak to them on this level as clearly as on the physical level.

Animals, however, do like some strong smells. For some dogs there's nothing like a bit of rotting flesh or manure to roll in, for some cats no clearer message than a tomcat's spray, but they are all highly selective about their odor preferences and will choose one smell over another just like a human. It is worth letting animals respond to an aromatic before you use it on them. With essential oils the pervasive odor will be with them intensely for many hours, maybe days, and if it gives them a "headache," what benefit is that for any other healing that could take place? Animals need their own smell; it is how they know who they are; it determines their personal space. Hairy, or in this case, furry, skin also absorbs essential oils more than hairless skin. You can reason with an animal regarding treatment just as you can reason with a person, and if animals feel palpable benefits to a hurt at the expense of temporary smell overload, they may tolerate it well. But if the smell really puts them off and they run from the room when you open the oil bottle, look for a substitute. Or choose a hydrosol.

Dogs and, even more so, cats respond very well to hydrosol treatments. The intensity of the odor and the period that it will last are greatly reduced from essential oils. As with humans, the diluted dose is the place to start, and then it can be increased or used neat if necessary. Hydrosols can be used internally and topically, on all the body parts. Applying neroli to a stressed dog's face relaxes the dog as quickly as it does people. You can use hydrosols for health care and for beauty, you can create psychological reactions and emotional ones; in fact, they work on animals just as they work on us.

There are limits, however. Hydrosols do not get rid of worms. However, a good diet, flea- and pest-prevention routines, and hydrosols used both topically and internally, as part of an animal's supplements, will go some way toward preventing infestation by parasites. Essential oils may be used with or without chemical vermi-fuges if your animal does become wormy.

Cats

Never use essential oils on a cat. The smell is far too strong, and even diluted, many of them are just too concentrated for a cat's skin and its terrain. If you wish to use aromatherapy on your cat, hydrosols are the safest choice.

Dilute hydrosols at child strength or less, one-half teaspoon of hydrosol per liter of water or one or two drops per dose for internal use. When giving a hydrosol to your cat in its water dish, make sure you provide an alternate water source so the animal doesn't become dehydrated if it won't drink the hydrosol. If it's still a no-go, try a different water or add two drops to a small bit of food. Cats are fussy, so it may not be easy.

You can also give the cat the two or three drops with an eyedropper directly in its mouth.

Here are dilution guides for acute and chronic phases of an illness:

Acute: One-half teaspoon per five hundred grams (one pound) of body weight, to be divided into six to eight doses, given at intervals throughout the day only until the condition clears up.

Chronic: One-quarter teaspoon per 500 grams (1 pound) of body weight, to be divided into two or three doses, given morning, noon, and night daily for three weeks. Reassess the condition at the end of a week off and repeat only if necessary.

Teeth and gum problems. If left to their own devices, most cats are very much the hunter. They will kill birds, mice, rats, even baby rabbits. It is their natural pattern of behavior, and they usually eat at least part of what they kill. One of the "joys" of cat ownership is the headless mice they bring as little presents. For many modern cat owners this is considered an undesireable trait: We'd rather Fluffy didn't kill birds, we'd rather that he or she not eat horrible dirty mice, we prefer the sanitized cat devoid of killer instinct, happy to sit in our laps and purr. I apologize to those this may upset, but cats are really just small tigers, and we should allow them to be what they are, not what we would make of them. Even house cats need to chew!

Gum disease, in humans and animals, is frequently the result of lack of chewing exercise, friction, and circulation in the gum tissue, coupled with residue of food that may be between the teeth. A cat's diet should be sufficiently varied to stimulate the mouth and gums and keep the cat healthy, but this is one of the most common problems facing pets today. Unless some changes to diet are made, no amount of hydrosol or anything else will cure gum disease. Allow the cat some chewing material, especially as the healing process progresses, and monitor the gum health carefully. Chewing will increase the circulation in the gums, help push out pus and infection, and rekindle the animal spark.

Gingivitis. Dilute immortelle hydrosol 50 percent with water and rub two or three drops on the gums four to six times a day every day for three weeks. If the condition is advanced, use the hydrosol undiluted. If there is a lot of discharge and/or bleeding from the gums, you could add 20 percent cypress, thyme (linalol or thymol), or tea tree waters; if there is a lot of inflammation, add 20 percent German or Roman chamomile or peppermint; and if the infection seems to be nonlocalized or spread throughout the body, add three to five percent Greenland moss or *Echinacea* to your immortelle base. If there is no visible difference in the condition of the gums at the end of ten days with a diluted hydrosol, repeat with a pure hydrosol mixture.

Digestive problems. Use three to five drops of undiluted hydrosol in the cat food daily for three weeks. Try coriander, peppermint, yarrow, fennel, or rosemary. Bad breath is usually a sign of digestive problems and diet imbalance.

Urinary tract problems. Use three to five drops of undiluted hydrosol in all meals and five drops in the water dish daily for three weeks. Try juniper berry, yarrow, cypress, sandalwood, basil, car-

rot seed, or oregano. If there is an infection, use winter savory, oregano, tea tree, or thyme CT thymol, but be careful with this last one; use it only in tiny dilutions, as it is hot to the tongue.

Respiratory problems. Put five to seven drops of hydrosol in the cat's food or rub ten to fifteen drops of undiluted hydrosol on the chest and abdomen two or three times daily for three weeks in addition to or replacing the food dose. Choices include *Eucalyptus radiata* or *globulus*, *Inula*, rosemary (verbenone is best, but cineole is okay), or bay leaf. Use a humidifier if the air is dry, and add one hundred milliliters of hydrosol to the water in the unit.

Clumping cat litter is not good for cats. Moisture makes the litter clump into cakes, easing the job of cleaning the litter tray, but if litter dust is inhaled, the moisture in the mouth, sinuses, and lungs can also make it cake, creating the possibility of litter balls in the airways. As if hairballs weren't enough.

Coat and skin care. Mist a fine spray of hydrosol over the animal's coat; usually two or three spritzes is enough. Smooth the hydrosol into the fur while gently massaging the muscles or brush it gently through the fur to distribute. Skin covered with hair absorbs hydrosols and oils faster than bare skin, and you do not need to soak the animal. If you do bathe your cat, add two to three tablespoons of hydrosol to the rinse water. Cedar is good for the coat and helps deter fleas. Rosemary gives a nice shine to the coat but may be a little too stimulating for cats unless you're ready for a tiger in your tank.

Cuts, scratches, and bites. Use pure lavender hydrosol from an eyedropper or cup to wash the affected area. If the cut looks septic, dilute hydrogen peroxide (3 percent topical) with 60 percent or more hydrosol, and wrap the cat in a blanket before applying the mixture; it may sting a bit. Use scarlet bee balm, thyme CT thuyanol, tea tree, or cinnamon. Some tomcats are extremely nasty when they fight and can do a lot of damage. Wash these types of wounds several times a day using the peroxide-hydrosol blend, gradually increasing the proportion of hydrosol as healing progresses.

Kitty odor. Few houses with indoor-only cats lack the pervasive odor of the litter tray. A mist of hydrosol can be directed over the litter every day after cleaning, and hydrosol can be used as a final rinse for the tray whenever it is washed. You can also use hydrosol as an environmental fragrance in cat areas and on their bedding. Essential oils are better disinfectants, but the smell is so strong they can deter cats from using their litter trays (quite undesirable). The odor of hydrosols is light enough that cats won't be offended, and the household will benefit.

Dogs

Desmond Morris calls the dog "the wolf in your living room," and he is right. If we have done a disservice to cats through our attempts to "domesticate" them, what then have we done to dogs? Behavior problems abound; dogs are on Prozac these days. Hip dysplasia from poor breeding selections is rampant, arthritis is normal, ear and skin infections are as antibiotic resistant in animals as in humans, and tooth decay has created a need for doggie toothbrushes and liver-flavored toothpaste!

Samoyeds and huskies belong in cold climates and can suffer greatly in hot or tropical conditions. Akitas were bred as fighting dogs, not house pets. Dalmatians are carriage dogs bred for running many miles a day, not sitting in the yard and visiting a local park. And pity the poor shar-pei. A gene pool of only several hundred animals has spawned the thousands of shar-peis in the world today, and you want to talk health problems! Shar-peis have skin problems and infections in their wrinkles, hearing problems and infections in their ears, eye problems that can require surgery to sew the eyelids back open. Their digestive systems are a mess, and food allergies are de rigueur. They are the victims of our indulgence; we created a fad for a rare dog and then fed that faddism by inbreeding, overbreeding, and stylized breeding. The first shar-pei I ever saw nearly twenty years ago was twice as big as they are today, more like a Labrador, and although wrinkled, it wasn't the extreme cuddly toy of today.

Just as with cats, our desire to "domesticate and sanitize" the dog has wreaked havoc on their lives. And the first area requiring attention is diet. Dogs are hunters too. Even sweet, mild-mannered dogs will turn into killers that can run down a deer if they are in a pack. The pack mentality may be the least understood aspect of dog care and training, but if you wish to work with natural healing in a dog, you must give it some thought. Generally speaking, you are their pack. You, the owner, are the alpha or leader of the pack, and although the underlings may kick up a fuss now and again, you call the shots. This is the key to obedience and respect when training, and a dog will do more for love of his pack than for cookies or rolled-up newspapers. Your dog will follow your lead if you embrace the pack concept, and dogs will happily do as you do, even taking medicines or allowing treatments to take place.

All that was said about diet for cats holds true for dogs as well. Dogs are carnivores. They have sharp fangs and grinding molars and will make short work of even knucklebones, happily gnawing away for hours. Their short digestive system is designed to handle volumes of raw meat, and feeding canned cooked food is nonsensical. Dogs don't know how to cook, so why cook their food? Just because we don't like raw meat or follow a vegetarian diet is no reason to force this on our beloved pets. We must feed an animal what it wants and needs, not what we want it to have, and there is no such thing as a vegetarian dog. However, not everyone is willing or able to search out raw, ideally organic meat for his or her dog, and non–meat eaters may find it distasteful to handle bloody bones or even minced raw burger. If you must feed your dog a kibble, choose a good organic one and supplement the dog's diet with raw beef bones so its teeth get a workout and don't rot in its head.

My neighbor's two-year-old Labrador developed epilepsy. The owners saw vets and even a neurologist, who prescribed lifelong medication and pooh-poohed the idea that it was possibly diet related. A simple change in dog food from a "scientific" kibble to an organic kibble supplemented with raw bones stopped the seizures, and the dog was symptom-free for six months, until she was fed one meal of the old scientific kibble. The next day she had a seizure, and the old kibble was thrown out for good. On her new diet, she was totally seizure-free for more than eight months and in the past two years has had only a few episodes. She is also thinner, happier, and better behaved, all around a happier puppy. Enough said.

Dogs are slightly less sensitive to essential oils than cats are, and although hydrosols are a better first choice, you can use diluted oils on a dog very effectively without harming it. With hydrolates, use one-half to one tablespoon per day for a medium-size (Labrador) dog and increase or decrease the dose depending on the size of the dog and the health problem. Toy dogs should be given one to one and one-half teaspoons per day, preferably diluted. Adjust your dose according to the animal's weight, just as you would with humans. A seventy-kilogram Newfoundland needs a higher dose than a thirty-kilogram Labrador, and a seven kilogram miniature schnauzer needs even less. Hydrosols may be used undiluted on dogs, although it is always best to start with a diluted treatment and increase the strength as need be, depending on the ailment.

Tooth and gum problems. Use undiluted immortelle hydrosol on the gums three to five times a day every day for three weeks. If there is a lot of discharge and/or bleeding from the gums, you could add up to 40 percent cypress, thyme (linalol or thymol), or tea tree waters. If there is a lot of inflammation, add 50 percent German or Roman chamomile or peppermint, and if the infection seems to be nonlocalized or spread throughout the body, feed one-half tablespoon of Greenland moss or *Echinacea* two or three times daily as well as the immortelle for the three-week treatment. If the treatment coupled with dietary rationalization does not make at least some difference in the condition of the gums at the end of three weeks, consult your vet.

Toothbrushes for dogs have been invented as a necessity to combat the effects of bad diet. Dogs' teeth and gums need lots of exercise, and feeding your dog raw meaty beef bones one or two times a week from puppyhood will save not only your shoes and table legs but your dog's teeth.

Digestive problems. Give one-half to one tablespoon of hydrosol per day, divided between water and food, for three weeks. Try coriander, peppermint, yarrow, fennel, carrot seed, oregano, basil, or rosemary. Bad breath is usually a sign of digestive problems and diet imbalance and must be addressed on all levels.

Diarrhea. Feed one-half tablespoon of undiluted cinnamon hydrosol (bark is best) every thirty minutes for four doses, then hourly for four doses. This usually does the trick, as the cinnamon not only calms the stomach and digestive tract but also helps kill any bacterial cause of the diarrhea. Live yogurt, one tablespoon three times a day, can help balance intestinal flora, and a dish of boiled white rice with or without cinnamon

water can also help stem diarrhea by absorbing excess fluid in the bowels. If the diarrhea is caused by stress or travel, use those remedies as described prior to departure or during the trip or stressful event. Many modern dog foods are designed to compact and firm a dog's stool, often by the addition of rice, making it easier for humans to clean up in poop-and-scoop areas. If you are switching your dog to a new food or a natural diet, the animal may experience diarrhea and/or more frequent bowel movements during the changeover and much larger bowel movements on a natural diet. Consider this a change for the better, since any diet that compacts and hardens stools is obviously doing something unnatural to the digestive system. You can surely imagine how you would feel on a diet that made your stools hard and dry.

Urinary tract problems. Give one-half tablespoon of hydrolate three times daily and one tablespoon of hydrolate in the water dish daily for three weeks. Try juniper berry, yarrow, cypress, sandalwood, or goldenrod. If there is an infection, use winter savory, oregano, scarlet bee balm, or thyme CT thymol. You can use a turkey baster to gently squirt hydrosol into your dog's mouth, then hold the jaws shut until the dog swallows, but don't choke the dog.

Respiratory problems. Give one tablespoon of hydrosol internally two or three times daily and rub two tablespoons of undiluted hydrosol on the chest and abdomen twice daily for three weeks. Choices include *Eucalyptus globulus*, *Inula*, rosemary (any), thyme (any), oregano, winter savory, or a blend. You can also use one or two drops of essential oil in the dog's bedding, or place a diffuser with a respiratory blend near where the dog sleeps at night. A good blend for dogs is equal parts ravensara, *Eucalyptus radiata,* and palmarosa, with just a few drops of patchouli or vetiver. Do not use a candle diffuser near pets, as it is a fire hazard.

Hot spots. Compress hot spots with lavender, German chamomile, and/or yarrow. This relieves the itching that makes dogs constantly lick a sore or spot. You can compress as frequently as you like, or bandage a compress in place to prevent licking and promote healing. Hot spots created by pressure sores from lying on pavement or hard surfaces should be compressed as well; try German chamomile, lavender, immortelle, witch hazel, and geranium. Provide some type of bedding or blanket for the dog to lie on to ease the pressure and promote healing.

Paw problems. For bruises or cuts on the pads from sharp stones, gravel, and the like, foot soak or compress with a mixture of 60 percent immortelle and 40 percent lavender. Keep the dog off its feet as much as possible. For burns from hot sand, pavement, or such, compress with lavender, or if very burned use lavender hydrosol to which one drop of lavender oil has been added. For salt damage from melting winter ice, wash the feet in clean water after every walk and spritz pads, between toes, and lower legs with lavender and Roman chamomile in equal parts. Depending on where you live, your dog's feet may be exposed to a variety of unnatural conditions. Be

aware of these potentially damaging surfaces, and at least once a week inspect your dog's feet and give them a little massage (they smell like corn chips). In places where large amounts of salt are used to keep streets and pavement free of ice, you may want to consider dog boots. As embarrassing as the boots may be to your dog, the dog will thank you for the protection, as salt can set up serious wounds that may take a long time to heal.

Shampoos. Dilute shampoo by 30 percent with hydrosol, then add an equal quantity of water in a plastic container and use as normal. Many pet shampoos are medicated for fleas or skin conditions, so choose the appropriate hydrosol and/ or essential oil to treat the condition. I combine four drops each of sea pine and cedar essential oils in a sodium-lauryl-sulfate-free shampoo, then dilute it with one-quarter cup each of cedar and rosemary hydrosols and one-quarter cup of water. I use the same hydrosols in the rinse water, and my dog really doesn't get fleas. You may wish to use a medicated shampoo at full strength and follow with a hydrosol–essential oil rinse instead.

Skunk. Go for the oils! Use ten drops of lemon, ten drops of pine (*Pinus pinaster* is best, but any pine will do), and twenty drops of lavandin. Add the oils to two tablespoons of shampoo with a little water and wash the dog well, leaving the shampoo on the coat for three to five minutes before rinsing. Towel dry and rub fifty to one hundred milliliters of pine or balsam fir hydrosol into the coat and brush it through. If you live in an area with skunks, keep a bottle of this blend on hand; it's nearly always late at night that skunk sprays happen, and you'll be in such a panic that you won't be thinking of looking up a recipe, just how to get rid of that SMELL!

Grooming. Between shampoos, keep Fido smelling sweet and looking sleek by regular brushing with hydrosols. Just mist the coat and brush the hydrosol through—this is really good for smelly dogs, and regular use may actually banish some of that doggie odor. All the tree waters are well liked by dogs, giving them a sense of green and a healthy natural smell that doesn't totally obscure their own odor.

Cuts and bites. Wash the wound with a 50 percent hydrosol, 50 percent hydrogen peroxide blend (use only 3 percent topical hydrogen peroxide). Use lavender, balsam fir, tea tree, or thyme linalol; add a chamomile if the cut is swollen or inflamed. All of these waters will also calm the dog, just as they calm us. Use rock rose if there is bleeding, and if the cut is deep or bleeding will not stop, pressure compress with one drop of *Cistus* oil and *Cistus* hydrosol together. If that doesn't work in five to ten minutes, call a vet, as an artery or vein may be damaged. Foot pads bleed copiously if cut and take a long time to heal, as walking continually splits them open; in these cases, use the hydrosols two or three times daily in a compress, followed by one drop of lavender oil, and keep walks short until healing is complete.

Behavior problems. Spray a gentle mist of hydrosol around the head from behind the ears, or spray your hands and wipe them over the dog's face once or twice; repeat three times a day. Don't spray anything directly at your dog's face; dogs hate that. Try neroli or linden for high anxiety, nerves, and stress states caused by travel or upset. For a dog that has long periods alone, use Roman chamomile, lavender, St. John's wort, or one of the conifer hydrosols; you could spritz an old T-shirt that carries your smell with the hydrosol and leave it in the dog's bedding so it feels the pack is close. Aromatic Tincture of melissa and German chamomile works as well as Rescue Remedy and can be used frequently without worry of an overdose. Tellington Touch or any kind of energy healing is highly useful in dealing with behavioral problems, as are the necessary components of plenty of exercise and lots of love and attention.

Housebreaking "accidents." I have not heard of a hydrosol that stopped a dog from messing in the house, although you could try peppermint, but hydrosols can help remove the odor if your dog does have an accident. Wash the area with warm, soapy water to which you have added one-half to one cup of hydrosol. Try oregano, tea tree, peppermint, pine, or a combination of these. Put paper on the wet area to blot up the excess moisture, and spritz a little more of the blend on the spot when it is almost dry. In these cases you may want to use essential oils, not just hydrosols. Problems in housebreaking may be behavioral, due to lack of attention to a dog's natural evacuation cycles, caused by insufficient exercise, or diet related, or they may indicate that there is some kind of health problem.

Birth and postpartum care. Five to seven days before delivery, add one tablespoon of clary sage hydrosol to the dog's morning feed and one table-spoon of Roman chamomile hydrosol to the evening feed. Other choices would be fennel or geranium for morning; linden, neroli, or rose for evening. Most labor will begin in the evening, so it helps to give relaxing, stress-reducing hydrosols at this time; morning choices are those that have possible hormone-related functions. During labor you could wipe the dog's face with chamomile or linden, preferably diluted 50 percent with water so the smell is less strong to the pups. There are also many homeopathic and herbal remedies that should be explored to make whelping as easy as possible for the bitch. Fennel hydrosol will help with milk production and flow postpartum, and sore teats may be washed or misted with German chamomile when the puppies start to grow teeth. Hydrosols are great for the mother's bath a few days after the birth and can be safely used to clean and disinfect around the puppies.

Birds

Birds love water, so hydrosols are a natural choice here. Leave a birdbath out for your birds at all times and add no more than one-eighth teaspoon hydrosol per five hundred milliliters (two cups) of water in the bath. Any birdbath should be broad and shallow to allow the birds to spread their wings and to prevent the risk of drowning. The old view that birds should always be caged has fortunately changed over recent years, particularly when it comes to anything larger than a finch. But even caged birds love a bath, and you can allow a mist of 10 percent hydrosol and 90 percent water to float gently down on birds even inside a cage. To watch them shower is such a joy; of all the animals, only elephants seem to love baths more.

Birds are mostly flock animals, although some mate and live only in pairs. No bird lives totally alone for its whole life, and keeping just one bird means that you must keep it company, become its flock. Living in a cage or being alone for many hours a day can stress a bird. It may pull out its own feathers, refuse to eat, become destructive or aggressive, and squawk continuously or never at all. However, knowing your animal will help you recognize these signs and deal with the stress factors before the bird becomes too ill.

Diet is also an issue; make plenty of water available, and stir birdseed with a paper towel wrapped around a chopstick to remove dust and "stuff." You can mist birdseed with hydrosol, but remember that if you leave it damp it will sprout, which your birds may like or not. Be sure that sprouting seed doesn't become moldy, which can readily happen and could be toxic to the birds. Feed good-quality birdseed, organic if possible, and supplement with cuttlefish, mineral blocks, and whatever your bird would naturally eat in the wild. It used to make me feel nauseated, but I gave my birds maggots from the local fishing store every couple of weeks, and they loved me nearly as much as their maggots.

Mites. Treat with a mixture of 20 to 25 percent hydrosol and 75 to 80 percent water. Use cedar, balsam fir, yarrow, or green myrtle. Birds from pet shops tend to pick up mites, which can cause skin irritations and feather loss.

Molting. Make a mix of 10 to 20 percent hydrosol with 80 to 90 percent water. Mist this gently over the bird two or three times a day or place it in a birdbath to be used as needed to calm skin and reduce itching. Try geranium, Roman chamomile, lavender, carrot seed, or linden. Hydrosol baths will help break down the coating on the new feathers, which your bird will greatly appreciate. Lots of birds will also want to be "scratched" when they are molting to help free the new feathers from their sheath, so go on . . . itch your bird.

Respiratory problems. Put two or three drops of hydrosol in the water dish or on the food daily for three weeks. One or two drops of hydrosol on a tissue wrapped around a chopstick can be used to stir the seeds to remove dust and pollens. Throw out and replace food daily if you put hydrosols on the seed. Use *Inula*, rosemary verbenone, green myrtle, or thyme CT linalol. You may place one drop of essential oil on a tissue and tuck it on the outside of the cage if the problem is not cleared up by hydrosol treatment, but do not put the tissue anywhere the bird can reach it.

Stress. Add three or four drops of hydrosol to the water dish, changing the water daily, for three weeks, and give daily mists with a solution of 40 percent hydrosol and 60 percent water. Use linden, neroli, lavender, angelica, or Roman chamomile. If the bird is so depressed that it is unresponsive, try cornflower, melissa, lemon verbena, St. John's wort, or purple bee balm (geraniol type). Try a different food, moving the cage or perch near a window, putting mirrors or toys in the cage, letting the bird fly loose, or consider getting another bird as company; in addition, give plenty of your own time, attention, and love.

Other Animals

Any mammal, from hamster to horse, can benefit from hydrosols. Always bear in mind the animal's weight in figuring a dosage. Acute conditions—anything that appears suddenly and severely—benefit from tiny doses at frequent intervals for a short period of time. Chronic or long-term conditions respond best to regular doses over a three-week cycle, with a week off in between to assess any changes that may have occurred in the condition.

Here is a guide for the daily dosage for small animals:

Acute phase: One-half teaspoon per five hundred grams (one pound) of body weight, to be divided into six to eight doses, given at intervals throughout the day only until the condition clears up.

Chronic phase: One-quarter teaspoon per five hundred grams (one pound) of body weight, to be divided into two or three doses, given morning, noon, and night daily for three weeks. Reassess the condition at the end of the week off and repeat only if necessary.

Amphibians and fish should never be treated with hydrosols, nor should hydrosols ever be added to their water habitat. The pH of hydrosols will alter the pH of the water and may cause serious harm to the creatures. Reptiles, likewise, should not be treated with hydrosols, although I have often wondered how a large snake would like a mist bath or scale shine with fairly neutral hydrosol like lavender or an exotic from their home country. Not being a snake owner, I guess I'll never know, but if you wish to try it, please use only a very diluted hydrosol, check with your vet or reference material to determine the normal pH of the snake's skin or scales, and do a patch test first, leaving at least twenty-four hours after application to gauge any negative effects.

Goats, ponies and horses, cows, and larger animals can all have hydrosols added to their drinking water, but always offer alternate untreated water sources to the animal so it does not suffer from dehydration if it will not drink the hydrosol. You can also "drench" larger animals, forcing them to drink a dose, just as you would a dog. Use a large plastic (not glass) turkey baster or squirt bottle and gently pour the liquid into the animal's mouth while you hold it open—be prepared to get a little wet and lose some of the dose—then hold the mouth closed while the animal swallows, but do allow it to cough if need be so it doesn't choke or get liquid into its lungs.

Check the profiles for the correct hydrosol to treat specific conditions, and remember that with larger animals it is safe to combine essential-oil treatments—topically, aerially, and even internally—with a hydrosol treatment. Larger animals, like humans, have much greater tolerance for the strength and potency of essential oils than do small mammals, cats, and even dogs.

One client cured "cough" in her cow herd with drenches of *Inula* hydrosol and an essential-oil blend diffused into the barn at night!

HOME AND HEARTH

Hydrosols, like all aspects of aromatherapy, can and should be a part of everyday life. For health, for the environment, for mood, for flavor, for spirit, and for fun, make your life more naturally aromatic. This is where many of my hydrosols go as they approach their best-before date.

Hydrosols around the house can be incorporated into cleaning products. Spritz on the dusting cloth and leave sweet-smelling shiny surfaces; it's even safe on polished woods. Add hydrosol to your glass cleaner, diluting it by 10 to 20 percent, and let the sun shine in. Pour one-quarter cup into clean toilet bowls and down the sink and tub drains to help deodorize. Clean the sink with baking soda and a cloth soaked in hydrosol instead of chemical cleaners. Add hydrosols and essential oils to floor-washing water. Throw one-half cup of hydrosol into the dishwasher with the detergent or into the rinse cycle of the laundry. Even houseplants can benefit from a tablespoon of hydrosol added to each liter of water; this is especially good for acid-loving plants like azaleas and violets. If a plant needs very alkaline soil or conditions, like a fig tree *(Ficus benjamina),* do not feed hydrosols, or check the pH chart before using.

Environments can be improved by adding hydrosols to humidifiers; whether it is cool or hot steam doesn't matter—just add three tablespoons of hydrosol per liter of water for a noticeable aromatic difference. If you don't have a humidifier, place bowls of water with hydrosols on radiators to achieve the same effect. In southern climes dehumidifiers and air conditioners may be more necessary then humidifiers. Dehumidifiers extract water from the air and deposit it in a pan below, so add some hydrosol to the water receptacle in the machine to prevent bacteria from growing and to reduce that musty smell. Central air conditioners also have water receptacles that can benefit from the same treatment. I once stayed in a tiny hotel in the Nevada desert that had a "swamp cooler." This ingenious device allowed water to trickle down a large flat surface while a fan blew at the surface from behind. It was fairly effective, given the forty-degree-Celsius temperature outside, at adding moisture to the cool air, but the odor was definitely of swamp. I poured a whole bottle of rosemary into the tank and received the double bonus of the stimulation of the rosemary and the coolness of the air. All the swampy smell went bye-bye.

Small candle-type diffusers or "burners" can be filled with hydrosols instead of water in the top; choose something that will complement your essential-oil selection for maximum synergy. Do not put hydrosols into the receptacle of nebulizer-type diffusers, as these are specifically designed for essential oils only. Fountains, so much a part of decor these days, are the perfect place to pour your hydrosols; they will give only the lightest of fragrance and won't, therefore, offend the overly smell conscious in offices or clinics, and they do wonders for balancing feng shui energy.

Put hydrosols in liquid soap dispensers, diluting the soap about 10 percent, and you'll have a much nicer fragrance, softer hands, and some natural antiseptic action as well. Why stop there;

why not make your own soap and use hydrosols instead of water in the recipe? They are less volatile than essential oils, so the soap won't lose its scent as rapidly, and while you'd never put neroli essential oil in soap, you can use the hydrosol and give deluxe soap new meaning.

The uses for hydrosols in the kitchen are almost endless, and I have included some culinary recipes in chapter 6. There are several aromatherapy cookbooks on the market, but the best ones I've seen, by Maria Kettenring (see the bibliography), are available only in German as of this writing. Hopefully some brilliant publisher will have them translated and published so we can all benefit.

If you cook with herbs, dried or fresh, you are already cooking with hydrosols in a manner of speaking. Cooking with the lid on a pot allows the steam rising off the food to condense on the inside of the lid and fall back into the dish. This water is in effect a hydrosol, as it contains the water-soluble aromatic components of the cooking ingredients and is a steam that condenses back into water, just as in distillation. When you cook with the lid off, you thicken a sauce by allowing the steam to evaporate instead of going back into the "soup."

Generally you can use hydrosols to replace all or some of the water in any recipe. For pastas and rice you may wish to add the hydrosol to the cooking water, or sprinkle a teaspoon or two on the cooked dish just before serving. Choose a hydrosol that will complement the flavors of your dish, and feel free to experiment—all the best chefs do. Some hydrosols, like melissa, lemon verbena, cardamom, angelica, sweet fern, sweet gale, and cinnamon, will work just as well in sweet dishes as in savory. Others, like rose, neroli, Roman chamomile, are best in desserts; and those like the herbs, for example, sage, rosemary, and thyme, work best in savory dishes only.

For vegetarians, hydrosols are a wonderful addition to the kitchen repertoire. Soups, sauces, stocks, and gravies can be greatly enriched by the addition of these concentrated flavors, and you will surprise even your nonveggie friends by the complexity of taste they add to any meal. I have used them in marinades for tofu, textured vegetable protein, and vegetables, and no salad dressing is complete for me without a little bay leaf hydrosol. Steaming over plain water pales by comparison with steaming over hydrosols, and the simplest of pasta dishes becomes gourmet with a sprinkle of hydrosol.

Using hydrosols in the kitchen is perhaps the most ancient of their applications. Persian, Turkish, Greek, Egyptian, and Roman cooking all made wide use of aromatic waters, and even today baklava is made with rose- or orange-blossom water, depending on the country you're in. You can even put hydrosols in the ice-cream machine for sorbets and granita—and don't limit yourself to the sweet ones; try a thyme linalol and melissa combination for a palate cleanser at a multicourse dinner. Your guests will be wowed, and it couldn't be easier.

Flavor beverages, too. Orange juice with a spritz of neroli is out of this world, and in a Buck's Fizz (see page 254), well, what can I say, try it today! All fruit and vegetable juices, fresh squeezed or not, can be enlivened with a hint of hydrosol. Again, it's up to you to experiment, although some suggestions are in the recipe section. Salt, pepper, Worcestershire sauce, and Tabasco are no different in concept from bay, thyme, coriander, or sage. A squeeze of lemon, or a dash of melissa? Why not put the hydrosols in your ice tray and add flavored ice to your drinks. The melting ice will enhance rather than dilute the beverage, and the ice cubes can be used for alcoholic as well as nonalcoholic creations. Oregano cubes in tomato juice, winter savory in a green mix of freshly juiced vegetables, peppermint in lemonade or herbal iced tea—go crazy. Gin and tonic with juniper ice cubes, clary sage ice in punches or white-wine spritzers; shake your martini with flavored cubes or drink cassis vodka on black currant hydrosol–flavored rocks! As more and more hydrosols become available and more and more people begin to experiment, who knows what gourmet treats these kitchen aids will inspire.

Food and drink are two of the great pleasures in life, so enjoy them, and don't worry if you allow a little indulgence from time to time. Keep a selection of hydrosols in your fridge and you will have a second spice rack full of flavors in the kitchen.

ESOTERIC

The esoteric and metaphysical uses of hydrosols are myriad and are perhaps worthy of their own chapter. In fact, there is probably more data published to date on the esoteric than therapeutic uses of these amazing waters.

Aromatherapy is at a crossroads in public acceptance, and it is often the association with the airy-fairy aspect that makes people discount essential oils and aromatics as viable health products. It is a shame, in some ways, that we feel we must have scientific approval for what we already know. Essential oils work and have been used for centuries for their properties. Many pharmaceuticals have been developed from essential oils or their constituents, and many products that we take for granted and use daily, including mouthwash and toothpaste, hair and body-care products, foodstuffs, beverages, even cigarettes, contain oils or aromatic compounds. But part of the desire to see the "modality" become truly a "profession" has come to mean that we must be validated by "the system," in this case science. Personally, I think it's somewhat of a mistake. Yes, we should learn our chemistry and science, and yes, we should be aware of the potential interactions between essential oils and pharmaceutical drugs and even phytomedicines, but I don't want the government or the drug companies telling me what I can and cannot do with my oils and hydrosols. I don't want to see the standardized-extract movement even think about aromatherapy. I don't want people or organizations that are not qualified to make decisions about aromatics making decisions that affect aromatics, unless it's to say they must be pesticide- and contaminant-free,

but we can do that through our peer-reviewed organizations, and the sooner the better.

There is no doubt that hydrosols, like essential oils, contain the life-force energy of plants. Even science accepts that water is energetic, so these products give us a double whammy on the esoteric side by being both water and plant in one. Try using a pendulum over a glass of plain water and then over some pure organic hydrosol. You'll be amazed. Desert white sage hydrolate is so energetic that it nearly pulls the pendulum from my hands, the swing is so strong, and yarrow water has a distinct flower-shaped spiral energy pattern unlike any other. Lavender water will cause a clockwise spin and lavandin a counterclockwise one, just like the respective oils. These aspects are just as real as the pH and chemical properties of the hydrosols and must be considered when working with them for healing.

Energy

The *Longman Dictionary of Contemporary English* defines energy as "the quality of being full of life and action; power and ability to do work or be physically active."

The quality of being full of life and action. Taken literally, we might not apply this characteristic to most objects, certainly not most inanimate or seemingly inanimate objects. But taken in a broader context and applied to, say, a glass bottle, where does this take us? The bottle is capable of action, it can "hold" liquid, and glass is actually a liquid itself, one that is moving at a very slow speed. So although it seems inanimate, glass is actually animate. From this view, a glass bottle can, therefore, have energy. Now, how can we determine whether hydrosols contain energy?

Some people who consider themselves sensitive can just hold a substance, or hold their hand over a substance, and feel energy. I once held my hands on either side of a liter bottle of fine lavender oil and was stunned by the "energy" coming off the bottle. A colleague with me said, "What do you think you're doing?" I told her, and she scoffed. So I said "You try it," and when she did, her face went very still, then exploded in an ear-to-ear grin as she exclaimed, "Oh, my, I've never felt anything like it." We all have the ability; we just don't always know it or use it. When I do trade shows, it is common for visitors to pass their hands over the bottles, feeling for the vibrations. If they like what they find, they will pick up and handle the bottles, absorbing the "vibes" through their hands, and last they will open and smell them. But by that point, for these folks at least, they have already determined the presence of the life force and "know" how much energy is waiting to be shared.

Hydrosols affect our health, even when used in tiny amounts. This could be construed as the power and ability to do work . . . as energy. Turning back to the idea of hydrosols as holograms and fractals, we can also see that they contain an energy in their physical structure. They have odor and taste, at the very least, and the chemicals contained in their makeup all have their own energy—and not just on the physical levels. This energy goes right down to the molecular and even subatomic level, so, for me at least, they have life, energy, on the most profound level.

Energy Work

Therapeutic Touch, Touch for Health, hands-on healing, Reiki, and many others are all different names for "energy work." I guess marketing has been applied to the esoteric world as much as any other, since this is possibly the first type of healing work that humankind ever practiced, and it is only in recent years that all the multitude of names have been applied. The principle is that the energy of the universe, God/Goddess, the Divine Force (more names), is allowed to flow through the body and hands of the healer into the client, and that this energy combines with the intention of both healer and client and manifests the healing process. When we were still at one with nature, we were far more in tune with the rhythms and patterns of the body and understood health as imbalances in the "spirit," or energy, realm. Modern ecologists, psychologists, anthropologists, and many other "ologists" are exploring these ideas and their relevance; meanwhile the nurses, holistic health practitioners, traditional healers, and shamans have never stopped doing it.

Hydrosols are a wonderful adjunct to use in all types of energy work. Because they come from plant material, they contain information about the rhythms and patterns of the planet as well as the plant. They are also imbued with the life force of the plant and are definitely "alive" in this respect, as are the essential oils. But hydrosols offer the benefit of having a much more subtle fragrance, which can be a major benefit given the hyperawareness of the senses that often accompanies illness or in hospitals and nursing homes. They are also water, one of the cornerstones of life; nothing and no one can live without it. And water has its own energy and connections to the rhythms of the earth and its human, animal, and plant inhabitants. Our bodies are primarily water, as is discussed elsewhere in this book, and our body's water content is a major force in our body rhythms.

Before you begin energy work, you will want to clear your own energy field; you can either mist the selected hydrosol through your "field" or place three drops on your hands and wipe down your energy body, releasing any "flotsam and jetsam" that could cloud your perceptions. To choose the appropriate hydrosol, you can refer to the profiles or allow intuition to play a part and sense what is the appropriate fragrance and vibration for the work you wish to conduct. Depending on your client, you may also use a pendulum or allow the client to participate in the selection process, which can give him or her a sense of empowerment through active participation in the healing. Once the appropriate hydrosol is selected, place one to three drops on the palm of your right hand, declaring the intention of the work you are about to do, asking for the help of the plant and its energy, and requesting permission from the client to ensure that all energy shifts will be appropriate and beneficial. Then commence in your usual fashion.

You will find your hands are more sensitive, more "tuned," and the client may feel the movement of energy far more clearly. Always work appropriately and with permission when you are shifting energy fields, as you can easily do as much harm as good if you are not careful.

You can also place one drop of hydrosol on specific points of the body during a treatment as you feel weakness or blocks that may be hard to clear. As you apply the hydrosol, make your intentions clear and afterward go over the area again; you should feel a significant difference. It is rare that you will need more than one drop of hydrosol, but occasionally you may use up to three drops; the idea is not to soak your client but to use the waters for their vibration, their energy, and the hologram of information in that energy. As you become used to hydrosols, you will find your own method and will come to know which waters resonate best with you and with certain types of health problems. After all, each person has his or her own resonance and every disease also has its own resonance. Often disease is the result of the loss of harmony or balance in the body that conflicting or nonharmonic resonances create. Energy work tries to restore the balance in the body.

Reiki is a form of energy healing where symbols are incorporated into the hands-on healing. The symbols carry specific meaning and are used in particular ways to rebalance the body. Hydrosols can make the symbols even more powerful. If we trace a pattern in the air with our fingers, we achieve one level of energy; to write it down achieves a much greater level of energy, activating the years of cellular memory that we hold from learning to write. However, Reiki practitioners consider it inappropriate to "write down" or commit to paper the secret symbols, so what to do? Write with hydrosols. Using the water as a paintbrush, even if we are writing in the air, adds a palpable energetic dimension, and one practitioner I know swears she can "see" the symbols she writes, floating in the air for many minutes after she paints them with the waters. You can also "write" your symbols with hydrosol on paper or on the body of the client and no record will remain after the fact.

If energy work is used to aid the passage into death, anointing the body is a wonderful ritual that can be done privately or with the help and permission of family. Nearly every culture has rituals surrounding death, and it is only a matter of creating the appropriate context for those concerned. Death is still the greatest fear for most people, and it is not uncommon for the dying to need permission before they let go, or to need help in taking the final steps toward release. I watched my mother dying of cancer after years of illness, and on what proved to be her last night, I sat with her for hours, using oils, crystals, and poetry to help her finally let go. She had her own reasons for holding on, but when I left her that night I felt quite sure that it was over, and her face, even in a coma, had relaxed from resistance into acceptance. After her death I poured the petals of a dozen roses over her body, and not only did they touch her spirit but they soothed mine as well. Sandalwood, rose, angelica root, sweet gale, linden, and cypress are some hydro-

sols to be considered for this purpose, but any hydrosol can be used if it is appropriate for the individuals concerned.

Whatever method of energy work you use, you will love the difference that these waters can make. It is in some ways no different from using holy waters, waters from sacred springs or wells, flower essences, gem elixirs, or any other water to which we have ascribed an energy or power. No, hydrosols are not holy water in a religious sense, but they can be "wholly" in a spiritual sense, or holy in a holographic sense, embodying the wholeness of life and the world in which we live. They carry the intention with which we imbue them and the knowledge and vibrations of their source; these are powerful tools that carry resonance for our use.

Geomancy, Feng Shui, and Dowsing

Geomancy comes from the Greek *gaie*, or *ge*, meaning "earth," which is where the word *Gaia* comes from, and *manteia*, meaning "divination." Geomancy is an extremely broad field and includes not only methods of divining past, present, and future but also methods of working with earth energy, ley lines, and concepts that could be included in feng shui. Wicca and magic, which are currently enormously popular (even the U.S. Army allows the practice of Wicca), include many aspects of geomancy and promote our relationship with Mother Earth and all of her inhabitants from all the realms and dimensions. Plants are an intimate means of connecting with earth energy, as is water, and each of these magical elements has its own realm of fairies, sylphs, gnomes, undines, and spirits of all kinds, so hydrolates provide a double connection when entering into this field.

Use hydrosols to mark energy lines in your home and garden; to create magic circles, zones of protection, or vortices for meditation, healing, safety, growth, and energy flow. Watch your plants flourish when you add a drop to their water or bathe them in a mist of dilute hydrosol for glossy, shiny leaves. You can even use hydrosols to help deter pests on houseplants by combining them with a little soapy water and washing affected parts.

Feng shui is big news at the turn of the millennium, and hydrosols can be a wonderful tool for this practice. Try assigning a specific water or create blends for each part of the ba'gua and use them to rebalance those areas of your space. Fountains are popular both for their feng shui properties and for their beauty and peaceful sound. Use hydrosols in fountains; they are safe for the pumps as well as the materials your fountain is made of, and if you have crystals in your fountain, they'll love the new addition. Hydrosols will not add so much fragrance that they offend the smell-free-zone types, but their energy will enliven the water and be enlivened in turn by the flow and movement within the fountain.

Any ritual that honors the earth or the seasons, such as at solstice, equinox, harvest festivals (Thanksgiving can have new meaning), May Day, and so on, can incorporate hydrosols. Water aids the fecundity of Gaia and all that she fosters, and the plant waters are a powerful symbol of her bounty and a wonderful gift to return to her in thanks. Rituals are very personal things, and if you begin to incorporate hydrosols, you will soon devise the most powerful way for your own meanings and intentions.

Water has also been a favorite medium for scrying, a method of divining or "seeing," much like using crystal balls. Scrying bowls are filled with water and the reflective surface stared at in a meditative state until the mirrorlike plane reveals its messages. How much more powerful to scry into angelica hydrosol, or perhaps white sage or . . . Find a water that will connect you to the appropriate energy and realm, whether tree, root, flower, or herb of sustenance; the more you work in this way, the more you will be guided.

Dowsing, or using a pendulum, is another form of geomancy and is an extremely fast method for testing the energy field of a substance. Anything can be used as a pendulum—a key on a piece of string, a pendant or necklace—but serious dowsers like to have proper pendulums, and there are hundreds of styles, designs, and materials in which they are made. There are even special pendulums for geologists that contain tiny hidden compartments, the idea being that you place a small amount of the substance that you are hunting inside the pendulum, thus tuning it specifically to seek out more of the same material. Sounds odd, perhaps, but I was turned on to these pendulums by a serious geologist who was as un–airy-fairy as you can get, and he swore by it. This type of pendulum can be interesting for aromatherapists, as it allows a drop of oil or hydrolate to be placed inside the pendulum prior to working with it, and you can tune your work to the individual or vibration that you need.

Pendulums can be used for answering questions, but only of the yes-no variety. If you wish to learn dowsing, there are many books and teachers out there.

Hydrosols are a powerful cleanser for pendulums, either before or after working. Used before, they will cleanse any previous attunements and remove patterns; they can also raise vibrations or tune the pendulum for the specific applications about to be undertaken. Used after working, hydrosols can eliminate any unwanted or negative energy that may have been picked up, a concern in healing work or space-clearing work. Periodically I like to wash my pendulums in hydrosols, just as a little treat. They are, after all, tools, and all tools work better when properly cared for.

Patricia Davis describes an excellent method of dowsing the chakras in her book *Subtle Aromatherapy*, and both oils and hydrosols can be used to realign and rebalance what the pendulum reveals. You can also dowse oils and hydrosols, and although you can use this as a spot check method for quality, it cannot replace buying from reliable sources and using all your senses and modern science to discern product integrity. If you spend time actually dowsing, you will find that each oil or hydrosol has a completely unique "energy print," much like a fingerprint. Some are elliptical, some circular; some are even figure eights and more complex spirals and patterns. They go clockwise and counterclockwise, back and forth, right to left, every which way the pendulum can swing, and in

every possible size of arc. One of my students plans to map the energy fields of aromatics and publish them, and by that point our understanding and acceptance of what these individual prints mean in terms of healing may carry as much weight as the properties ascribed to the chemical functional groups do today. As Schnaubelt says, "We know further that the oils' inherent natural complexity gives them the ability to heal. So, while we profit from the complexities of essential oils, our trusted scientific reductionist instruments cannot sufficiently understand these complexities."[7] Embracing the energetic aspect of both oils and hydrosols expands, rather than reduces, our vision of what they are and what they can do for us.

In my classes I always get out the dowsing rods and pendulums at some point. I try to make it fun and offer the demonstrations as information and experience that can be merely a parlor trick or yet another healing tool—after all, you can't offend people by carrying on in ways that threaten their own belief structures, now can you? It is always a wonderful experience to watch as people realize that their own energy field may extend for thirty feet or more—it gives riding the bus a whole new dimension!

Dowsing rods, sometimes called L-rods, are diagnostic tools for energy fields and evolved from the old Y-stick used in water witching. Most water witches are men, and the favored tool is a Y-shaped branch, preferably of ash or witch hazel wood. Accounts of water witching date back as far as we have records, and I wonder if water witches were put to death as often as healing witches—probably not. The two prongs of the Y are held in the hands, with the main branch pointing straight ahead. As the witch approaches the underground spring or water source, the stick will point sharply down at the ground, indicating where the well should be dug. Believe it or not, this is still how many wells are located today, simply because it works.

L-rods can also be used for finding water but have their best application in measuring the energy field of a person, place, or thing. Dipping the rods in hydrosol, applying hydrosols to the palms of the hands, or just applying it to the tips of the rods are some of the most obvious ways to marry the two, and as coat hangers are a favoured medium for making L-rods and are usually steel, the vibration of the metal can be raised to a higher frequency by the use of plant waters. Hold the rod loosely in one hand by the short end of the L, perpendicular to the client's body and about 6 to 8 inches away. Slowly move it from the head down to the feet, watching for any movements in or out of the rod as it scans the field. Again, use the methods of drop anointing described in Energy Work (page 204) to rebalance blocks or unevenness that show up.

As will be described in the section on crystals, hydrosols are wonderful for distance work, being able to create a web of energy across time and space, so pull in the extra help that hydrolates can offer. If the person you are working with has the same hydrosols on hand, that person can anoint his or her body at that end while you use the waters as appropriate at your end, creating a nonlocal and profound connection.

Shiatsu and Acupuncture

Now that institutions like the Stanford and Harvard medical schools are teaching acupuncture and shiatsu, I suppose they should be elevated out of the esoteric section, but they deal with energy, or chi, in the body, and so here they remain. Elements of traditional Chinese medicine (TCM), both these methods are concerned with a complex system of energy points on the body and the pathways (meridians) of energy, or chi, that connect the points. The systems are ancient, and the points have been mapped and accepted for around five thousand years. Hydrosols and oils can be used to stimulate the points and meridians as effectively as finger pressure or needles. When combined with physical pressure or the insertion of acupuncture needles, hydrosols can create an active synergy in the treatment. You may wish to trace the meridians between points with hydrosols after the needles are inserted or the points are stimulated by pressure. The meridians form connecting highways throughout the body, and using an eyedropper or your finger with the appropriate hydrosol to trace the path is powerful and simple. Oils are less appropriate for this purpose because of their potency and cost, but you can do it with the water.

One concept that TCM practitioner Miriam Erlichman and I have dubbed aromapuncture involves applying just one drop of hydrosol at a time to acupuncture points without using any pressure or needles—just one drop of water touched to the skin on the point. I have undergone a number of aromapuncture sessions and can say that they are some of the most powerful treatments I have ever had. During the first, one drop of *Inula* applied to a lung point gave me the instantaneous sensation of breathing the freshest air imaginable, of my lungs seeming to expand far beyond their physical capacity. Black spruce applied to the adrenal points on the abdomen sent electric currents throughout my body, and Erlichman actually asked if I was feeling the electricity *she* was feeling. I have had visions bordering on hallucinations from other points and always feel incredible for days afterward. Although there is no needle involved, we decided to call the treatment aromapuncture because the energy is passing into the skin as though it were a needle, and sometimes the sensation from the hydrosol is so sharp and intense that it feels as if a needle were inserted.

As was mentioned in the section on TCM, you must know your plants to replace Chinese herbs with hydrosols, but we cheated a little sometimes, using *Angelica archangelica* instead of *A. chinensis* and neroli, or bitter orange blossom (*Citrus aurantium* var. *amara* flos.), instead of immature fruit (petitgrain), as is recommended in the Chinese materia medica, and still had wonderful results. I would urge anyone who practices TCM to experiment with these methods. Don't use the needles at first, just the waters, so you can be sure that they are causing the effects felt by the client. Erlichman has been practicing TCM for seventeen years and is a devout lover of hydrosols, so the concept was easy for her to grasp. At a recent conference in Vancouver, Hong Jin of the Oregon College of Oriental Medicine presented a paper on herbs used on acupoints to treat common illnesses that discussed topical application of herbal pastes for everything from arthritis to asthma, so the aromapuncture method is really not too far out.

Flower Essences and Gem Elixirs

The Bach flower essences were the first and remain the best known, but plant essences now abound and there are specialty products from every region of the world. Whether they are the Australian bush, Canadian forest, South African, or Pacific Northwest essences, the concept is the same in every case. These are vibrational healing liquids made by floating plant material on pure water in the sunlight and then diluting this product (usually with alcohol for stability) and bottling it for use.

Analyzed, these substances contain fewer identifiable components than homeopathics, if that's possible, and yet they contain memory and vibration, which science does not choose to measure. And like homeopathics, which are also memory and vibration, they work. You need never try any essence other than Rescue Remedy to know just how effective these are, and placebo effect be damned, they work just as well on animals, children, plants, and crystals. My dog passes out for hours if I give her just three drops of Rescue Remedy, and I never go to a wedding or funeral without it; it's a lot more subtle than a spray of hydrosol, and the bottle can travel up and down the rows quite unnoticed, leaving calm and/or smiles in its wake.

Flower essences work happily with hydrosols, essential oils, and aromatic tinctures. They can be added to drinking water with the chosen hydrolate so that together they work their magic through the day. They can also be combined in topical treatments such as compresses, baths and sitz baths, and so on. I would like to see flower essences made with hydrosols instead of plain springwater, using the same plant material for both or creating combinations that work synergistically. If only I could grow rock rose in Canada, I would float the flowers on the hydrosol and go happily to heaven.

Gem elixirs or essences are not a new thing but have hit the mainstream in the last few years. The most famous book on the subject is the two-volume set by Gurudas, which details many methods of both making and using gem essences. Just as flower essences can be combined with hydrosols, so can gem elixirs, and as always the synergy is more powerful than the individual components, and that can really be something.

You can make your own gem essences with water or hydrosol and will find many books to help you link the gems with the appropriate plant waters and healing dimensions. Simply place the clean gem or crystal in a jug of hydrosol and water and leave it in the sun or moon for twenty-four hours, or until the desired vibration is achieved. You can also look at astrological influences, combining plants and gems that are ruled by the same planet or associated with the same star sign. You may choose to link them by their healing properties—peridot for the adrenal glands with black spruce hydrosol, garnet with

sage for circulation and the gonads—or by their colors: amethyst with lavender, celestite with cornflower, citrine with goldenrod or linden, depending on the exact hue of the stone. We are in a realm without rules here. Perhaps the country of origin is the link: tourmaline or quartz from Madagascar with cinnamon or geranium hydrosol, labradorite with Labrador tea *(Ledum groenlandicum)*. Talk to the crystals, listen to the waters; they will lead you on a journey of discovery. Then send me a card and let me know what you learn, and share it with the world. We are all magicians at heart.

Crystals

Of course, gem elixirs are made with both crystals and hydrosols, but there is so much more that you can do when you bring rocks and water together. Rocks, for as heavy, hard, and unyielding as they seem, are easily wrapped by the liquid flow of water; rocks are worn down by water, and the movement of water around rocks adds force and energy to the flow of the water in return. Did you know that water is colder on the downside of a large rock? The energy created by the flow of water around the obstacle in its path improves its "health" and lowers the temperature; four degrees centigrade is the healthiest water temperature.[8] Think about this in terms of healing energy and our ideas about fractals and chaos. Water and rocks have a symbiotic relationship in my mind and represent two of the elements, or nature spirits: water and earth.

So crystals and hydrosols have a symbiotic

relationship that works on many levels. Both are alive, both have consciousness, and both are capable of providing enlightenment and healing. When one thinks of the long history of crystals as objects of power and talismans connecting the earth and the heavens, it is also reasonable to assume that crystals and aromatics of all kinds may have been used in combination for millennia.

Cleansing crystals. When you first acquire a crystal, it is always a good idea to cleanse it, to remove any "other" energies the stone may be carrying. It is generally accepted that crystals carry the memory of every person who has ever touched them and also the memory of their existence, including how they were removed from the earth. Although it would be nice if all rock hounds gently removed their finds from the ground, it is a fact that many crystals are "found" in less than gentle ways, and that can leave an unhappy vibe in the stone. Then it is sold from dealer to dealer until the day it comes to you, and although some of the hands may have treated the crystal with love and respect, others have not, and it is really important that you start by healing the crystal before you use the stone for your own healing or for healing others.

Solar-dried sea salt is a wonderful cleanser for most crystals. You can use one tablespoon of salt with enough hydrosol or hydrosol and water to cover the stone; leave it to rest in this bath for twenty-four hours to one week, until it feels "lighter" when you lift it out. (*Note:* Some crystals should not be put into sea salt, as it will damage the structure of the stone, for example, se-

lenite, amber, galena, and some of the softer crystals.) If the crystal comes from someone who has already begun the healing, you can bathe it in pure hydrosol without the salt, perhaps put it in the sunlight or under a full moon to add those energies to the mix. A crystal that comes with specific information already programmed may need only a light cleansing so that "fingerprints" are removed but not the data. In this case dilute your hydrosol with distilled water or springwater 50:50 and pour a stream gently over the crystal while you turn it and rub it, consciously seeing the prints disappear but leaving the vibration refreshed and accessible.

As described in the discussion of pendulums, you may also need to cleanse crystals after certain types of work to get rid of unwanted energy and to recharge the crystal's own forces. Depending on the situation, an overnight bath in pure hydrosol may be more than enough, but you can safely leave your crystal soaking for several days if needed. Many hydrosols can be used for cleansing, and you can consider the specific energies and personality of the stone when looking for a sympathetic water. Some to consider are clary sage, white sage, angelica root, rose, sweet fern, balsam fir, cypress, myrtle, St. John's wort, and exotics like lotus. The more heavy-duty the cleansing and healing required, the longer it will take and the more focus and intention will be required. Hydrosols add a powerful aspect, however, and you may find that cleansing will actually take less time in plant waters than in springwater.

Awakening crystals. Sometimes our presence alone will cause a crystal to wake up, a sure sign that you are to be the new guardian of this particular consciousness. However, sometimes we know a crystal is for us or is gifted but it requires a little help to awaken from its slumber. Chanting, singing bowls, and bells are classic ways to wake a sleeping crystal and work on awakening our consciousness to boot. Hydrosols can also be used, either in combination with sound or on their own. Try placing some hydrosol in your singing bowl; let it warm up first, as cold water stops the bowl from singing. As you start to work the bowl, the resonance of the tone will cause the hydrosol to fountain up in the center, as though it were dancing. The crystal can be anointed with the charged water or placed beside the bowl so the sound waves can travel through and around it. Be patient when you start to work with hydrosols and singing bowls; it takes a while to master the knack of creating sound with water in the bowl, but it is worth the effort for the beauty of the event and the new range of tones your bowls will produce. You can also drink the hydrosol after charging it with sound, but be sure your singing bowl is clean and of a good quality; crystal singing bowls are best for charging hydrosol for consumption.

To awaken a crystal with hydrosol alone, place some in a clean glass bowl and wet your hands in it frequently while rubbing, squeezing, and massaging the crystal. Talk to it, explore all the surfaces and facets both inside and out, keep dipping your fingers and rubbing in more hydrosol, using the energy of the plant as a second voice, added to your own, and calling for the crystal to wake up: "Join us, come and play, we're waiting for you." You can perform this on crystals already awake and in your keeping, and you may be surprised when new glimmers, rainbows, and light appear inside the stone even while you work.

Tuning crystals. Most tools are designed with a certain function in mind, and that is also true with some crystals. However, all crystal energy can be tuned to a specific vibration or focused to a desired intention; that is part of their magic. When tuning crystals for healing, you will want to choose your stones and the hydrosols for their specific health properties. Rose quartz and rose hydrosol for the heart is an obvious example. You may want to meditate or dowse for appropriate choices before you begin or allow intuition and your own knowledge to guide you in your selections. Sit with the crystal and the hydrosol, speak to them both, explaining what you need, being clear about your intentions and seeking permission for the work and the requested help. You may wish to develop a ritual of attunement, dipping the crystal several times and holding it to your forehead, adding your own energy and receiving guidance from the earth and water. You may find that just one to three drops of hydrosol placed on the crystal and rubbed over its surface will suffice, or use any other method that seems right for you personally. Intention is the name of the game here, and your intentions will be exponentially magnified by both the crystal and the hydrosol, so do be careful what you ask for—you will probably get it.

If you are trying to tune in to a specific vibration, there are a few ways this can be done. One method, which will also provide information that can then be used for other purposes, is to create a vibration scale and then dowse the hydrosol and crystal to see where they fit on the scale. A high-vibration crystal will raise the vibration of the hydrosol, and vice versa. Generally crystals with a low or weak vibration are not used for healing, but a hydrosol with a resonance as high as the crystals will, when combined, create a synergistically amplified vibration that is greater than the sum of the two individual parts. A bar or circle marked from one to ten is the simplest measurement scale. You hold your pendulum over the scale while you hold the item in the other hand and ask to be shown its vibration point. You can make a note of the vibration of hydrosols, which may also tell you if they start to go off or if you buy an inferior batch. When you combine a higher vibration with a lower one, either they will meet in the middle somewhere or the lower one will come up to the point of the higher one. You can also tune several crystals to each other in this manner.

You can tune additional information into the crystal from the hydrosol. If you find you "fall asleep" when you meditate, put rosemary or sage hydrosol on an amethyst crystal and hold it while you meditate; you will remain more alert in your altered state. A friend of mine used to correct me whenever I mentioned meditation; he'd say, "You mean nap, don't you?" So I explained about the rosemary-amethyst combination, which led him to stop teasing about napping and start calling me crazy.

If you are part of a group meditation, the members of the group could use sweet gale hydrosol to anoint themselves and their crystals. Sweet gale creates energetic webs and will link all the participants in a positive and loving manner. A crystal matrix for global healing and positive change can be built in this manner. This is a wonderful practice if the group is not all together in one location, as it will provide yet another link across time and space. I think of sweet gale as the WWW of hydrosols, a worldwide web that has nothing to do with the Internet.

Healing with crystals. You may pursue any of the methods described in this section and combine them with crystals in healing sessions. Hydrosols are an unobtrusive but powerful adjunct to the work, whether they are placed on the healer, the healing tools, or the client or just kept nearby. I like to bathe or mist my crystals briefly before using them in healing to charge them up and create a protective field around them and, through them, myself. The day starts better after a little shower. Again, make sure you match the vibration of the stone and the chosen water, by virtue of either their properties, their colors, their astrological associations, or their personality.

There are many books on crystals and crystal healing, and practitioners are popping up all over. Use these resources and your own intuition when exploring the connections between earth and water; they have loud voices, these elements, and will speak volumes if you open your ears and your heart.

And now I hope you will know what to do with your hydrosols.

SIX

Bubble Bubble— The Recipes

It is easy to imagine one of the Cro-Magnon women mentioning to her friends
that her favorite recipe for roast leg of bear used cypress wood
and dried leaves from a thyme bush.
James V. Kohl and Robert T. Francoeur, *The Scent of Eros*

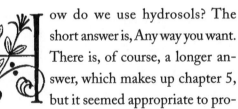ow do we use hydrosols? The short answer is, Any way you want. There is, of course, a longer answer, which makes up chapter 5, but it seemed appropriate to provide some proper recipes also. They cover a whole gamut of applications, from the purely pleasurable to the highly therapeutic.

Hydrosols can be used individually or mixed into blends in exactly the same way that you blend with essential oils. In combinations they create synergies and have increased properties and strength, just like the oils. The aromas of the less-sweet varieties can be dramatically improved by the addition of equally appropriate but sweeter-smelling waters. Although they are not normally incorporated into aromatherapy massage, hydrosols have their place even in this arena. If massage is your primary practice, you can use the hydrosols to compress specific areas before and during the bodywork, use them as a spritz to cool the client during hot weather, wash the feet before a reflexology session, or as described in the monographs in chapter 3 for various other modalities.

Short forms used in the recipes:

A.H.: aromatic hydrosol
E.O.: essential oil
V.O.: vegetable (or carrier) oil
gm: gram
kg: kilogram
ml: milliliter (30 ml equals approximately 1 ounce)

THERAPEUTIC RECIPES

The Head

HEADACHES

50 ml A.H. peppermint
50 ml A.H. Roman chamomile
100 ml water (if headache is severe, omit
      water)

Take 2 teaspoons undiluted hydrosol orally; add remainder to the water and compress forehead and nape of neck simultaneously with cloths soaked in blend. Lie down for 15 to 20 minutes. You can add 2 to 4 drops E.O. peppermint to the blend for migraines.

The Eyes

TIRED OR BLOODSHOT EYES

A.H. chamomile (Roman or German), green
      myrtle, or cornflower

Spritz the hydrosol directly into eyes from a safe distance, keeping eyes open. I have put these hydrosols into sterilized dropper bottles and put 2 or 3 drops in each eye at a time. I prefer chamomile for everyday use; myrtle for irritation from pollution, dust, and so on; and cornflower for computer eyes.

CONJUNCTIVITIS (PINK EYE)

5 ml A.H. Roman or German chamomile

Place in eye cup and bathe eye, blinking several times. Throw away hydrosol and disinfect eye

cup after each use. Do not use the same water for each eye; conjunctivitis is very contagious. *If the eye is swollen shut:* Put the hydrosol on a cotton pad and place it on eyelid; change every 10 minutes until swelling is reduced and eye can be opened. Usually takes less than an hour.

A sterilized eyedropper can be used to drip a few drops of hydrosol into the eye.

BLACK EYE

30 ml A.H. immortelle

Put 5 ml A.H. on a cotton pad and apply to site of impact; repeat every 5 minutes for 6 applications. Follow with:

5 ml A.H. immortelle
5 ml A.H. German chamomile or yarrow
5 ml Greenland moss

Soak a pad with the blend and place on eye. Wrap lightly with a dry cloth and leave in place while you lie down for at least 30 minutes. Replace the pad frequently.

Homeopathic remedy of *Ledum palustre* (a relative of Greenland moss) can be taken as well; this is particularly good if there is a puncture wound associated with the black eye.

Ear, Nose, and Throat

NOSEBLEED

10 ml A.H. rock rose

Put 5 ml rock rose on a cotton ball and hold on outside of nose near the bridge. Put 2.5 ml of rock rose on each of two cotton balls and place one in each nostril.

If nosebleed is a result of a blow to the face or head, use A.H. immortelle on bridge of nose and 1 drop immortelle E.O. on site of impact.

SINUS CONGESTION

60 ml A.H. winter savory, oregano, or balsam fir
2 to 5 drops E.O. *Eucalyptus globulus,* thyme
    CT thuyanol, ravensara, rosemary
    verbenone, or oils appropriate to the
    condition.

Put 30 ml A.H. into a clean, nonmetallic bowl, pour on 30 ml boiling water, add your essential oils, tent your head with a towel, and inhale the steam and vapors for 3 to 5 minutes. Keep your eyes closed, as the vapors are strong. Repeat as needed up to four times a day. You can also snuff a few drops of hydrolate into each nostril between inhalations.

Place remaining 30 ml A.H. into 1 liter of water and sip throughout the day.

Additionally:

5 drops E.O. *Eucalyptus radiata*
5 drops E.O. *Ravensara aromatica*

Combine oils and apply neat to front, back, and sides of chest and soles of feet between inhalations and at bedtime.

5 ml A.H. thyme CT linalol or purple bee balm
    (*Monarda fistulosa*)
5 ml A.H. German chamomile
1 teaspoon honey

At bedtime drink a tea with the two hydrosols and honey.

When the sinus congestion is completely solid, with no drainage and no effect from blowing the nose, use the following method: Take two small squares of construction paper or blotting paper and place 1 drop of E.O. rosemary CT verbenone, elecampane, or *Eucalyptus globulus* on each paper square, then roll them into small tubes and insert gently in each nostril while lying down. Try to inhale through the tubes (although you may not actually be able to breathe through your nose); keep the tubes in place for 10 to 15 minutes.

EARACHE

Never put A.H. or E.O. directly into the ear. Place on a cotton ball and insert the cotton ball into the ear. Depending on the nature of the earache, one of the best methods is to use 1 drop of oil on a cotton ball in the ear and compress of hydrosol around the outside of the ear, across the sinus, and on the neck.

1 drop E.O. spike lavender, *Eucalyptus radiata,*
    or thyme CT thuyanol

Put oil on a cotton ball, insert in ear, and change hourly for the first day, three times a day thereafter, until better. For children, use only *Eucalyptus radiata* or *Lavandula angustifolia.*

50 ml A.H. spike or true lavender, bay laurel,
    green myrtle, or a combination of the
    three
50 ml hand-hot water

Combine A.H. with water and use to dampen

compress. Compress around ear, down the neck, across the sinuses, and on all areas that are tender. Repeat at least five times the first day and three times a day for three days after.

Ear infections can be serious, and it is worth checking with a health-care practitioner if the problem persists for more than a few days. Ear candling or coning is an effective adjunct to home treatment and E.O. can be put into the candle as part of the treatment. Antibiotics are the standard allopathic treatment for earaches, especially in children, but they are rarely successful and should be a last resort.

SORE THROAT

15 ml A.H. cypress
15 ml A.H. ti tree
15 ml A.H. eucalyptus or green myrtle
15 ml A.H. Roman chamomile or lavender

Combine hydrosols. Use 10 ml diluted in 30 ml water as a gargle; repeat throughout the day. You may add $1/4$ teaspoon of sea salt to each gargle if you desire.

Schnaubelt recommends 1 drop of cypress oil to be taken orally and repeated whenever the soreness returns. Cypress tastes rather awful, and you may find washing down your drop of oil with the anti-inflammatory sweetness of A.H. Roman chamomile helps—both the throat and the flavor.

You may also compress the throat with the same blend as is used for gargling: Apply a cold compress and wrap throat lightly with a scarf or wool sock; the compress will heat up against the skin. Leave in place for 15 to 30 minutes.

TONSILLITIS

50 ml A.H. bay laurel
15 ml A.H. oregano or winter savory
15 ml thyme CT thymol or scarlet bee balm

Combine 20 ml of the bay laurel with the other two hydrosols. Use 10 ml of this mixture diluted in 30 ml water as a gargle; repeat throughout the day. You may also take $1/2$- to 1- teaspoon sips of this blend undiluted orally throughout the day. Dilute the remaining 30 ml A.H. bay laurel in 1 liter water and consume it throughout the day.

In addition, use the following rub:

5 ml E.O. palmarosa
5 ml E.O. bay laurel

Use 5 to 7 drops of this blend undiluted and rub outside of throat, on the underedge of the chin, and on area under ears and down the neck. Repeat after each gargle. If the skin is sensitive, dilute E.O. in equal amount of sesame oil or virgin coco-crème.

SWOLLEN LYMPH NODES

30 ml A.H. bay laurel

Dilute in 1 liter of water and sip throughout the day. Repeat daily for three weeks. Consume at least 1 liter of plain springwater each day in addition to your hydrosol water to help flush the system. If you see and feel absolutely no reduction in the swelling of the nodes within five to seven days, start applying 1 drop of E.O. bay laurel to the thoracic duct area under each collarbone three times a day. You may also consider a series of weekly aroma-massage treatments as a supportive measure. If the condition still does not improve after four to five days of the dual treatment, consult your health professional.

Regardless of where they appear in the body—armpit, throat, breasts—swollen lymph nodes are a sign that your body is overtaxed. Take some rest, boost your immune system, eat well, and think about what may be causing the problem. I have seen the bay treatment clear up all sorts of swollen lymph nodes in less than one month, even in clients slated for surgery, but it is always advisable to work with your health practitioners in tandem, and don't ignore what could be a warning sign of a bigger problem.

Respiratory Conditions

The best general-tonic hydrosols for the respiratory system are eucalyptus, elecampane, balsam fir, and the thymes and bee balms.

COLDS AND FLU

10 drops E.O. *Eucalyptus radiata*
10 drops E.O. sweet orange
7 drops E.O. palmarosa
3 drop E.O. cinnamon bark
2 drops E.O. thyme CT thuyanol or linalol
1 to 2 teaspoons emulsifier* (soy lecithin, Labrasol, or similar)
$^1/_2$ teaspoon honey (acacia or manuka is best)

50 ml A.H. balsam fir, green myrtle, eucalyptus, or black spruce
30 ml A.H. *Echinacea*

Put all ingredients in a 100 ml bottle, adding the oils and emulsifier first, then the honey, and finally the hydrosols, one at a time, and shaking after each addition. Depending on which emulsifier you use, you may need more or less than 2 teaspoons, and regardless, it will separate after 15 to 30 minutes or so. Shake before each use.

Use as a cough syrup and tonic for colds, coughs, and flu. Each of the hydrosols mentioned adds its own benefit; black spruce stimulates the immune system, as does balsam fir, which is also mucolytic, as is eucalyptus, which also works in synergy with the E.O.

*If you cannot get an emulsifier, make the blend without it and shake vigorously before use.

ALLERGIES

30 ml A.H elecampane

Dilute in 1.5 liters water and drink throughout the day every day for three weeks at the beginning of allergy season. Also use foot soaks every night before bed with 1 cup Epsom salts; 30 ml A.H. elecampane, *Eucalyptus globulus,* or rosemary CT verbenone; and 3 drops E.O. white spruce. There are many essential oils that can be of benefit to allergy sufferers, although white spruce works for most people. It is best to work with an aromatherapist to come up with the perfect blend for each individual.

BRONCHITIS

50 ml A.H. elecampane
OR
30 ml A.H. elecampane *and*
20 ml A.H. cinnamon bark

Dilute in 1.5 liters water and drink throughout the day. In addition, take 1 tablespoon of pure elecampane hydrosol three times a day during acute stage. The following rub should also be used:

5 ml E.O. palmarosa
2 ml E.O. rosemary CT verbenone
2 ml E.O. black spruce
1 ml E.O. hyssop variety *decumbens* (Do not substitute *Hyssopus officinalis,* which can be toxic. If you can't get *decumbens,* use *Eucalyptus dives* or *E. globulus* instead.)

Combine oils and apply 15 to 30 drops at a time, undiluted, spread over the front, back, and sides of chest, using the entire 10 ml in one 24-hour period. This is called living embalming.

You may also make a steam of the following ingredients:

30 ml boiling water
30 ml A.H. oregano or winter savory
5 to 7 drops each *Eucalyptus radiata* and lemon eucalyptus

Pour boiling water over hydrosol in a nonmetallic bowl, add oils, and tent head with a towel while inhaling vapors for 5 to 10 minutes. Keep eyes closed. Repeat three times a day during acute stage.

You may also use the cough syrup described under Colds and Flu (page 219). French aromatherapists from Valnet to Franchomme, Penoel, and Baudoux also recommend suppositories for acute respiratory conditions. It is the fastest and most effective method for getting powerful essential oils to the lungs. Many European companies sell ready-made suppositories for asthma, acute infections, and so on. Check the supplier list for sources.

SMOKER'S COUGH

10 ml A.H. Scotch pine
10 ml A.H. black spruce
10 ml A.H. green myrtle or peppermint

Combine hydrosols and add to 1.5 liters water; drink throughout the day. May also be taken by the teaspoon during a coughing fit. Smoke less or quit.

Digestive System

The best general-tonic hydrosols for the digestive system are basil, cinnamon, Greenland moss, fennel, anise, cardamom, coriander, and peppermint.

GINGIVITIS AND RECEDING GUMS

20 ml A.H. immortelle

Dilute 10 ml in 100 ml water and use as a morning mouth rinse after brushing and flossing teeth; repeat at night. Do not swallow the rinse, and use it all every time. Repeat daily for as long as required. Receding gums may take several months to respond, but immortelle will have a positive effect. If the gingivitis is severe, use immortelle combined with mastic *(Pistacia lentiscus)* hydrosol in a 70:30 dilution; add 10 to 30 ml water and rinse for 60 seconds each time, three times a day.

INDIGESTION

5 ml A.H. peppermint
200 ml water

Combine and sip slowly. Repeat if necessary.

GAS OR BLOATING

5 ml A.H. cinnamon bark or leaf
5 ml A.H. fennel or basil
200 ml water

Combine and sip slowly.

HALITOSIS

30 ml A.H. peppermint

Take ¼ teaspoon at a time several times per day to a maximum of 30 ml per day. Repeat daily for seven days. Consider the cause. This works even for pets!

CANKERS AND MOUTH ULCERS

50 ml A.H. thyme CT thymol or
    scarlet bee balm

Use 5 ml at a time and hold in mouth around canker or ulcer; spit out after 60 to 90 seconds. Repeat five or six times a day until healed.

LACK OF APPETITE

30 ml A.H. Clementine petitgrain

Dilute in 1.5 liters water and drink throughout the day. If done daily for three weeks, followed by one week off, this can help reestablish healthy eating habits. Has been extremely effective for AIDS and cancer patients at all stages of the illness and treatments. I have *never* been so famished as when I drank petitgrain; I could think of nothing but food, to the point of distraction.

EXCESS APPETITE

30 ml A.H. sage

Dilute in 1 liter water and drink throughout the day. If done daily for three weeks, followed by one week off, this can help reestablish a more balanced approach to food. Sage also helps the body deal with the effects of poor diet. AVOID if hypertensive.

VOMITING

5 ml A.H. cinnamon bark

Dilute in 200 ml water and give by the teaspoon. Vomiting causes dehydration, and the cinnamon helps the stomach accept fluids. It works better than stale Coke or ginger ale. If the body won't keep down the cinnamon-water combination at first, use ¼ teaspoon of the straight hydrosol every 15 minutes for four to six doses and then try again with the diluted version.

For vomiting caused by motion sickness, use peppermint instead of cinnamon.

DIARRHEA

15 ml A.H. oregano or cinnamon bark

Take the undiluted hydrosol every 15 minutes for four doses; repeat if necessary. If the diarrhea is stress related, try basil, chamomile, or melissa hydrosol.

LIVER CONGESTION

15 ml A.H. immortelle
7 ml A.H. Greenland moss
7 ml A.H. yarrow
1 drop E.O. lemon

Dilute in 1.5 liters of water and sip throughout the day. Repeat daily for three weeks, then reassess the condition. Useful after an illness, for a hangover, or when quitting an addiction (such as cigarettes or alcohol).

CONSTIPATION

15 ml A.H. coriander
15 ml A.H. yarrow

Dilute in 500 ml water and drink in half a day. If necessary, repeat and combine with the following:

15 drops E.O. basil
15 drops E.O. coriander or cumin

Combine and take 1 drop internally and apply 7 to 10 drops undiluted to abdomen in clockwise massage after each meal.

COLIC, COLITIS

30 ml A.H. basil or tarragon
1 teaspoon manuka or acacia honey (optional)

Dilute in 1 liter of water and sip throughout the day. An effective antispasmodic, this works best in the three-weeks-on, one-week-off cycle, but the condition must be monitored closely and dosage should be adapted to the individual concerned. Basil is not a cure but can be a helpful part of treatment for all these conditions.

Colic and colitis may be indications of more serious health conditions, and it is worth doing a test dose first. Dilute $1/2$ teaspoon hydrosol in 100 ml water and sip over a 2-hour period; you will know before the time is up if your condition will respond favorably. However, as coconut macaroons have been showing positive results for controlling diarrhea in some colitis sufferers, why not basil? Consult with your health professional for any home treatment and: If in doubt, don't.

Circulatory System

The best general-tonic hydrosols for the circulatory system are sage, artemesia, immortelle, rosemary, bay, and witch hazel, but this is very dependent on whether the application is topical or internal and whether you want to increase or decrease circulatory activity.

CELLULITE

30 ml A.H. juniper berry and/or cypress

Dilute in 1.5 liters water and drink throughout the day. Repeat daily for three weeks; take one week off and repeat.

Dry brushing of the legs should be done daily, ideally morning and evening, along with a scrub every other day using coarse sea salts (on wet skin) to which you add ¹/₂ teaspoon carrier oil and 2 or 3 drops of E.O. juniper berry, grapefruit, or cypress.

Topical

10 ml E.O. lemon eucalyptus
5 ml E.O. immortelle
5 ml E.O cypress
2 ml E.O. juniper berry
2 ml E.O. sage
1 ml E.O. peppermint

Dilute in 25 ml vegetable, sesame, or hazelnut oil or in 25 ml of an unscented gel or lotion; apply two or three times a day every day.

Use all the treatments simultaneously for best results.

CIRCULATION STIMULANT

30 ml A.H. sage

Dilute in 1.5 liters water and drink throughout the day. Repeat daily for three weeks; take one week off and repeat. Do not use sage hydrosol if hypertensive.

RAYNAUD'S PHENOMENON

Raynaud's phenomenon is caused by spasms in the arterioles, resulting in a severe loss of circulation in parts or the whole of the fingers and toes, which can become quite severe. It is aggravated by cold weather, smoking, and immune depletion. Use both treatments for best results.

30 ml A.H. sage

Dilute in 1.5 liters water and drink throughout the day. Repeat daily for three weeks; take one week off and repeat. Do not use sage hydrosol if hypertensive.

15 ml A.H. peppermint

Dilute in 250 ml lukewarm water and soak the affected parts for 10 to 15 minutes, twice daily, every day until condition starts to improve.

VARICOSE AND SPIDER VEINS

10 ml A.H. witch hazel

Soak a cotton pad in the hydrosol and compress the veins for 10 to 15 minutes three or four times a day every day. Be absolutely certain that you are using a preservative-free true hydrosol. The witch hazel for sale in drugstores contains from 1 to 30 percent alcohol by volume, and this will aggravate, *not* ameliorate, the condition. This is safe to use in pregnancy.

HEMORRHOIDS

Hemorrhoids are varicose veins of the rectum and can be internal or external.

30 ml A.H. yarrow
30 ml A.H. cypress
30 ml A.H. witch hazel
10 ml A.H. German chamomile

Combine hydrosols; add 50 ml of blend to a sitz bath (2 liters) of hot water and 50 ml to a sitz bath of cold water. Sit in the hot bath for 1 minute, then sit in the cold bath for 30 seconds. Alternate between the two baths, spending longer in each one with each repetition and increasing the temperature difference (making the hot bath hotter and the cold bath colder) each time. Repeat daily. The same hydrosol combination can be used in a spray bottle and misted onto the rectum or used as a wet wipe after every bowel movement to cleanse and soothe the tissue.

A raw peeled garlic clove with one drop of mastic oil can be used as a suppository for hemorrhoids and is very effective in combination with the sitz baths. Yoga and Kegel exercises will strengthen the pelvic muscles and may help resolve the problem.

CHILBLAINS

The minor frostbite of chilblains can be quite painful and damage the skin.

A.H. lavender
A.H. rosemary CT cineole or camphor

Spray hydrosols directly on affected area and wrap in a dry tea towel. Apply *very* gentle squeezing massage to the area to stimulate circulation and help relieve the pins-and-needles feeling. Repeat the hydrosol application every 5 minutes until condition stabilizes, then apply every 30 minutes for four or five applications to help heal the tissue damage.

The Skin

The best general-tonic hydrosols for the skin are rose, geranium, rock rose, neroli, yarrow, and the chamomiles—but really, nearly every hydrosol has an application in skin care, and there are so many skin conditions that it is impossible to make generalizations.

BROKEN CAPILLARIES

A.H. rock rose

Spritz onto affected area two or three times a day, every day. If the condition is very severe, compress the zone instead. Some people find rock rose too strong on its own and combine it with equal portions of cornflower, frankincense, or neroli.

ACNE

Use all three acne recipes concurrently for best results.

25 ml A.H. winter savory or thyme CT thymol
25 ml A.H. yarrow

Combine hydrosols in a nonmetallic bowl and pour in 100 ml of hot water. Tent head with a towel and steam face for 10 to 15 minutes. Immediately afterward spritz on hydrosol of neroli, chamomile, or St. John's wort and allow to air dry. Repeat two times a week.

A.H. yarrow, rosemary CT verbenone, and/or thyme CT linalol

Any or all of these hydrosols should be used as a twice-daily cleanser and toner for acneic skin. Soak a cotton pad and gently pat the skin after washing with your regular cleanser; allow to air dry.

30 ml A.H. yarrow or wild carrot seed
1 drop E.O. peppermint

Dilute in 1.5 liters water and drink throughout the day. Repeat daily for three weeks; take one week off and repeat. This alone will do wonders for the skin.

ECZEMA AND PSORIASIS

Eczema and psoriasis are two very different conditions, but both seem to benefit to varying degrees from the following treatments. In holistic health terms they are both considered symptoms of some other underlying condition, often related to the respiratory tract. In fact, some types of psoriasis have been directly linked to staph infections of the lungs. However, anything that can bring some relief to sufferers is worth trying. Use both "healing" recipes simultaneously for best tresults.

For Itching

A.H. yarrow

Spray generously or pour over the area as required. Quite dramatic relief.

For Healing

A.H. sandalwood or rosemary CT verbenone

Soak a cotton pad with the hydrosol and compress the area. This helps promote healing of the raw skin underneath so it is less painful when the top layers come off.

15 ml A.H. elecampane or eucalyptus
15 ml A.H. melissa

Dilute in 1.5 liters water and drink throughout the day. Repeat daily for three weeks; take one week off and repeat as required. Skin conditions and respiratory conditions are considered "brother and sister," and elecampane is one of the best respiratory-system waters. Melissa helps reduce stress, which can aggravate both eczema and psoriasis.

BURNS

E.O. lavender
A.H. lavender

Apply E.O. directly to the burn; soak cotton in hydrosol and compress on top. Repeat every 5 minutes according to severity of burn. The hydrosol adds a significant cooling effect and works synergistically with the famed properties of the oil. For very severe burns you can use German chamomile hydrosol with the lavender oil. Continue until healing is complete to minimize scar tissue.

BRUISES

E.O. immortelle
A.H. immortelle or peppermint

As in the burn treatment, apply one drop E.O. to the site of the bruise and compress with cotton soaked in the hydrosol. The combined synergy of the oil and the hydrosol compress is phenomenal, although the hydrosol works well on its own. If you do not have immortelle, peppermint is also effective but much less dramatically so.

CUTS AND WOUNDS

A.H. witch hazel

Apply to a cotton pad and place directly on the damaged tissue. Leave in place for 10 to 15 minutes, refreshing with a new cotton pad once or twice. A year ago a friend fell off a ladder and came into the house with four separate wounds, the skin cut and grazed raw and already visibly swelling. We applied a different substance to each wound: A.H. witch hazel, A.H. peppermint, A.H. immortelle, and E.O. peppermint. The witch hazel was the instant success, giving pain relief and reducing swelling on contact. Immortelle reduced the swelling and pain but was less effective on the wound. The peppermint hydrosol had a good initial effect, but it didn't last long and had to be reapplied frequently. The peppermint oil took some time to act but eventually provided pain relief deeper into the tissue than the hydrosol and worked best on the pain in the underlying bone. The next day the verdict was that witch hazel was the winner.

SCARS

A.H. immortelle

Spritz hydrosol onto scar and then apply the following essential-oil blend while still moist. This is also great for stretch marks, which may cover a larger area than normal scars, and seems to speed up the process with old scar tissue and keloids.

2.5 ml E.O. immortelle
2.5 ml V.O. rose hip seed
5 ml V.O. hazelnut

Combine and use only 1 drop, or the smallest amount that will cover the scar, four to six times a day, every day. Results are usually visible in the first week or two. Tiny amounts repeated frequently are part of the key to success with scar tissue.

RADIATION

A.H. niaouli (*Melaleuca quinquinervia CT viridiflorol*)

Computer users should keep this by their desk. Spritz directly onto face, arms, and chest at regular intervals throughout the day; you can spray it right onto your clothing. Take regular breaks away from your computer screen. Anyone undergoing radiation treatment for cancer can use this hydrosol on all areas except the actual site of the cancer; it will not interfere with the treatment and will dramatically reduce tissue damage in the areas treated. Patients are always told not to apply anything to the skin before radiation treatments because some substances will increase the likelihood of burning and tissue damage. Niaouli hydrosol, totally invisible and nongreasy, will help prevent the burning and damage.

Reproductive System

The best general-tonic hydrosols for the reproductive system are sage, clary sage, rose, and St. John's wort, but as in skin care, the applications are so many and varied that you must really look at what you need and what hydrosol will do the specific job best for you.

PMS

Women are affected by PMS in vastly different ways. Choose any three of the hydrosols listed and combine for your personal needs. The "synergy of three" hydrosols in combination works better than any single hydrosol, but use what you have in a pinch. Use both recipes together for best results.

A.H. clary sage (for mood and cramps)

A.H. rose (for mood and excess heat)

A.H. sage (for cramps and circulation/cold)

A.H. cypress (for water retention)

A.H. geranium (for balance)

A.H. St. John's wort (for mood and insomnia
and as a general tonic)

Take 10 ml of each of your three selected hydrosols (30 ml total), dilute in 1 liter of water, and drink throughout the day. If PMS is a regular phenomenon, start drinking your hydrosol blend three to five days before your period is due and continue until it is over. The same hydrosol blend may be used to compress the abdomen and lower back for pain relief.

¼ to ½ teaspoon V.O. evening primrose,
borage seed, or rose hip seed

1 drop E.O. niaouli

Combine and take internally daily to balance the essential fatty acids in the body.

Although chocolate and sugar will suppress your immune system and are said to aggravate PMS, I find the occasional chocolate truffle flavored with essential oils works wonders!

MENOPAUSE

10 ml A.H. peppermint

10 ml A.H. sage

10 ml A.H. rose

To balance your hormones and your mood, dilute in 1 liter of water and drink throughout the day. Repeat daily for three weeks, take one week off, and repeat as required. It tastes a bit strange, so you may wish to alter the ratio to your preference, but again, the "synergy of three" adds a certain plus to the effects.

HOT FLASHES

1 part A.H. peppermint

1 part A.H. clary sage or rose geranium

Combine hydrosols in a spray bottle and keep on hand. Spritz directly on face, wrists, and back of neck when hot flashes occur.

There are many recipes for topical and internal essential-oil blends for menopause, but the simplest is to use *Vitex agnus-castus*, the chaste tree leaf or berry, oil. One drop taken daily is showing quite promising results in reducing the effects of menopause. Unfortunately, I have yet to find a hydrosol of *Vitex*.

FIBROIDS

All three treatments are to be used in conjunction.

Topical

5 ml E.O. immortelle
5 ml E.O lemon eucalyptus
5 ml E.O. cypress
20 ml V.O. foraha *(Calophyllum inophyllum)*
65 ml V.O. sesame

Apply two times a day to lower abdominal region and sacrum; repeat daily for three weeks.

Douche

20 ml A.H. rock rose
20 mlA.H. immortelle

Dilute in 50 ml distilled water and douche every morning.

Pessary

2 ml E.O. lemon eucalyptus
4 ml E.O. immortelle
5 ml E.O. geranium
6 ml E.O. rock rose
8 ml E.O. cypress
100 gm cocoa butter

A pessary is a vaginal suppository. Blend the five essential oils. Melt the cocoa butter over very low heat until it is only three-fourths melted. Remove from heat and swirl pot to melt the rest. Leave to sit for a moment. Lay out three sheets of waxed paper. If you cradle the waxed paper in a paper-towel tube cut in half lengthwise, it's easier to form the roll. Now stir the oil blend into the cocoa butter, which should just be setting at the edges. Pour a third of the mixture slowly onto each sheet of the waxed paper and leave to harden. Store the wrapped pessaries in the freezer. Cut into one-inch pieces; you should get twenty-one pessaries from this amount of mixture, seven from each of the three rolls. Use one suppository every night for three weeks, then take a week off during menses.

I have seven clients who have "cured" their fibroids with this treatment. It takes anywhere from two to six cycles, depending on the individual, but it worked for all of them. A new medical treatment for fibroids involves injecting a chemical into the femoral artery, temporarily cutting off circulation to the uterus and the fibroids, which are then "passed" vaginally. The treatment requires hospitalization for twenty-four to thirty-six hours and is described as very painful. The aromatic treatment causes no pain and no excessive discharge, but I believe it works in a similar way owing to the pH and astringent, cicatrisant properties of the rock rose and the "dissolving" properties of some of the oils.

ENDOMETRIOSIS

Use both the douche and topical treatment together.

Douche

15 ml A.H. rock rose
15 ml A.H. rose
30 ml distilled water

Combine hydrosols and water and use as a douche every day between your periods.

Topical

1 part E.O. blend customized to client
1 part V.O. foraha *(Calophyllum inophyllum)*
1 part V.O. St. John's wort maceration

A large number of oils can benefit endometriosis sufferers, beginning with classics like sage, clary sage, geranium, lavender, and rose. However, everyone experiences different symptoms. One client used wintergreen, niaouli, lemon eucalyptus, marjoram, blue tansy, and sage to ease the intense spasms and cutting pains she had from ovulation to menses. She based her blend on one for pain in childbirth. It is important, whatever oil blend is used in conjunction with the hydrosol douche, that both treatments be done regularly so results can be monitored and attributed to the correct remedy.

Endometriosis is a painful and potentially serious medical condition that can affect women from menarche to menopause. Current medical treatments include surgery (sometimes repeated), hormone therapies, promoting early onset of menopause, pregnancy (when appropriate), and the use of heavy painkilling medications. If you wish to use this or any other natural protocol, talk to your health professional, keep notes on what you do and the effects or benefits you feel, and don't give up if it doesn't work the first month. Valerie Worwood commenced a trial on endometriosis and aromatherapy several years ago, but fewer than 30 percent of the participants kept up the protocol, and so the results are inconclusive. The more real-life data that can be compiled, the more likely that scientific investigation will be

instituted. This is one area where I would be very happy to see clinical trials take place.

THRUSH AND VAGINITIS

Use both treatments together.

Douche

15 ml A.H. rosemary CT verbenone
15 ml A.H. German chamomile
15 ml A.H. lavender
15 ml bay laurel
100 ml warm distilled water

Combine hydrosols and water and use as a douche two times a day. If the condition is severe, you may wish to douche with the hydrosols undiluted for the first two days, then add water for the remainder of the treatment. I have one client who used straight undiluted sandalwood hydrosol with great results, and you may wish to experiment with this.

Internal Treatment

1 teaspoon organic kefir or live yogurt
2 drops E.O. ti tree

Take a tampon (preferably of organic, unbleached cotton) and roll it in the yogurt–ti tree mix and insert. Replace the tampon every 2 to 3 hours for three to four days.

JOCK ITCH

A.H. German chamomile or witch hazel

Spritz all over the area and allow to air dry completely. Repeat two or three times a day as required.

Renal System

The best general-tonic hydrosols for the renal system are juniper berry, balsam fir, black spruce, peppermint, petitgrain, cypress, yarrow, sandalwood, and elder.

WATER RETENTION

30 ml A.H. juniper berry or cypress

Dilute hydrolate in 1 liter of water and drink daily; repeat for three weeks. You can alternate between the two hydrosols to relieve the monotony of just one flavor or combine the two in varying amounts to suit your taste. They are both very diuretic, and you will notice that for the first five to ten days you will be visiting the bathroom frequently. However, your body will come to a new balance, and the effect after three weeks is wonderful. This can be used on an as-needed basis thereafter or for occasional water retention as a result of hormone imbalance or lifestyle.

CYSTITIS

30 ml A.H. winter savory
15 ml A.H. sandalwood
15 ml A.H. balsam fir
1 drop E.O. lemon

Dilute in 1 liter water and drink throughout the day. Repeat daily for seven days, then stop. You may also take Aromatic Tincture of dandelion and cypress.

GOUT

Use both treatments concurrently for best results.

Internal Treatment

50 ml A.H. juniper berry or cypress or a
    combination
2 drops each E.O. lemon and grapefruit

Dilute in 1.5 liters water and drink daily for three weeks. Ideally you should drink 1 liter of plain water in addition to the flavored water to help flush the system.

Topical

2 ml E.O. juniper berry
2 ml E.O. immortelle
3 ml E.O. wintergreen (the real thing, not
    synthetic methyl salicylate)
3 ml E.O. basil or rosemary CT cineole
25 ml V.O. St. John's wort infused in olive oil

Apply very delicately to the affected parts as required for pain.

PROSTATE PROBLEMS

It is unbelievably difficult to get men to "test" things, or maybe it's just difficult because the suggestions are coming from a woman. Women seem to be the big experimenters when it comes to health. However, three male clients who were experiencing signs of normal age-related prostate inflammation all found their symptoms improved using this recipe. I would say it's experimental but worth trying.

15 ml A.H. Greenland moss
15 ml A.H. rosemary CT verbenone

Dilute in 1.5 liters water and drink throughout the day. Repeat daily for three weeks; take one week off and repeat as required. One of the men who had the most problems also took saw palmetto and pygeum in a capsule, and perhaps this is a "synergy of three" for this problem.

Nervous System

The best general-tonic hydrosols for the nervous system are melissa, neroli, both chamomiles, linden, and St. John's wort.

ANXIETY AND STRESS

10 ml A.H. melissa
10 ml A.H. sweet fern
10 ml A.H. Roman chamomile or linden

Combine the hydrolates and add to 1 liter of water or take undiluted ¼ teaspoon at a time, followed by a few sips of water. The sweet fern is an impressive system tonic and prevents the chamomile from causing sedation. Some people experience a laxative effect from melissa, but I believe this is because it relaxes us and allows the release of everything stress makes us hold.

CAFFEINE JITTERS OR EXAM NERVES

5 ml A.H. neroli

Add the neroli to a glass of water and sip slowly. The effect is usually palpable within two to three minutes. You can mist the neroli on your face at the same time, or instead, if the nerves are not too bad.

MENTAL CHATTER

5 ml A.H. angelica root

Add the angelica to a glass of water and sip slowly. This is extremely good for those who spend too much time thinking or in their head. It will ground you and slow down your mind at the same time.

DEPRESSION

1 5ml A.H. St. John's wort
15 ml A.H. *Echinacea*
5 ml A.H. rose

Combine the hydrosols in 1 liter of water and drink daily for three weeks. Although the jury is still out on whether St. John's wort hydrosol has the same intensity of effect as the macerated oil when used for depression, this combination seems to strengthen resolve, improve general well-being, and give a sense of calm and hope. The rose makes you feel valued. Not a bad start.

Muscular System

For most problems affecting muscles, tendons, ligaments, and joints, the essential oils are of more use than the hydrosols. However, compresses and baths both can be useful methods of hydrotherapy, and hydrosols are an obvious adjunct in all water treatments. As was stated earlier, many health conditions are the result of chronic long-term dehydration of the body, and drinking plenty of water should be a part of any protocol dealing with muscular or joint complaints.

Refer to the hydrosol monographs for more information, and always consider the synergistic effects you can achieve using the same plant in both essential oil and hydrolate form.

ARTHRITIS

Use both treatments together for best results.

A.H. goldenrod

Compress the affected area with either hot or cold hydrosol, depending on which provides the best relief.

Topical applications of essential oils in conjunction with the hydrosol are very beneficial for arthritis. I make a trademarked synergy-of-three called Moose Grease containing goldenrod, black spruce, and Scotch pine essential oils in an ointment base that is neither heating nor cooling, just very pain relieving and anti-inflammatory.

15 ml A.H. goldenrod
10 ml A.H. juniper berry
5 ml A.H. peppermint

Dilute in 1 liter water and drink throughout the day. Repeat daily for three weeks; then take one week off.

ACHES AND PAINS

30 ml A.H. black spruce
30 ml A.H. Scotch pine

Soak a cotton pad or cloth with the hydrosols and apply to the area. Cover with a piece of plastic wrap and then wrap or cover with a wool cloth and bandage it in place; leave on for 30 minutes. Body heat will warm up the compress, and the heat will be held in by the plastic and wool.

LOTIONS AND POTIONS

Unless otherwise noted, all these preparations should be used at once or stored in the fridge and used within the advised time, usually less than three weeks if there is no alcohol added. Many of the recipes make only enough for one treatment.

DEODORANT #1

This recipe, from *Forum Essenzia* (1999), the German aromatherapy magazine, is by Dorothea Hamm. It is appropriate for both men and women.

2 drops E.O. bergamot
2 to 3 drops E.O. grapefruit
2 drops E.O. green myrtle
2 to 3 drops E.O. vetiver (Vetiveria zizanioides) or sandalwood
2 drops "essence" of iris
80 ml A.H. rock rose
20 ml ethyl alcohol (optional emulsifier/ preservative)

Combine all ingredients in a spray bottle and shake well before use. Both vetiver and sandalwood inhibit the growth of odor-forming bacteria. Many people do not like to use alcohol on the skin, and if you choose to leave it out, you may wish to add a few drops of an emulsifier or soya lecithin to help disperse the oils in the hydrosol.

DEODORANT #2

If you prefer a powder deodorant to a wet or spray deodorant, try this version.

200 gm baking soda
50 gm rice powder
50 gm corn starch
8 drops E.O. petitgrain
5 drops E.O. vetiver
3 drops E.O. palmarosa

Put half the baking soda in a mortar and pestle or a glass bowl. Add the essential oils drop by drop, mixing them in well and making sure you crush any beads that form. Put the oil-and-soda mixture in a large jar and add the remaining baking soda and other powders and shake well. Store in a dark-colored jar with a tight-fitting lid. Apply with a sea sponge or powder puff.

My aesthetician and colleague, Simone Zrihen of Aroma-Terrapeutics, makes amazing beauty products. A major fan of hydrosols in skin care, she has formulated a complete body-care system that will keep you glowing from head to toe. All the recipes should be customized to your individual needs, and she suggests using only organic essential oils and organic, preservative-free hydrosols—naturally.

HAIR PACKS

Base

3 ounces white clay
1 ounce sage powder
1 ounce Rhassoul clay (volcanic ash from Morocco)
20 drops each of neem oil, nettle tincture, and horsetail extract

Mix together, then add ingredients listed below for your personal hair color and type.

Dark Hair

4 tablespoons base
2 drops E.O. thyme linalol
2 drops E.O. bergamot
1 drop E.O. palmarosa in 2 tablespoons extra-virgin olive oil

Combine essential oils and base. Add Dark Hair Rinse (page 234) 1 tablespoon at a time to create paste. Use a soft brush to apply to scalp and hair. Leave on for a minimum of two hours or overnight (cover hair with plastic wrap and towel). Use Dark Hair Rinse for the final rinse.

Light Hair

4 tablespoons base
2 drops E.O. German chamomile
2 drops E.O. lemon
1 drop E.O. ylang ylang in 2 tablespoons sunflower oil

Combine essential oils and base. Add Light Hair Rinse (page 234) 1 tablespoon at a time to make paste. Use a soft brush to apply to scalp and hair. Leave on for a minimum of two hours or overnight (cover hair with plastic wrap and towel). Use Light Hair Rinse for the final rinse.

Problem Scalp

4 tablespoons base
2 drops E.O. wintergreen
2 drops E.O. lavender
1 drop E.O. rosemary cineole in 2 tablespoons
rice bran oil

Combine essential oils and base. Add Problem Scalp Rinse 1 tablespoon at a time to create paste. Use a soft brush to apply to scalp and hair. Leave on for a minimum of two hours or overnight (cover hair with plastic wrap and towel). Use Problem Scalp Rinse for the final rinse. (If you cannot obtain real wintergreen essential oil, use goldenrod instead.)

RINSES

Prepare only as much rinse as you'll need for one use—more for longer hair and less for shorter hair.

Dark Hair

40% A.H. rosemary verbenone
25% A.H. sage
25% A.H. lavender
10% apple cider vinegar

Light Hair

40% A.H. German chamomile
25% A.H. nettle or nettle tea
25% A.H. cedarwood
10% apple cider vinegar

Problem Scalp

40% A.H. frankincense
25% A.H. neroli
25% A.H. orange mint
10% apple cider vinegar

EYE COMPRESSES

Excellent for computer strained eyes, redness, irritation, and crow's feet. Soothes and gives new sparkle to eyes. Soak two round cotton pads with the hydrosol and leave on eyes for 10 to 15 minutes while you lie down with your feet up. Use any of the following hydrosols—fennel seed, German chamomile, Roman chamomile, rose, cornflower, clary sage, or elder flower.

FACE PACKS

The basics are easy; it's the specifics that are complex. That's what makes a really great aesthetician worth her weight in gold. Every face will need different treatment, from area to area and from week to week. The T-zone is frequently oily, but the rest of the face may be sensitive and dry. Winter may cause broken capillaries, while summer sun can cause freckles or wrinkles. Get to know your skin and give it what it needs when it needs it, just like the rest of your body. Aromatherapy offers so much scope for custom treatments that you can certainly come up with some fabulous combinations that will keep you looking "gorgeous, dahling" all year-round.

These face packs remove the dead cells on the topmost layer of the skin and stimulate circulation. Add the essential oils and other oils to the base, then blend in the hydrosol 1 tablespoon at a time to create a smooth paste. Massage the pack gently into the skin with a circular motion and leave on for 10 to 15 minutes. Rinse with lukewarm water and spritz with hydrosol.

Base

1½ ounces wholemeal organic soy flour
½ ounce sweet almond flour
½ ounce orris root powder
½ ounce powdered oats or oat flour

Combine the base ingredients in a glass container and mix well. You may add up to 1 ounce of clay to the face-pack base, selecting the type appropriate for your skin, or add 1 teaspoon to the amount used in an individual recipe if you do not wish to use clay every time you use the packs. Some people find clays too drying for their skin with regular use, but a once-a-month treatment provides extra-deep cleansing when necessary.

Clay Types and Their Actions

Blue: Healing and cell regenerating, antiphlogistic. For acneic and sensitive skin.
Green: Controls sebum production. For oily skin.
White: Detoxifies and balances. For delicate skin.
Red: Cleansing and toning. For all skin types except very dry.

Dry Skin

4 tablespoons base
1 teaspoon castor oil
4 teaspoon avocado oil
1 teaspoon helio-carrot oil
1 500-mg evening primrose oil capsule

2 drops E.O. rosewood
2 drops E.O. clary sage
1 drop E.O. patchouli
A.H. linden blossom

Oily Skin

4 tablespoons base
1 teaspoon castor oil
4 teaspoons St. John's wort-infused oil
1 teaspoon wheatgerm oil
1 500-mg capsule borage oil
2 drops E.O. sweet orange
2 drops jasmin sambac absolute
1 drop E.O. benzoin
A.H. neroli

Mature Skin

4 tablespoons base
1 teaspoon castor oil
4 teaspoons hazelnut oil
1 teaspoon wheatgerm oil
2 drops E.O. palmarosa
2 drops E.O. rose geranium
1 drop rose otto
A.H. rose

Acneic Skin

4 tablespoons base
1 teaspoon castor oil
3 tablespoons jojoba oil
1 teaspoon vitamin E oil
2 drops E.O. bergamot
2 drops E.O. grapefruit
1 drop E.O. sandalwood
A. H. lemon verbena

BREAST MISTS

Combine all ingredients for your formula in a spray bottle. Keep mists refrigerated. Do not use mists or massage oil if breast-feeding or pregnant; only Roman chamomile hydrosol should be used on the breasts when breast-feeding.

For the Active Woman

50% A.H. peppermint
25% A.H. sweet gale
25% A.H. orange mint

Daily Use and Mature Skin

50% A.H. rose geranium
25% A.H. rose
25% A.H. frankincense

Daily Use for All Ages

50% A.H. lavender
25% A.H. fennel seed
25% A.H. sandalwood

During PMS and Menopause

50% A.H. sage
25% A.H. cypress
25% A.H. angelica root

Uplifting and Toning

50% A.H. black spruce
30% A.H. peppermint
20% A.H. frankincense

BREAST MASSAGE OIL

90 ml apricot kernel oil
10 ml olive oil or helio-carrot oil

2 drops E.O. rose geranium
2 drops E.O. frankincense
1 drop E.O. clary sage
1 drop E.O. lemongrass

Blend all ingredients in an opaque glass bottle. Put a little massage oil on both hands and, using both hands at the same time, very gently rub each breast with circular movements, moving outward toward the underarms. Your left hand should be moving clockwise around the breast and your right hand counterclockwise. Do this gently after your bath or shower. Then mist with your choice of breast mists.

Benefits: Brings superb tone to breast tissue, stimulates lymphatic circulation, and promotes healthy well-being for the whole body!

LEG AND FOOT MISTS

Sports

50% A.H. ti tree
25% A.H. sage
25% A.H. cypress

Achy or Heavy

50% A.H. rosemary
25% A.H. witch hazel
25% A.H. fennel seed

Rejuvenation

50% A.H. thyme linalol
25% A.H. lavender
25% A.H. sweet fern

Sweaty

50% A.H. elder flower
25% A.H. peppermint
25% A.H. clary sage

FOOT POWDER

4 ounces white clay
4 tablespoons corn starch
2 tablespoons boric acid
1 tablespoon rice flour
1 tablespoon orris root powder
10 drops E.O. peppermint
5 drops E.O. ti tree
5 drops E.O. lavandin abrialis or grosso
5 drops E.O. lemon

Mix dry ingredients, then add essential oils. Use a mortar and pestle or fork to make sure the essential oils are thoroughly mixed into the powders.

Store in a glass jar or glass shaker. With small dusting puff or cotton balls massage into the feet, or dust socks and shoes with it. Use one of the leg mists and let dry before dusting with the powder for maximum results. The powder will keep well at room temperature.

BODY MISTS

Calming

50% A.H. rose
25% A.H. coriander seed
25% A.H. lavender

Cleansing

50% A.H. juniper berry
25% A.H. wild Canadian ginger
25% A.H. basil

Refreshing

50% A.H. *eucalyptus globulus*
25% A.H. orange mint
25% A.H. balsam fir

Romantic

50% A.H. neroli
25% A.H. rose
25% A.H. vetivert

SIMPLE FACE SCRUB

1 tablespoon pin oatmeal
1 tablespoon (approximate) A.H. to suit your skin type
1/8 teaspoon V.O. avocado, apricot kernel, or hazelnut

Put oatmeal and oil in a small bowl. Add hydrolate drop by drop until a paste forms. Apply to face with a gentle circular motion, avoiding eye area. Rinse thoroughly with warm water and follow with a spritz of cold hydrosol.

SIMPLE BODY SCRUB

You will want to stand in the tub while you do this, as the salt gets everywhere.

1/2 cup coarse gray sea salt (sometimes called Celtic sea salt)
1/2 cup cornmeal

2 teaspoons sesame oil

2 to 3 tablespoons A.H. rosemary, lavender, elder flower, or melissa

Combine salt, cornmeal, and oil; add hydrosol blend and allow to rest for 10 minutes. Wet your skin, either with water or hydrosol, and apply scrub using circular motion starting with the right foot up to the hip, then the left foot to hip, arms up to shoulders, and torso from neck down to hips. Rinse with cool to cold water, the colder the better. You may wish to tie the salt scrub into a cheesecloth if you find it too hard to work with it loose.

CUCUMBER TONER

1 large English cucumber

250 ml A.H. witch hazel, rose geranium, elder flower, linden, or lavender

Scrub the cucumber to remove any wax on the skin and run it through a juicer. Combine cucumber juice with hydrolate and store in the fridge. Apply using a cotton ball with gentle dabbing motions; use within one week. If you do not mind alcohol on your skin, you can add 30 ml vodka or grain alcohol to the blend, which will double the shelf life.

SIMPLE WITCH HAZEL TONER

100 ml A.H. witch hazel

2 teaspoons dried, or a large handful of fresh, sage, finely chopped

Pour hydrosol over herbs and allow to infuse in a warm place for 2 to 3 hours. Strain into a ster-

ilized bottle. This is exceptionally good when your skin is exposed to sun or wind.

YARROW TONER

100 ml A.H. yarrow

100 ml A.H. rose or neroli

25 ml A.H. witch hazel

25 ml vegetable glycerin

3 drops E.O. clary sage or yarrow

Combine all ingredients in a sterilized bottle and shake well. This is great for damaged or sensitive skin and for balancing the complexion; use clary oil and neroli water for oily skin or the T-zone.

CITRUS SPLASH

In Turkey you are often offered a splash of lemon cologne to wash and refresh your hands and face before a meal in a restaurant. It is a lovely custom, and one restaurateur showed me how they made their own by macerating fresh lemons in grain alcohol—simple! This is my version.

2 whole organic lemons

2 whole organic limes

500 ml vodka or 40 proof alcohol

10 drops organic E.O. lemon

10 drops organic E.O. lime

500 ml A.H. neroli

Chop fruit coarsely and place in a widemouthed jar, pour the vodka over the fruit, and leave to macerate for five to seven days, shaking the jar frequently. Strain the mixture, squeezing the fruit to extract all the liquid, then pour through a paper coffee filter. Add the essential oils and shake vigorously; add the hydrosol, shake again, and store in a sterilized bottle. May be used as a body splash or cologne or to "wash" hands or face and is just divine in hot, humid weather. Offer it to your guests before dinner and make them feel really special.

EXFOLIATING FOOT SCRUB

In England a slang name for feet is dogs, which tells you how little attention some people give to these all-important parts. Love your feet and treat them kindly; they will reward you, and you may notice your circulation improve as well.

1/4 cup cornmeal, ground adzuki beans, or ground lentils
2 teaspoons castor oil
1 to 2 tablespoons each A.H. peppermint and sage

Put the meal, beans, or lentils and the castor oil in a small bowl; add the hydrosol drop by drop until a thick paste is reached. Don't make it too wet. Let stand 10 minutes to swell, and add a little more hydrolate if it is too dry. Soak feet in warm water, then massage the paste in, paying particular attention to the heels and calluses. Wrap your paste-covered feet in plastic bags and lie down with legs elevated for 15 minutes, then rinse off in cool to cold water. Both sage and peppermint have odor-reducing properties and improve circulation while softening skin; castor oil works better than anything on calluses.

SIMPLE SCRUB SOAP

This is an easy cheat that is fun to make and use, good for the "dogs" and hard-working hands.

2 bars (125 gm each) good-quality pure-olive-oil soap*
50 ml A.H. lavender, rose, geranium, chamomile, or whatever is appropriate
1 small loofah sponge

Grate the soap on the fine side of a grater, the side you use for Parmesan cheese or chocolate. The finer you grate it, the better your finished soap will be. Place in a heavy-bottom saucepan, add the hydrosol, and heat over a low flame. Meanwhile, use a serrated knife to slice the loofah crosswise into one-half-inch-thick pieces. The loofah must be dry or you won't be able to cut it. Line an eight-inch-square baking dish with plastic wrap so that it hangs over at both ends and cover with the loofah slices, fitting them in as snugly as possible. Stir the soap mixture until all the soap is melted; you may add essential oils at this point if desired. Pour the liquid soap over the loofah slices and cover the dish with a heavy board to keep it clean while it sets, which may take a day or more. Turn out onto a board and cut into pieces so that each soap contains one slice of loofah.

*You can substitute the same amount of a glycerin soap for the olive-oil soap; this gives the finished product more intrigue, as the transparency of the soap allows you to see the formation of the loofah inside. Olive-oil soap is opaque, and you lose the visual effect but not the benefit.

IN THE KITCHEN

Some of the recipes in this section have been reprinted, with permission, from the two books by Maria M. Kettenring, *Aromakuche*. If you can read German, order them today; they are the best aromatherapy cookbooks in the world. For now you may find the first one, published in 1994 by Joy Verlag, of more use, as it comes packaged with a beautiful wall chart, "The ABC of Aromakuche," listing herbs by their Latin names (fortunately these are universally understood) and suggesting appropriate types of recipes where the essential oils *and* hydrolates can be used. For instance, lemongrass *(Cymbopogon citratus)*, both essential oil and hydrosol, is good in soups, appetizers and sorbets, salads, vegetables (particularly steamed), tofu, dips and condiments, Asian recipes such as stir-frys and curries, fish dishes, desserts, and beverages.

Hydrosols in the kitchen are a boon for the vegan, vegetarian, and meat eater alike; all you need is a love of food to enjoy their benefits. I no longer have the time to make stocks to keep on hand; I use hydrosols instead—in everything from sauces, soups, and gravies to main courses and desserts. I am providing only a limited number of recipes, as ideas; Maria's books are more complete than anything I can attempt. However, if nothing else, I hope you will get the idea that aromatherapy is as at home in the kitchen as it is in the clinic, and good nutrition is, after all, part of our well-being.

Soups

BASIC STOCK

Use 100 ml of hydrosol for every 2 liters of water when making stock. This assumes that you will be cooking your ingredients for one hour or more, whether your dish is vegetable or meat based. With fish stocks, which are usually cooked for only 15 to 20 minutes, add 2 to 3 tablespoons of hydrosol per 2 liters of water in the pot.

Soups being made without a "stock" as a base will be greatly improved by the addition of 1 to 2 tablespoons of hydrosol per liter of soup. The classic kitchen herbs, thyme, rosemary, sage, marjoram, oregano, bay, dill, and basil, all produce hydrosols that will give your soup the same depth of flavor that a stock would normally supply. Others, such as melissa, clary sage, coriander, and cardamom, are also worth trying. As a vegetarian for twelve years, I was always frustrated that no amount of miso or vegetables could give my soups the complexity of flavor I like. Now, even though I eat organic meat, I tend to use hydrosols more often than stock or broth.

MUSHROOM SOUP

500 gm mushrooms
2 tablespoons butter
2 tablespoons olive oil
1 large onion, finely chopped
1 or 2 garlic cloves, crushed
sea salt
freshly ground black pepper or 2 drops E.O.
    black pepper

750 ml water
1 tablespoon A.H. bay leaf
1 tablespoon A.H. thyme CT thymol

Rinse mushrooms and chop coarsely. If you are using exotic varieties like shiitake, remove stems and soak separately in a small bowl with the hydrosols. Melt butter and oil in a large pot; add onion and garlic, a pinch of sea salt, and a few grinds of fresh pepper; cover pot and allow to steam and sauté for 5 to 7 minutes over medium heat. Remove lid and stir until onion is translucent and soft but not brown. Try to prevent all the fluid that has accumulated in the pot from evaporating, as it adds flavor. Throw in the mushrooms, reduce the heat to low, and stir. All the liquid will be absorbed at first, but as you cook them the mushrooms will give it back; you can add more butter or oil if you need it. After 3 to 5 minutes, add the water and hydrosols and cover the pot. If you have soaked the mushroom stems in the hydrosols, remove them and strain the hydrosol for sand before adding to the pot. Turn the heat back up to medium for 10 minutes, stirring occasionally. Test for flavor and adjust seasoning to taste. I partially puree this soup with a hand blender and serve it with a dollop of yogurt and lots of fresh parsley.

COLD NECTARINE-MELON SOUP

1 ripe galia or honeydew melon
4 ripe nectarines
2 teaspoons A.H. peppermint
2 drops E.O. green pepper
1 tablespoon acacia honey

Peel and deseed the melon; wash and pit the nectarines and cut into pieces. Puree the melon and nectarines with the peppermint hydrosol in a food processor until smooth. Add the green pepper oil and sweeten with honey to taste. Chill for at least 20 minutes. Serve in chilled glass bowls garnished with fresh mint leaves. (From *Aromakuche*.)

"CREAM" OF CARROT SOUP

5 cups water or stock
1½ teaspoons sea salt
4 medium carrots, peeled and coarsely chopped
1 small parsnip, peeled and coarsely chopped
1 large Spanish onion, peeled and coarsely chopped
3 teaspoons fresh ginger juice or 1 tablespoon A.H. wild ginger
1 tablespoon A.H. cinnamon
4 drops E.O. black pepper

Bring water or stock to boiling; add salt and chopped vegetables; reduce heat and simmer uncovered for 20 minutes. Allow to cool, then puree. Add ginger juice or hydrosol, cinnamon hydrosol, and pepper oil and check seasonings. Serve garnished with fresh chopped parsley or cilantro. (From Miriam Erlichman.)

MISO-GINGER SOUP

1 Spanish onion, diced

1 tablespoon toasted sesame oil

6 cups water

1 stick kombu seaweed, washed

2 stalks celery, including leaves, thinly sliced

2 medium carrots, thinly sliced

6 garlic cloves, minced or pressed

2 tablespoons grated fresh ginger

1 teaspoon Dijon mustard

2 heaped tablespoons barley or rice miso

2 tablespoons A.H. wild ginger

2 tablespoons organic tamari

2 tablespoons lemon juice

1 tablespoon umeboshi plum vinegar

1 teaspoon brown rice vinegar

1 teaspoon sea salt

1 bunch spring onions, chopped (for garnish)

Sauté Spanish onion in sesame oil until translucent and a little browned. Add one cup of the water and the kombu and simmer for 5 minutes. Add rest of the water, the cut-up vegetables, and the fresh ginger and simmer for 30 minutes. Add remaining ingredients, except spring onion, and stir over low heat until miso is dissolved; the miso must not boil. Remove kombu, garnish with spring onions, and serve. (From Miriam Erlichman.)

Vegetables

Steaming vegetables preserves their vitamins but makes them more difficult to flavor. If you steam them, try adding 1 to 2 tablespoons of hydrosol to the steaming water or sprinkle 1 tablespoon over the cooked vegetables as soon as you take them from the pot.

"ORANGE" CARROTS

500 gm carrots (organic)

4 tablespoons water

2 teaspoons butter

2 drops E.O. sweet orange

$1/2$ tablespoon A.H. Clementine petitgrain

sea salt

Organic carrots can be just scrubbed and not peeled, then cut into batons 1 inch long and $1/4$ inch square. Put all the ingredients except the salt into a heavy-bottomed pot with a lid, add a pinch of salt, cover and cook over low heat for 5 to 10 minutes. Check periodically to make sure all the water does not evaporate and to test for doneness. There should be almost no liquid left in the pot by the time the carrots are cooked. Serve with parsley sprigs or chopped chervil.

MINTED PEAS

1 cup frozen peas

2 to 3 tablespoons water

1 teaspoon A.H. peppermint

sea salt

2 teaspoons butter

Put peas, water, hydrosol, and a pinch of salt in a pot, cover, and cook over low heat for 3 to 5 minutes. Check for doneness—the time will vary depending on whether the peas are petit pois or large; do not let the peas cook dry. Drain any water left over and add the butter.

This recipe is great with lamb. Frozen peas are a fact of life for many people, and this will make them taste really fresh.

AFGHANISTAN CREAMED SPINACH

1 kg fresh spinach
1 large onion, peeled and finely chopped
5 teaspoons organic sesame oil (not toasted)
sea salt
$1/2$ cup water
1 tablespoon A.H. cardamom
5 drops E.O. cardamom
5 drops E.O. cumin
2 egg yolks, beaten
100 ml heavy cream or crème fraîche

Wash and clean spinach, place in a pot while still wet, cover, and cook over medium heat until just wilted. Drain. Brown the onion in the sesame oil with a pinch of sea salt. Mix the water with the remaining ingredients and cook over gentle heat until thickened, stir in spinach and onion, and serve with plain boiled rice. (From *Aromakuche.*)

Salads

POTATO SALAD

1 kg new or any waxy, firm-textured potato
    (try Pink Fir Apple potatoes)
sea salt
1 tablespoon A.H. sage, bay laurel, or thyme

1 tablespoon olive oil
Freshly ground pepper or E.O. black pepper
spring onions or shallots
mayonnaise
yogurt (optional)

New potatoes should be scrubbed but the skins left on, as they contain valuable vitamins. Cut potatoes into cubes and place in a large pot with sea salt and plenty of water. Cook until just done; do not overcook, as the latent heat will continue the process after they are drained. Drain off water and immediately sprinkle the hot potatoes with the hydrosol. Place potatoes in a large bowl and stir in the olive oil and pepper; leave to cool completely. Meanwhile, finely chop the spring onions and add to bowl with enough mayonnaise or mayonnaise and yogurt to achieve a creamy texture, but do not stir so much that you break up the potato cubes. Freshly chopped chives will add color and taste, if you have them.

Choose your potatoes wisely, as many are genetically engineered.

TABBOULEH

$1/2$ cup bulgur wheat
2 teaspoons A.H. peppermint
1 teaspoon A.H. melissa or lemon verbena
sea salt
1 large bunch parsley (1$1/2$ cups chopped)
3 medium tomatoes, finely chopped
1 small onion or 3 spring onions, finely
    chopped
olive oil
fresh lemon juice or E.O. lemon

Put the bulgur in a large bowl, add the hydrosols and a pinch of sea salt, and cover completely with water. Leave to soak for 1 to 2 hours. Drain well and fluff with a fork. Mix chopped parsley, tomato, and onion into bulgur. Add olive oil to taste and plenty of fresh lemon juice. If using lemon essential oil, taste after each drop is added; it's easy to add too much.

SALAD DRESSING

You can add hydrosols to any dressing recipe or store-bought brand. Add no more than $1/2$ teaspoon at a time and taste after each addition.

Basic Vinaigrette

1 tablespoon red-wine or cider vinegar
$1/2$ teaspoon A.H. of your choice (bay laurel, thyme, tarragon, dill, wild ginger are good options)
$1/2$ teaspoon Dijon mustard
4 to 6 tablespoons extra-virgin olive oil, the finer the better
sea salt and freshly ground black pepper
pinch of sugar
1 garlic clove, peeled

Place all ingredients except garlic in a bottle, put the lid on, and shake like crazy or use a blender. Taste and adjust flavors. Put the peeled garlic clove in the bottle and refrigerate for several hours. You may then remove the garlic if you wish.

Main Dishes

Essential oils and hydrosols are delicious added to meat recipes, either during cooking or in the gravy or sauce.

ROAST CHICKEN

1 whole organic chicken
2 organic carrots, scrubbed and chopped
1 small onion, unpeeled and chopped
1 leek, washed, trimmed, and chopped
A.H. marjoram or thyme CT linalol
A.H. sage
1 lemon, halved, juice squeezed and saved
sea salt
freshly ground pepper or E.O. black pepper
2 garlic cloves, crushed
butter

Wash and dry the chicken inside and out. Place carrots, onion, and leek in the bottom of your roasting pan and pour 2 tablespoons of each hydrosol over them. Pour lemon juice over chicken, covering all the surfaces, and place lemon pieces inside the bird. Rub salt, pepper, and the garlic into the skin and place breast side up on top of vegetables in the pan. Dot surface with butter and place in 350°F oven. After 20 minutes baste chicken with pan juices or extra hydrosol; repeat every 20 minutes and cook until leg juices run clear (approximately 25 minutes per pound at 350°F). When chicken is cooked, remove pan from oven, place on a heated serving platter, and tent lightly with foil, but allow room for steam to escape so the skin stays crisp.

To make gravy, pour off all but 1 tablespoon of fat from the pan, sprinkle in 1 tablespoon wholewheat or spelt flour, and cook, scraping up the brown bits and vegetables. Add 1 glass red wine, 1 tablespoon of each hydrosol, and approximately 250 ml water or stock, stirring continuously over medium heat until desired consistency is reached. Strain gravy into a heated jug and serve with the chicken.

MOCK VENISON MEATBALLS

500 gm extra-lean ground organic beef or
    buffalo meat
1 garlic clove, minced
1 egg
1 tablespoon wheat germ
3 drops E.O bay laurel
3 drops E.O juniper
1 drop E.O. rosemary CT cineole
sea salt
freshly ground pepper or E.O. black pepper
sesame or sunflower oil, organic
1 large red onion, cut in half and then into
    thick slices
2 tablespoons A.H. juniper berry
1 tablespoon A.H. bay laurel
3 tablespoons A.H. wild ginger
3 tablespoons dry red wine

Combine the meat, garlic, egg, wheat germ, and essential oils, adding just a pinch of salt but a generous amount of pepper. Form into small meatballs no larger than a walnut. Heat a heavy-bottomed skillet over medium-high heat and add 1 tablespoon organic sesame or sunflower oil.

Fry the meatballs in small batches, shaking the pan to keep them round. Add oil as necessary between batches. When all the meatballs are cooked, pour off any extra oil and add 1 tablespoon fresh oil and the onion; cover with a lid and allow the onion to steam and sauté for 5 minutes. Remove lid and stir, scraping up any brown bits on the bottom of the pan; cook until onions are translucent. Add the hydrosols and the dry red wine, making sure the bottom of the pan is scraped clean. Bring to a boil and cook for 5 minutes, or until reduced by half. Add meatballs and immediately reduce heat to low; simmer for 15 minutes, covered. Serve over fat egg noodles and garnish with a spoon of sour cream and plenty of finely chopped fresh parsley.

This is my favorite meal when it's twenty below zero outside. By changing the hydrosols and essential oils and using virgin coco-crème as your oil, you can turn this into an equally delicious Asian or curry dish.

STEAMED SALMON

$^1/_2$ cup A.H. blend (melissa, dill or tarragon or
    both, and petitgrain)
$^1/_2$ cup water
1 salmon fillet (4 to 6 ounces), preferably wild,
    per person
sea salt
freshly ground pepper
1 drop E.O. lemon per fillet
1 spring onion per person, trimmed and cut in
    half lengthwise

Put hydrosol blend and water in a pot large enough to hold your steamer rack; you may need more or less hydrosol depending on the size of your pot. Wash and dry fish and sprinkle both sides with salt and pepper and the drop of lemon oil. Place the spring onion with its cut side up in the rack and the salmon with its skin side down on top of the onion. Arrange all the fish in the steamer, being sure to leave enough room for steam to circulate around the fish. You may need two pots if you are cooking for more than three or four people. Cover pot with aluminium foil and a lid and place over high heat. Begin timing as soon as you hear the water come to boiling, allowing 10 minutes per 1 inch of thickness of the fish (therefore a half-inch-thick fillet requires just 5 minutes).

Remove pan from heat when time is up and carefully remove the lid and foil; be careful, as the steam escaping is *very* hot and can burn. Check for doneness and serve with butter, a wedge of fresh lemon, and finely chopped chervil or flat-leaf parsley.

Vegetarian Main Dishes

MEDITERRANEAN ROAST

2 small zucchini

sea salt

4 large peppers (2 yellow, 2 red), cut in half lengthwise, deseeded but stems left on

1 medium red onion, cut into eighths so the sections are still attached at the stem end

14 sun-dried tomatoes in olive oil

16 large black olives (kalamata are best), pitted and coarsely chopped

16 large pimento-stuffed green olives, coarsely chopped

8 medium garlic cloves, peeled and coarsely chopped

6 large Roma tomatoes, finely chopped or 28-ounce can cooking tomatoes, drained and chopped

1 tablespoon each A.H. thyme, bay laurel, and oregano

freshly ground pepper

2 tablespoons extra-virgin olive oil flavored with 2 drops E.O basil

Cut zucchini in half lengthwise and scoop out seeds so they become little "boats." Salt lightly and leave upside down to drain for 30 minutes, then rinse and pat dry. Place zucchini boats, pepper halves, and onion into a large roasting pan. Place 1 sun-dried tomato in each pepper half; coarsely chop the remaining sun-dried tomatoes and sprinkle some into zucchini boats and the rest on top of onion. Sprinkle chopped olives and garlic evenly over all the vegetables.

Combine Roma tomatoes and hydrosols and spoon into pan around, not on, the vegetables (if using canned tomatoes add $1/2$ teaspoon brown sugar). Sprinkle everything with a little salt and pepper and drizzle with the basil-flavored olive oil. Bake for 1 hour uncovered at 325°F; do not stir, as the vegetables must remain upright. Serve at room temperature with French bread, watercress salad, and a dry red wine. Tastes like Provence.

LENTIL AND SPINACH TIMBALES

300 gm yellow or red lentils

1 liter water

2 tablespoons A.H. marjoram or oregano

1 tablespoon A.H. savory

1 tablespoon A.H. sage

sea salt

2 eggs

handful fresh parsley, very finely chopped

1 small onion, finely diced

2 tablespoons olive oil

160 gm spinach

150 ml (approximately $1/2$ cup) white sauce
    made with equal parts milk and bay leaf
    or thyme hydrosol

1 garlic clove, minced

90 gm cream cheese

handful fresh bread crumbs

freshly ground pepper

Wash and drain lentils. Boil with 1 liter water, hydrosols, and a pinch of salt; cook, covered, for 30 minutes or until just soft. Drain off any remaining water and puree; allow to cool completely. Beat in one of the eggs and the fresh parsley. Sauté onion in olive oil until lightly browned; add spinach, remove from heat, and stir while latent heat wilts the spinach. Cool. Combine white sauce, nutmeg, salt and pepper, cream cheese, the remaining egg, and bread crumbs with spinach; puree until smooth. Place a layer of lentils in a lightly oiled loaf pan or individual ramekins; follow with a layer of spinach, and repeat layers, ending with lentils. Place pan in a larger baking dish and add hot water to halfway up the sides; bake at 350ºF for 1 hour for a large pan or 20 to 30 minutes for individual dishes, or until a knife inserted comes out clean. Allow to sit for 15 minutes after removing from the oven, then carefully turn the cakes out of the pans. May be served hot or at room temperature with seasoned tomato sauce or a spicy salsa and salad.

Sauces and Dips

THAI GREEN CURRY PASTE

2 teaspoons coriander seeds

$1/2$ teaspoon cumin seeds

3 to 4 green chilis (jalapeño or ristra), or just 1
    habañero, according to taste

2 teaspoons salt

4 teaspoons brown sugar

3 inches fresh ginger root, peeled, or 3 drops
    E.O. ginger

1 medium onion, peeled and quartered

3 garlic cloves, peeled

7 drops E.O. lemongrass

3 drops E.O. lime

1 cup fresh cilantro

1 cup fresh basil

$1/4$ cup fresh peppermint or apple mint

$1/2$ cup fresh arugula

$1/2$ tablespoon A.H. coriander

1 tablespoon A.H. cardamom

$1/2$ tablespoon A.H. lemon verbena

Dry-fry the coriander and cumin seeds in a hot skillet until fragrant. Grind chilis, salt, and brown sugar into a paste in a food processor; add seeds, ginger, onion, garlic, and essential oils and grind until smooth. Add the greens all at once and process until a smooth paste is achieved, adding the hydrosols while the machine is running. This can be kept in a jar in the fridge for several weeks.

To use, add 5 tablespoons of paste to $1\frac{1}{2}$ cups coconut milk and cook your curry in this sauce. Hydrosols may, of course, be added to the curry sauce during cooking.

CREAMY TOMATO SPREAD

500 gm pressed, dry cottage cheese
2 or 3 ripe fresh tomatoes, peeled
3 green onions
1 teaspoon each A.H. basil, thyme linalol, and carrot seed

Combine all ingredients in a food processor and pulse until blended well. Season to taste with salt and pepper. Serve chilled. Do not substitute regular creamy cottage cheese for the pressed, dry variety, or it will be more like soup than a spread.

Grains and Pasta

All grains and pastas benefit from additional flavorings. They are, after all, usually considered a vehicle for whatever they accompany, providing the starch/carbohydrate element of the meal and (historically) filling you up in case there isn't enough of everything else to go around. Add hydrosol to the cooking water or sprinkle the cooked food with hydrosols after draining and use a fork to distribute them thoroughly.

I am providing one pasta recipe, but there are already thousands out there, so play with hydrosols in your own favorite recipes; you will be blown away by the extra zip they add.

ROBERTO'S PASTA

In my former career one of my favorite colleagues was based in Milan, and he introduced me to both arugula and this recipe. I'm sure it has a proper name, I just don't know what it is. It is best made in early summer, when both the sage and the peas are fresh, but using the hydrosol will allow you to have the flavor of fresh even in winter.

$\frac{1}{2}$ box spaghettini (use a good-quality Italian brand to avoid genetically modified wheat)
4 tablespoons olive oil
2 garlic cloves, peeled and minced
1 cup fresh or frozen peas, blanched for 30 seconds
15 large fresh sage leaves, cut lengthwise into fine slivers
2 tablespoons A.H. sage

Cook spaghettini until just al dente in plenty of water with a generous pinch of sea salt. In a frying pan, heat olive oil and sauté garlic until it is browned. Throw in the peas, sage leaves, and hydrosol; cover and cook over medium heat for 2 to 3 minutes. Add spaghettini; toss and serve at once with freshly grated pecorino romano cheese and lots of freshly ground black pepper.

SAGE RICE

1¹/₂ cups water
1 cup white basmati rice
sea salt
1 teaspoon A.H. sage

Bring water to boiling; add rice, a pinch of salt, and hydrosol; cover and reduce heat to very low. Cook for approximately 20 minutes. (From Miriam Erlichman.)

MOROCCAN SWEET COUSCOUS

This recipe can be served as a dessert but usually accompanies a tagine, or Moroccan stew, of chicken, prunes, and the ubiquitous olives. The dishes work extremely well together.

500 gm couscous
1 liter boiling water
sea salt
1 tablespoon A.H. cardamom
¹/₂ tablespoon A.H. cinnamon leaf
125 gm Thompson golden raisins
100 ml cream
2 tablespoons sugar
2 tablespoons unsalted butter
3 tablespoons A.H. rose

Put couscous in a bowl and pour the boiling water over it; stir once, add salt and hydrosols, stir again, and cover with a tight-fitting lid or foil until cool. Drain off any remaining water and fluff couscous with a fork. (Alternatively, you can mix the hydrosols into the dry couscous, then steam it in a cheesecloth-lined steamer over the

water for approximately 15 minutes.) Meanwhile, soak raisins in the cream, stir in the sugar and rosewater, and set aside. Add the butter to hot couscous and slowly pour on the cream mixture; a large fork or rice paddle works best to stir this. Serve in a broad low dish garnished with edible flowers and toasted pine nuts.

Desserts

BAKLAVA

It sounds more complicated than it is, and the taste of homemade baklava, containing real rose- and neroli waters, is beyond compare. Use an approximately 10 x 12-inch baking dish.

1¹/₄ cups unsalted butter
1 package frozen phyllo pastry, defrosted
2 cups finely chopped walnuts or pistachios
3 teaspoons ground cinnamon
3 tablespoons dry bread crumbs

Syrup:
1 cup sugar
³/₄ cup water
1 tablespoon fresh lemon juice
¹/₄ cup honey (wildflower or orange blossom)
3 tablespoons A.H. rose
3 tablespoons A.H. neroli

Melt butter over low heat. Lightly grease a 10 x 12 rectangular baking dish with some of the melted butter. Unroll phyllo pastry and have a damp tea towel handy to cover the sheets you're not working on. Working quickly, use a pastry brush to coat a sheet of phyllo with the melted butter; lay it in the baking dish, making sure it hangs over the end and goes up the sides. You may find, depending on the exact measurements of the dough, that you will have to stagger the sheets around the edges to ensure that the phyllo always goes over one end and one side each time; it just makes for a neater finished product. Repeat until you have six layers of buttered phyllo in the bottom of the dish. Sprinkle one-third of the walnuts, 1 teaspoon of cinnamon, and 1 tablespoon of bread crumbs over the phyllo. Layer in another four sheets of buttered phyllo and top with one-third of the walnuts, 1 teaspoon cinnamon, and 1 tablespoon bread crumbs. Add four more sheets buttered phyllo and the remainder of the walnuts, cinnamon, and bread crumbs; then add another six sheets of buttered phyllo. Fold the overhanging edges of dough onto the top, brushing any dry bits with butter. Add four more sheets of buttered phyllo on top, tucking them down the outside of the pastry to make a neat bundle. Score the top few layers with a sharp knife in a diamond pattern; this prevents the phyllo from breaking up when you cut it after baking.

Bake at 350°F for 30 minutes, then reduce heat to 300°F and cook 30 minutes more, or until top is golden. Remove from oven.

To make the syrup: Put sugar, water, and lemon juice in a small pot and bring to a boil. Boil rapidly for 5 minutes, then remove from heat and stir in the honey and hydrosols. Pour warm syrup over warm baklava and allow to cool completely. Yum, yum!

MELISSA CHEESECAKE

This could just as easily be made with lavender, rose, neroli, lemon verbena, cardamom . . . let your imagination run wild.

4 tablespoons unsalted butter
1 cup graham cracker crumbs
350 gm cream cheese
350 gm cottage cheese
³/₄ cup sugar
150 ml sour cream
3 tablespoon A.H. melissa
4 eggs
1 small bunch fresh melissa leaves, stems
    removed and discarded, finely chopped
grated zest of 1 lime (optional)

Melt butter. Put cracker crumbs in a springform pan and make a well in the center. Pour in the melted butter and mix well, then press the buttered crumbs into bottom and 1 inch up the sides of the pan; refrigerate for 20 minutes. Combine cream cheese, cottage cheese, sugar, sour cream, and hydrosol in a large bowl. Beat on low speed with a hand mixer; overbeating will cause the cake to crack. Add the eggs two at a time and mix until just blended. Stir in melissa leaves and lime zest, if using, pour into prepared pan, and bake for 1¼ hours at 275°F. Turn off oven and allow cake to sit in oven for 15 minutes before removing. It may seem slightly jiggly in the very center, but it will set; allow to cool completely. Remove springform ring, glaze top of cake with Melissa Honey Curd (recipe follows), or serve with fresh fruit salad sprinkled with melissa hydrosol.

MELISSA HONEY CURD

500 ml honey (linden blossom is nice)
4 eggs plus 2 yolks
2 lemons
3 tablespoons A.H. melissa
5 drops E.O. melissa

In the top of a double boiler lightly beat the whole eggs and the two yolks. Grate the zest from the lemons and squeeze out the juice. Turn on heat and add honey, lemon juice and zest, and the hydrosol. Keep the water underneath at a low simmer, stirring frequently until the mixture thickens and will coat a spoon. Remove from heat, stir in the melissa oil, and pour immediately into hot sterilized Mason jars and seal. Will keep for about one month sealed, seven to ten days in the fridge after opening.

COOKED FRUIT

Fresh fruit salad is lovely sprinkled with some hydrosol, but fruit poached or baked with hydrosols is equally exciting. Use any standard recipe and just add 1 to 2 tablespoons of your chosen hydrosol to the liquid in the recipe.

Baked apples work well with A.H. cinnamon.

Poach pears or apples with melissa, verbena, or wild ginger.

Bake bananas with geranium or clary sage, or be adventurous and use something savory.

SORBET OR GRANITA

This is the first thing people think of making with hydrosols. You can cheat on the recipe, but this will make a real sorbet that tastes quite as good as any of the gourmet brands on the market . . . better, even. It works best with an ice-cream machine, but you can do it by hand too.

$4^1/_2$ cups white sugar
$1/_4$ cup water
$1/_2$ lemon, juiced
$1/_2$ cup A.H. lavender, rose, neroli, geranium, or petitgrain, or a combination to your taste
1 cup fruit pulp (optional)
3 egg whites, whipped until peaks form (optional)

Prepare the sugar syrup by putting $4^1/_2$ cups white sugar in a heavy-bottomed, high-sided saucepan; add $1/_4$ cup water and stir to liquefy sugar. Bring slowly to boiling, stirring occasionally until all the sugar is dissolved. Stop stirring at this point and let the sugar boil until temperature reaches 220ºF on a candy thermometer, the soft-ball stage. Remove pan from heat and allow syrup to cool completely. Once syrup is cold, stir in lemon juice and hydrosol and pour into your ice-cream machine. Alternatively, pour into a wide bowl and place in the freezer, checking it every 30 to 40 minutes and beating it to break up the crystals. This gets quite difficult the firmer it freezes, but beating the sorbet will give it a nicer texture. Freeze until firm. You may add up to 1 cup sieved fruit pulp to the syrup before putting it in the ice-cream machine, as desired. A creamier "ice" can be made by beating 3 egg whites until stiff and folding into the mixture with the hydrosols just before freezing. In this case you will get significantly better results in an ice-cream machine.

Beverages

AFTER-SCHOOL PUNCH

Kids love special drinks; it makes them feel grown-up, and they really get into things like sprigs of herbs or flavored ice cubes, which last long after the glass is empty.

$1/2$ tablespoon A.H. peppermint

1 tablespoon A.H. clary sage

1 tablespoon A.H. linden

2 teaspoons honey (optional)

1.5 liters springwater

Combine hydrosols, honey, and water; serve chilled with sprigs of fresh mint or ice cubes made with diluted peppermint hydrolate. This "punch" is a good pick-me-up when the kids come home from school and need energy for play, homework, or other activities.

ICED "TEA"

1 cup A.H. melissa or lemon verbena

2 tablespoons A.H. clary sage

2 tablespoons A.H. purple bee balm

1 tablespoon A.H. peppermint

2 liters springwater

Combine all ingredients in a large jug; you may add honey, but most people find this does not require any additional sweetener. Serve over ice cubes with a sprig of fresh herb, or for a really special touch, freeze borage flowers in ice cubes and put one in each glass. Caffeine-free, of course!

ROSE ICED TEA

1 cup fresh mint leaves, chopped

1 organic orange, sliced

1 organic lemon, sliced

1 cup English Breakfast tea, brewed twice normal strength

1 tablespoon A.H. rose or rose geranium

2 tablespoons maple syrup

1 liter (32 ounces) springwater

Put mint leaves in a jug and use a wooden spoon to bruise them against the sides. Add remaining ingredients and stir well. Refrigerate for 8 hours or overnight and serve over rose hydrosol ice cubes. (From Miriam Erlichman.)

CINNAMON OAT MILK

3 cups water

2 heaping tablespoons rolled oats (fine)

1 heaping tablespoon barley flour

2 tablespoons maple syrup

1 teaspoon real vanilla extract

$1/2$ teaspoon Celtic sea salt

2 teaspoons A.H. cinnamon

Combine ingredients in a blender and blend on medium speed until smooth. Refrigerate for several hours. Makes a delicious beverage and can be used to substitute for milk in a dairy-free diet. (From Miriam Erlichman.)

GARDEN COCKTAIL

2 stalks celery

1 green pepper, seeded

4 ripe tomatoes, cored

2 large carrots

1 teaspoon A.H. coriander

1 tablespoon A.H. bay laurel

Run all the vegetables through a juicer, add the hydrosols, stir and enjoy.

HANGOVER HELPER OR LIVER CLEANSE

1 large red apple, cored

2 red beets

1 carrot

2 to 3 stalks Swiss chard, or a small bunch of spinach

1 inch of ginger root

1 teaspoon A.H. Greenland moss

1 tablespoon A.H. wild ginger or sweet gale

Run the apple, the vegetables, and ginger through a juicer, stir in the hydrosols, and sip slowly.

KIDNEY CLEANSE

2 whole limes, peel removed

2 large pears

1 large apple

2 teaspoons A.H. elder flower

1 teaspoon A.H. yarrow or petitgrain

Run the fruit through a juicer, stir in the hydrosols, and serve with juniper ice cubes.

GOOD-MORNING TONIC

1 tablespoon A.H. rosemary CT cineole or camphor

1 teaspoon A.H. peppermint

1 teaspoon honey (acacia or manuka)

$1/2$ teaspoon A.H. black spruce

Add hydrosols to an 8-ounce glass of room-temperature or warm springwater, add honey, and drink this first thing when you get up in the morning every day for three weeks. Rise and shine!

SLEEPY-TIME TEA

1 tablespoon A.H. German chamomile

1 teaspoon A.H. angelica

1 teaspoon honey

1 slice of fresh lemon

Put hydrosols and honey in a mug, fill with hot, not boiling, water, and add the lemon slice. You can also add German chamomile hydrosol to hot milk but omit the lemon. This is especially good for people with peptic ulcers. Good night.

WHITE-WINE PUNCH

1 bottle dry white wine (75 cl)

3 tablespoons A.H. clary sage

2 tablespoons A.H. melissa or lemon verbena

2 tablespoons A.H. orange mint or elder flower

1 liter soda water or sparkling mineral water

small bunch fresh melissa leaf, chopped

10 borage leaves, very finely chopped

borage flowers or rose petals to garnish

Combine wine and hydrosols and chill well. Pour into a serving jug or punch bowl and add soda or sparkling water; garnish with flowers. Alternatively, you can place one borage flower or one rose petal in each compartment of an ice-cube tray and make floral ice cubes, or fill a tube-cake pan with flowers and a blend of hydrosols and water and freeze, so that you have a floral ice ring to float in the punch bowl. Using hydrosols instead of water to make ice means your beverage is not diluted as the ice melts; in fact, the flavor gets better.

BUCK'S FIZZ

Brut champagne or sparkling wine
freshly squeezed orange juice
A.H. neroli

Fill champagne flutes one-third full with orange juice; add two or three spritzes ($^1/_4$ teaspoon) of neroli, and top up with the champagne. Even sparkling wines become deluxe in this combination.

MIRIAM'S MARTINI

2 ounces Bombay gin per martini
1 teaspoon A.H. rose geranium per martini
1 ounce dry vermouth per martini

Have all ingredients well chilled. Place in a cocktail shaker of crushed ice, shake well, and strain into chilled martini glasses. Garnish with a twist of lemon. My assistant Jessica replaces the vermouth with hydrosol and uses vodka for her martinis; either way these are quite fantastic 'tinis.

MARGARITA

$1^1/_2$ ounces gold tequila
$^1/_2$ ounce triple sec or Grand Marnier
1 ounce freshly squeezed lime juice
1 teaspoon each A.H. neroli and lemon
    verbena

Combine all ingredients in a cocktail shaker or blender with plenty of crushed ice. Shake well or blend until slushy, and serve in salt-rimmed glasses. (From Miriam Erlichman.)

HOME AND GARDEN

When I teach classes for the home practitioner, I often recommend using essential oils and hydrosols to make home cleaning products. So many people suffer from environmental sensitivities and chemicals are so prevalent in every aspect of our daily lives that I feel it is very worthwhile to look for ways to reduce direct contact with toxins whenever possible. Replacing chemical home cleaning products with natural substances is easy and fun, and they work virtually as well in most cases.

There are some buts, however, and sometimes the most surprising things can happen. A case in point was when one of my students came into class and related the story of how she cleaned her bathroom sink and taps, then deodorized them by placing one drop of undiluted palmarosa oil on each tap handle and leaving it overnight to work. Work it did! In the morning when she tried to turn on the taps, the Lucite handles fractured into a dozen pieces in her hands. It seems that the terpene content in the oil reacted with the terpenes used in the manufacture of the plastic and changed the chemical structure, making it brittle and fragile. Her husband, who also attended the class, had brought the "evidence" and spent the entire evening ribbing me about the "safety" of essential oils. As my friend Lucie says, "Never judge an experiment," just learn from it.

TUB AND TILE CLEANER

I use this on sinks, taps, stove tops—just about anywhere you would use a powder or cream cleaner in the house.

small box baking soda
1 cup salt
10 drops E.O. palmarosa or ti tree
10 drops E.O. lemon
A.H. winter savory, ti tree, or oregano, or a
    combination

Combine baking soda, salt, and essential oils in a glass bowl and mix thoroughly. Sprinkle the cleaning powder over the surface, wet a cloth with the hydrosol, and use a little elbow grease. The mix is gritty enough to remove bath residue but will not scratch the surface. Rinse well for a clean shine.

TELEPHONE SPRITZ

40 ml ethyl alcohol (not rubbing alcohol) or
    overproof vodka
5 drops each E.O. thyme, palmarosa, lemon-
    grass, and peppermint
80 ml A.H. ti tree or thyme CT thymol, or a
    combination

Combine alcohol and essential oils in a 120 ml spray bottle; shake well. Slowly add the hydrosol and shake again. The alcohol will help the oils disperse in the waters for a short period before they separate again. Spritz the mix on your telephone handset, dial—the whole phone—and wipe off with a clean, dry cloth. I also use this on my computer keyboard: Spray the cloth, then wipe the keys with it; don't spritz the board directly.

HUMIDIFIERS

100 ml A.H. of your choice

Add the hydrosol to the humidifier every time you add water. It will drastically reduce the musty smell that can come with increased humidity, and if you choose something like oregano, thyme, savory, or one of the more antiseptic hydrosols, you not only have a nice odor but kill germs as well.

COMPOST

Any hydrosols that are past their best-before date or have developed a mold or off odor can be poured into the compost heap or diluted in water and used to feed the plants. Compost making actually requires a certain amount of thought, skill, and work, and years ago I was given a tip by an old Yorkshire farmer. He used to urinate in his compost pile to speed up the decomposition process. The acidity of urine is extremely beneficial to compost, although he specified, and I have since seen it in old books, that it must be only male urine, as female is too acidic. You can imagine how well it went down with male friends when I asked them to "help" with my compost!

Hydrosols, being acidic in nature, also work, and as they become more alkaline as they degrade, you never have to worry about the level of acidity. It's also much less embarrassing.

Sources and Resources

The biochemical make-up of plants, for instance, is notoriously variable geographically—and plant chemicals have provided a great many of society's medicines and industrial products.
Paul Ehrlich, in *The Gaia Atlas of Planet Management*

Hydrosols are already available from most aromatherapy product distributors, and more companies are selling them all the time. Hydrosols are also available from some good health food stores and natural pharmacies, but always ask if they contain preservatives if they are not cold stored. However, for the biggest and best selection of premium quality hydrosols you may find that the Internet and mail-order sources are your best choice. The companies listed in this index (some only on-line) all sell hydrosols of therapeutic grade, and a year or two from now there will be tens of dozens more. So don't despair if your corner shop doesn't have them yet; they will one day soon.

Acqua Vita
85 Arundel Ave.
Toronto, ON M4K 3A3
(416) 405-8855; fax (416) 405-8185
www.hydrosols.com; e-mail: info@acqua-vita.com
Founded by Suzanne Catty in 1995, Acqua Vita offers a comprehensive variety of aromatherapy services, including health consultations, aromatic massage, reflexology, and vibrational healing.

Education is offered through workshops, lectures, and full-time courses and via correspondence. Acqua Vita teaches a two-hundred-hour in-class "Aromatic Practitioner" certification program, which is offered (without the bodywork module) as a home-study course. The "Layman Practitioner" course is a thirty-hour program designed for the nonprofessional user of aromatherapy. Advanced and specialist classes and weekend distillation workshops are also available.

Acqua Vita offers a selected range of certified organic and wild-crafted essential oils, Aromatic Tinctures, synergies, and products and over forty hydrosols at both retail and wholesale.

SUPPLIERS

North America

Natures Gift
www.naturesgift.com
Offers a broad range of essential oils and hydrosols, mostly organic, via the Internet. A fun and personal Web site.

Natural Extracts of Australia
1727 North Dillion Street
Los Angeles, CA 90026
(323) 660-7914; fax (323) 660-7922
e-mail: melaleuca@earthlink.net
U.S.-based broker of therapeutic-grade essential oils.
Able to supply hydrosols in very large quantities.

Original Swiss Aromatics
P.O. Box 606
San Rafael, CA 94915
(415) 479-9120; fax (415) 479-0119
www.pacificinstituteofaromatherapy.com
Offers a wide range of organic and wild-crafted essential oils and skin- and body-care products, including many rare species for therapeutic use. Through Pacific Institute of Aromatherapy offers education, home study, and conferences. Director Kurt Schnaubelt, Ph.D., is the author of two books on clinical aromatherapy.

Prima Fleur
1525 E. Francisco Blvd., Suite 16
San Rafael, CA 94901
(415) 455-0957; fax (415) 455-0956
Distributor of organic hydrosols produced by the California-based Aromatic Plant Project. Also offers a wide selection of essential oils and skin-care products. Wholesale mail order only.

Rae Dunphy Aromatics
1910 Bowness Rd. NW
Calgary, AB T2N 3K6
(403) 283-8889; (800) 563-8938;
fax (403) 283-2996
e-mail: raedunphy@home.com
Offers a comprehensive range of primarily organic essential oils; some hydrosols, diffusers, and base oils; excipients and gels. Retail and wholesale.

Scents of Knowing
P.O. Box 1159
Haiku, HI 96708
Phone/fax (808) 573-6733; (800) 457-0480
www.scentsofknowing.com;
e-mail: scentoknow@aol.com
Distiller of native Hawaiian species of plants for hydrosols and essential oils. Also offers hydrosols, attars, and ruhs from India. Specialist in vibrational aspects of aromatherapy. Offers education.

Sensory Essence
P.O. Box 87
Island Lake, IL 60042
(847) 526-3645; fax (847) 487-1971
e-mail: jan.salko@woldnet.att.net
Organic and wild-crafted hydrosols and essential oils, including some rare species. Mail order only.

Solstice Botanicals
11080 Franz Valley Rd.
Calistoga, CA 94515
(707) 942-5607; fax (707) 942-0211
www.aboutlavender.com;
email: lavenderdc@aol.com
Grower of organic plants mostly from European stock and producer of organic hydrosols. A small list but of good quality, and new varieties are added each year.

White Lotus Aromatics
801 Park Way
El Cerrito, CA 94530
Fax (510) 528-9441
www.members.aol.com/somanath/fragrant.html;
e-mail: somanath@aol.com
Offers a select range of essential oils, absolutes, ruhs, attars, and some hydrosols traditionally distilled in India. Also offers educational trips to distillation projects in India.

A Woman of Uncommon Scents
P.O. Box 103
Roxbury, PA 17251
(717) 530-0609; (800) 377-3685;
fax (717) 263-6347
e-mail: 75730.1510@compuserve.com
Wholesale bulk organic and wild-crafted essential oils and hydrosols for professionals.

Europe

Avicenna
Unit 80, Spindus Rd.
Speke Hall Industrial Estate
Liverpool L24 1YA U.K.
Offers a small range of organic and wild-crafted hydrosols, essential oils, and distilled tinctures grown and produced in the United Kingdom and Lebanon. For the herbalist, a broader range of standard tinctures and fresh and dried herbs is available. A hydrosol specialist, Avicenna also offers education.

D'Oyles
5 Jarratt St., Kingston Square
Hull, East Yorkshire
HU1 3HB U.K.
44 (01482) 581 776; fax 44 (01482) 581 774
Offers a wide range of chemotype-specific, organic, and chemical-free hydrosols and essential oils, plus prepared aromatic medicinal products in gels, capsules, and suppositories for the professional practitioner. Also offers education.

The English Chamomile Company
36 High St.
Northwold, Thetford,
Norfolk, IP26 5LA U.K.
Phone/fax 44 (1366) 728 922
www.chamomile.co.uk;
e-mail: chamomile@dial.pipex.com
Roman chamomile essential oil and hydrosol.

Essentially Oils
8–10 Mount Farm
Churchill, Chipping Norton
Oxfordshire OX7 6NP U.K.
44 (1608) 659 544; fax 44 (1608) 659 566
www.essentiallyoils.com
e-mail: essentially.oil.ltd@dial.pipex.com
Wide range of essential oils, some hydrosols and ancillary aromatherapy products. Interesting newsletter available by subscription.

Florial
42 Chemin des Aubepines
06130 Grasse, France
33 (493) 778 819; fax (33) (493) 778 878
www.florial.com; e-mail: info@florial.com
Certified organic and wild-crafted essential oils and hydrolates. Reliable service by mail order.

Miron Glass
Badenerstrasse 21
CH-8953 Dietikon, Switzerland
41 (01) 740 6969; fax 41 (01) 740 0880
U.S. office: 2485 N. Beachwood Drive
Los Angeles, CA 90068
(323) 467-0558; fax (323) 467-5558
e-mail: mironusa@aol.com
Supplies dark violet glass bottles.

Phyto-Aroma Organic International
c/o AYUS GmbH
Weinstrasse 60
77815 Bühl
Germany
33 (4) 90 64 13 78; fax 49 (7223) 901 383
www.aroma-seminar.de
e-mail: phyto-aroma@t-online.de
One of the largest collections of essential oils, mostly organic and wild. Also many hydrosols, including unusual varieties. Education offered by Malte Hozzel at the Provence seminar center.

Prima Vera Life
Am Fichtenholz 5
D-87477 Sulzburg, Germany
49 (83) 76 80 80; fax 49 (83) 76 80 839
Extensive range of organic and wild-crafted
essential oils as well as some hydrosols, carrier oils,
and a huge range of aromatherapy products. Offers
yearly conferences and "AromaKuche" classes with
Maria Kettenring.

Asia

Dianna Olivia Lim
Singapore
e-mail: aromaart@pacific.net.sg
Distributor of essential oils and hydrosols, primarily from India. Mail order only.

Healing Plants / SM Alternatives
17 Lyndhurst Terrace, ground floor
Central, Hong Kong
H.K.S.A.R. China
e-mail: parisem@netvigator.com
Holistic practice offering aromatherapy treatments
and a variety of essential oils, hydrosols, blends, and
products, primarily organic.

Australia

Bush Sense
P.O. Box 285
Blaxland NSW, Australia
61 (2) 4727-6707
e-mail: bushsense@mail.com
Mark Web, author of *Bush Sense: Australian
Essential Oils and Aromatic Compounds*, is a bio-
chemist, botanist, and distiller. He offers a select
range of exceptional quality indigenous Australian
essential oils and hydrosols as well as education
programs.

INFORMATION RESOURCES

American Botanical Council
P.O. Box 144345
Austin, TX 78714-4345
(512) 926-4900; fax (512) 926-2345
www.herbalgram.com
e-mail: custserv@herbalgram.org
Publisher of the excellent magazine *Herbalgram*
and purveyor of hundreds of books on
phytomedicine, plants, aromatherapy, and ethno-
botany. Associated with the Herb Research
Foundation.

Herb Research Foundation
1007 Pearl St., Ste 200
Boulder, CO 80302
(303) 449-2265; fax (303) 449-7849
www.herbs.org
An excellent resource for all things plant related.
Education director Mindy Green is the author of
two books on aromatherapy. Associated with the
American Botanical Council.

Aromatic Plant Project
219 Carl St.
San Francisco, CA 94117
(415) 564-6785; fax (415) 564-6799
The APP coordinates the organic growing and
distilling of native species in several parts of the
United States. Their hydrosols are offered for sale
exclusively through Prima Fleur. Director Jeanne
Rose, author and a long-time advocate of hydrosols, prepares a quarterly newsletter and provides
weekend workshops in distillation and
aromatherapy.

DISTILLATION EQUIPMENT

Extractor
Francis Mainguy
305 rue Principale
Grondines, Quebec
Canada G0A 1W0
(418) 268-8671; fax (418) 268-3406
e-mail:extractor@globetrotter.net
Offers efficient and affordable small-scale home
distillation units in a variety of sizes for North
American consumers. Also offers worldwide
consultant service, design, and construction of
large-scale stills for commercial aromatherapy
businesses.

Stove Stills
Robert Pappas
3043 Elisa Court
New Albany, IN 47150
(812) 945-5000; fax (603) 506-2536
www.essentialoils.org
Offers two sizes of home distillation units for the
North American hobbyist as well as worldwide
GCMS analysis service of essential oils.

HYDROSOL ANALYSIS

Laseve
Départemente des sciences fondamentales
University of Quebec at Chicoutimi
555, University Boulevard
Chicoutimi, Quebec
Canada G7H 2B1
(418) 545-5011 x2332; fax (418) 545-5012
www.uqac.uquebec.ca/laseve

AROMATHERAPY INTERNET

Newsgroups

www.egroups.com/invite/kercher
list@idma.com

On-line Information

www.davidsuzuki.com
Independent environmental foundation run by
David Suzuki

www.fda.gov
Legal information from the U.S. government on
natural products

www.herbs.org
The Herb Research Foundation

www.libraries.uc.edu/Lloyd
Herb reference library

Conversion Chart

1000 milliliters = 1 liter

1 liter (946.4 milliliters) = 32 ounces = 1 quart (1.06 quarts liquid)

30 milliliters (29.6 milliliters) = 2 tablespoons

5 milliliters (4.9 milliliters) = 1 teaspoon (3 teaspoons = 1 tablespoon)

250 milliliters (236.6 milliliters) = 1 cup

500 milliliters (473.2 milliliters) = 1 pint

30 grams (28.35 grams) = 1 ounce

1000 grams = 1 kilogram (1 liter of water weighs 1 kilogram)

1 kilogram = 2.25 pounds

(As a rough guide you can make grams = milliliters)

To convert degrees Celsius to degrees Fahrenheit, multiply the Celsius temperature by 1.8 and add 32.

0 degrees C = 32 degrees F (freezing)

100 degrees C = 212 degrees F (boiling)

Notes

Chapter 1

1. Michael Talbot, *The Holographic Universe* (New York: HarperPerennial, 1991).

2. Dorothy L. Severns, "Chaos and Fractals in Aromatherapy: The Non-linear Dynamics of Essential Oils," in *Proceedings: Third Aromatherapy Conference on Therapeutic Uses of Essential Oils, October 30–November 1, 1998,* ed. Kurt Schnaubelt (San Francisco: Pacific Institute of Aromatherapy, 1998), p. 85.

3. Ibid., p. 86.

4. Ibid., p. 89.

5. Kenny Ausubel, *Seeds of Change: The Living Treasure* (San Francisco: HarperSanFrancisco, 1994).

6. Lucette Laflamme et al., "Effects of Organic and Conventional Production Systems on Yield and Active Ingredient Concentration of Medicinal Plants."

7. Joanna Blythman, "No, Prime Minister," *Manchester Guardian*, June 5, 1999.

8. Ausubel, *Seeds of Change.*

9. Jenifer Kahn, "The Green Machine," *Harper's* (April 1999): 70–73.

10. Ibid.

11. Joanna Blythman, "No, Prime Minister," *Manchester Guardian*, June 5, 1999.

12. Garrison Wilkes, "Genetic Erosion," in *The Gaia Atlas of Planet Management,* ed. Norman Myers (London: Pan Books, 1985).

13. Ibid.

14. Steven Martyn and Kim Elkington, personal correspondence, February 2000.

15. Douglas Adams and Mark Cawardine, *Last Chance to See* (London: William Heinemann, 1990; Pan Books, 1991).

Chapter 2

1. David Suzuki, *The Sacred Balance* (Vancouver: Greystone Books, 1997).

2. Ibid.

3. Ian Urquhart, "Brace Yourself for a Water Fight," *Toronto Star*, January 10, 2000.

4. Ibid. Ian Urquhart notes that Canada discharges as much pollution directly into its waterways (7 percent) as it treats (7 percent), while the United States treats (13 percent) a little more than it dumps (11 percent). In fact, the province of Ontario and the state of Pennsylvania are the two biggest polluters of the Great Lakes, with combined air and water pollution per annum of 36,532,706 kilograms and 26,340,987 kilograms, respectively. One out of every three Canadians and one out of every seven Americans depend on the Great Lakes for water.

5. Douglas Jehl, "Tampa Bay Looks to the Sea to Quench Its Thirst," *New York Times*, March 12, 2000.

6. Paul C. Bragg, N.D., and Patricia Bragg, N.D., *Water: The Shocking Truth,* rev. ed. (Santa Barbara, Calif.: Health Science, 1998).

7. Suzuki, *Sacred Balance.*

8. Martin Mittelstaedt, "How Bad Is Canada's Water Problem?" *Globe and Mail* (Toronto), January 11, 2000, sec. A, p. 14.

9. Ibid. Martin Mittelstaedt remarks, "A 1993 Health Canada study suggests current THM guidelines of a maximum 100 parts per billion do not adequately protect against cancer. In a 1997 Health Canada report on the risks of drinking water, 60% of the experts consulted said bladder cancer was 'possible' while 40% said it was 'probable.'" In the United States the EPA has lowered the maximum allowable THMs in U.S. drinking water to 80 parts per billion, a ruling that will affect about 140 million Americans in the next four years. The EPA based its ruling on cancer rates found in lab animals and has also demanded that all American water utility companies send their customers water-quality reports containing information about THMs. Other research has suggested that the high estrogen levels found in tap water in many developed nations may have a link to the increase in diseases, particularly breast and prostate cancers. Problems of male infertility and reduced sperm count may also be linked to this high estrogen content, which is a result of nearly forty years of pharmaceutical hormones' being excreted by animals and humans.

10. Nicolaas van Rijn, "What We Have Is All There Is," *Toronto Star,* January 11, 2000.

11. Michael A. Mallin, "Impacts of Industrial Animal Production on Rivers and Estuaries," *American Scientist* 88 (January–February 2000): 26–37.

12. Ibid. Fecal coliform bacteria are another measure of water pollution. "The N.C. Division of Water Quality uses 200 colony-forming units per 100 milliliters (200 CFU/ 100 ml) as the state standard for safe human contact with water bodies. The spill incidents caused very high fecal coliform counts in the receiving streams—including a remarkable 3.4-million-units measurement in the New River following the June swine-waste spill." As if that weren't enough, although spills from waste lagoons are illegal and can be penalized, it is legal and normal practice for the waste to be disposed of by application to "sprayfields." These are land areas adjacent to the farms onto which the concentrated feces and urine is sprayed; the fields usually grow a cover crop such as Bermuda grass. Unfortu-nately, once saturated with either water or nutrients, or as a result of normal rainfall, the soil can no longer hold or bind the waste and this pollution then makes its way into local water supplies. See Mallin, "Impacts of Industrial Animal Production."

13. Robert Root-Bernstein and Michele Root-Bernstein. *Honey, Mud, Maggots, and Other Medical Marvels* (New York: Houghton Mifflin, 1998).

14. Ibid.

15. Ibid.

16. Deni Bown, *Encyclopedia of Herbs and Their Uses* (London: Dorling Kindersley, 1995).

17. Ibid.

18. Dawnelle Malone, "Killer Spices," *Herbalgram* 46: 16.

19. Joe Nasr, personal correspondence, November 5, 1999. Nasr, of British distiller Avicenna, also makes aromatic tinctures, which he calls distilled tinctures: "These are produced by distilling half the total amount of an aromatic herb in spring water to produce a volatile oil-rich aromatic water [hydrosol]. The remaining herb is then cold macerated in a solution of its aromatic water and alcohol. This process ensures that a gentle and adequate amount of the volatile components of the plant are present in the tincture alongside the water soluble components not present in pure essential oils." Avicenna supplies distilled tinctures of dill, caraway, fennel, geranium, and aniseed.

20. Donna Karan Cosmetics provided the following product recall information.

PRODUCT
Nectar Watermist a non alcohol body spray made from natural distilled water extracted from blossoms of orange trees packaged into .5 ounce, 4 ounce, 8 ounce and 16 ounce glass bottles. Recall #F-807-7.

CODE
The codes under recall consists of all product codes shipped prior to July 28, 1997 and includes the following items:

4 oz. Nectar WaterMist   Item #FG-8120D-00   Packaging Lot #s 71611, 71621, 71631;

8 oz. Nectar WaterMist   Item #FG-8123D-00   Packaging Lot #s 71641, 71651;

8 oz. Nectar WaterMist (tester)   Item #PG-7427D-00   Packaging Lot #s 71641, 71651;

Bulk lot #s 0.5 oz Nectar (tester) sample Item #PG-7421D-00   Packaging Lot # 7F09A (only given to sales reps);

Dramming/Nectar bulk (3 x 16 oz.)   Item #PG-7740D-00   Packaging Lot # 7F09A.

MANUFACTURER
Allure Cosmetics, San Leandro, California Herba Aromatica, Hayward, California (importer of scented floral water).

RECALLED BY
The Donna Karan Beauty Company (DKBC) New York, New York, by telephone visit and fax beginning on July 28, 1997, followed by letter on August 1, 1997. Firm-initiated recall ongoing.

DISTRIBUTION
California, New York, Washington state, Oregon, Virginia, Pennsylvania, Maryland, New Jersey, Massachusetts, Connecticut, Florida, Minnesota, Illinois, Wisconsin, Indiana, Michigan, Texas.

QUANTITY
Item #FG-8120D-00 – 3,606 units – 4 oz Nectar   Item #FG-8123D-00 – 1,967 units – 8 oz Nectar   Item #PG-7427D-00 – 713 units – 8 oz Watermist   Item #PG-7426D-00 – 4,028 units – 5 oz Nectar   Item #PG-7440D-00 – 65 units – Dramming bulk (3 x16 oz) were distributed.

REASON

Product is contaminated with Burkholderia cepacia, a pathogen.

FDA, *Recalls and Field Corrections: Cosmetics—Class II* (FDA Enforcement Report, September 17, 1997).

An Australian distiller, Bill McGilvary, was enlisted as a consultant on the product and its recall. He says, "The Burkholderia was present in the hydrolats as received, and most of the hydrolats were recovered by ultra filtration and subsequent preservation. If they had been properly looked after and managed during transit and storage, the problem would not have occurred." McGilvary, private correspondence, May 1999.

21. Greg Farrell, "Bottling Botanical Essences," *USA Today*, date unknown 1999.

22. In an article in the *Journal of Essential Oil Research* titled "Extraction and GC/MS Analysis of the Essential Oil of *Achillea millefolium* L. Complex," researchers discuss the following distillation parameters: "We observed that several monoterpenes appear in the first two fractions; after 60 minutes, they mostly vanished. On the other hand, the concentration of chamazulene, which is less than 0.3% in the 0–15 min intervals, is higher than 30% in the 30–120 min interval and its concentration remains approximately 20% after 240 mins. The concentrations of sabinene, camphor and beta-thujone decreased steadily as a function of time while that of eugenol increased from 0.19 to 9.3% after six hours. . . . The most productive interval in oil production is obtained during the first 15 mins: 755 mg of oil is then collected (70% of the total obtained after six hours). After 60 min., the concentration in chamazulene reaches its maximum value of 34% while the total yield in recovered oil already reaches 83% of the total essential oil extracted after six hours." Jean-Marie Hachey, et al., "Extraction and GC/MS Analysis of the Essential Oil of *Achillea millefolium* L. Complex," *Journal of Essential Oil Research* 2 (November/December 1990): 317–26.

A skilled distiller armed with this knowledge can select the best part of the distillation for hydrosol collection based on the content of water-soluble chemicals coming off the still. One can also see how this information would be used in industrial distillation when the desired end product is the isolated compounds of chamazulene. Industrial distillation would most likely be stopped after a sixty-minute run, whereas therapeutic distillation would continue for the full six hours.

Chapter 3

1. A case in point is sassafras oil, which causes huge debate in the aromatherapy world. Two completely different plants both have the common name sassafras: *Ocotea pretiosa,* and *Sassafras albidum,* so already we have a problem. However, the oil is our concern, and the concern with the oil is a chemical (phenol-methyl-ether) called safrole, which is metabolized into a toxin in the liver of rats. As Kurt Schnaubelt says, "After calamus and sassafras oils were fed to rats for a period of twelve months carcinogenic effects were

observed. These experiments should be viewed as curiosities, and one need not panic at the sight of a bottle of sassafras oil. Validity of these experiments with respect to normal human use is limited because they rely on massive over-doses." (*Advanced Aromatherapy* [Rochester, Vt.: Healing Arts Press, 1998].) The calamus oil in the test referred to contained high levels of beta-asarone.

Then consider the work from Bastyr University, described by naturopath Joseph Pizzorno in his book *Total Wellness* (Rocklin, Calif.: Prima Publishing, 1998). It shows that although safrole is metabolized into a hepatotoxin in the liver of rats, it initiates phase I liver detoxification in humans. Since nicotine also initiates phase I liver detoxifica-tion, it becomes clear that the suggestion of internal use of low doses of sassafras oil as an aid in quitting smoking makes sense. We can't always apply the finding and effects of experiments on animals to humans, nor can we assume that the effects a substance has in isolation compared with those that it has in its natural form and combinations, such as in a hydrosol or essential oil, are the same. Sassafras may not be an everyday oil, but it is very useful in treating gout and kidney stones and detoxifying the body when giving up tobacco.

2. Living embalming is a French aromatherapy practice in which twenty drops or more of undiluted essential oil are applied to the entire surface of the skin except the mucous membranes and face. Using nondermocaustic but powerfully antiseptic and antiviral oils like palmarosa, tea tree, ravensara, or thyme CT thuyanol, this procedure can be repeated several times in one day and can usually stop an infection before it takes hold.

3. Ear candling, or auricular coning, is an ancient practice in which a cone or hollow candle is used to introduce smoke into the ear canal and create a vacuum that then draws out the smoke and whatever else may be in the ear channel. Samples of ear cones made of clay have been found in Egyptian sites, and many aboriginal tribes around the world use smoke blown into the ear canal as a way of healing ear problems.

Chapter 4

1. Rudolphe Balz, *The Healing Power of Essential Oils* (Twin Lakes, Wis.: Lotus Light, 1996).

2. Jean Valnet, M.D., *The Practice of Aromatherapy* (Rochester, Vt.: Healing Arts Press, Rochester VT, 1990).

3. Ibid.

4. Ibid.

5. Ibid.

6. Hitoshi Masaki et al., "Active-Oxygen Scavenging Activity of Plant Extracts," *Biological Pharmacy Bulletin* 18, no. 1 (1995): 162–66.

Chapter 5

1. Masaki et al., "Active-Oxygen Scavenging Activity of Plant Extracts."

2. K. Knobloch and H. Strobel, "Effective Concentrations of Essential Oil Components to Scavenge Oxygen Radicals and Inhibit

Lipoxygenase Turnover Rates," *Planta Medica* 59, supplement 7 (December 1993): A669.

3. K. Masaki, T. Atsumi, and H. Sakurai, "Protective Activity of Hamamelitannin on Cell Damage of Murine Skin Fibroblasts Induced by UV Irradiation," *Journal of Dermatological Science* 10 (1995): 25–34.

4. C. A. J. Erdelmeier et al., "Antiviral and Antiphlogistic Activities of *Hamamelis virginiana* Bark," *Planta Medica* 62 (1996): 241–45.

5. H. C. Korting et al., "Anti-inflammatory Activity of *Hamamelis* Distillate Applied Topically to the Skin," *European Journal of Clinical Pharmacology* 44 (spring 1993): 315–18.

6. U. Kastner et al., "Anti-edematous Activity of Sesquiterpene Lactones from Different Taxa of the *Achillea millefolium* Group," *Planta Medica* 59, supplement 7 (December 1993): A669.

7. Kurt Schnaubelt, *Advanced Aromatherapy* (Rochester, Vt.: Healing Arts Press, 1998).

8. Olof Alexandersson, *Living Water* (Bath, England: Gateway Books, 1990).

Glossary

Absolute: highly fragrant plant extract obtained through the use of chemical solvents or enfleurage (fat extraction) as opposed to steam distillation. Primarily used for expensive floral material, such as rose or orange blossom, and for those plants or flowers that cannot be steam distilled, such as jasmine, hyacinth, and carnation.

Acneic: relating to acne

Adaptogenic: in aromatherapy this refers to an oils, ability to adapt to the needs of the body and/or change its effects according to dosage

Aerophagia: swallowing of air

Antioxidant: substance that inhibits oxidation and captures free radicals

Astringent: able to draw together soft organic tissues

Alkaloid: colorless, complex, usually bitter substances found in plant material, containing nitrogen and usually oxygen. Most commonly found in alcohol extracts of the plant.

Asthenia: lack or loss of strength, general debility, when you just don't seem to care much about anything

Attar: hydro-distillation of plant material into a base of sandalwood oil, usually found in India and performed with expensive flowers and substances difficult to steam distill

ADD: Attention Deficit Disorder

ADHD: Attention Deficit Hyperactivity Disorder

Aromapuncture: term coined by Suzanne Catty and Miriam Erlichman to describe the application of hydrosols to acupuncture points in the body without the use of pressure or needles

Aromatic Tincture: term coined to describe the preparation of tinctures using alcohol combined with hydrosols

Ayurveda: from the Sanskrit *Ayur* (life) *Veda* (knowledge or science). A system of health maintenance and care practiced in India based on Vedic text that are more than 4000 years old. Ayurveda is based on three main constitutional types and provides a philosophy of diet, health care, lifestyle, exercise, and spirituality designed to keep the individual in a state of balance and good health.

Beta-asarone: a chemical from the functional group ketones, which has liver toxic (hepatotoxic) effects

Carrier oil: also called a base oil or simply a carrier. Usually a nonvolatile fatty oil from natural sources that is used to dilute essential oils before application or ingestion, for example, sesame, olive, sweet almond, or coconut

Carminative: substance that promotes the release of gas from the stomach or intestinal tract

Cholagogue: a substance that promotes the release of bile from the gallbladder

Cicatrisant: stimulating the healing of wounds or scar tissue

Cohobation: a term used in distillation to describe the recycling of the distillate waters (hydrosols) back into the still to maximize the extraction of the dissolved essential oil molecules

Couperose skin: redness of the face (primarily the cheeks and nose) caused by numerous spider veins appearing on the surface or visible through the top layers of the skin

Chemotype: term used in aromatherapy to describe chemical anomalies within plants of the same genus and species that are created as a result of environment, geography, and numerous naturally occurring variables.

Dermocaustic : substance causing irritation to the skin

Decoction: in herbal medicine, a product made by the boiling of herbs in water

Distance healing: term used in energetic healing, most commonly reiki, to describe healing work conducted on an individual from a distance

Diuretic: substance that increase the flow of urine and removes water or fluids from the body

Emetic: substance that promotes vomiting

Expectorant: substance that promotes the expulsion of mucus from the respiratory tract

Free radical: a particularly reactive atom that has one or more unpaired electrons. Often used to describe oxygen molecules with unpaired electrons that contribute to the aging process.

Fractionated: a process, often chemical, that separates a substance into different fractions; to facilitate their use as isolates or to change the structure of the original substance eg: citrus oils are often fractionated to remove their monoterpene content, making them less volatile and therefore less likely to evaporate in bottles during storage or for sales. Fractionated citrus oils are more likely to cause issues of dermocausticity.

Frictions: a term in aromatherapy used to describe the application of essential oils, usually undiluted, by rubbing on specific parts of the body without massage. Term used by Nelly Grosjean to describe her blends, which are formulated specifically to be used in this manner.

Functional group: term used to describe groups of chemicals according to their structure; a characteristic reactive unit of a chemical compound especially in organic chemistry

Hepato: a prefix that refers to the liver, that is, a hepatostimulant is a liver function stimulant; a hepatotoxin is a substance toxic to the liver.

Hemostatic: to stop bleeding

Herbaceous: of herbs or green plants, resembling fresh herbs or plant material in smell or taste

Homeopathy: philosophy of medicine devised by Samuel Hahnemann and based on the principle that "like cures like." One uses a remedy that would normally cause specific symptoms to cure those same symptoms. Homeopathy uses only infinitesimal doses of substances to achieve healing, the more dilute or lower the dose the stronger the potency.

Hydrophilic: water loving, attracted by or to water

Infusion: in herbal medicine, the preparation of a substance made by steeping plant material in water, alcohol, or rarely oil, without the addition of heat, to extract active principles

In vitro: literally "in glass," describing laboratory tests conducted on isolated tissue, outside the living body; in an artificial environment

In vivo: literally "in the living," describing effects or tests on living bodies, animal or human

Ketone: a chemical functional group with a carbonyl group attached to two carbon atoms. In aromatherapy, ketones are considered unsafe by some. However, there are hundreds of different ketones some of which do have serious issues of toxicity, others of which have no issues of toxicity.

Lipophilic: fat or lipid loving, attracted by or to fatty substances

Living embalming: in aromatherapy also called "aromatic perfusion." A protocol that advises the application of quantities of undiluted essential oils over large areas of the body, excluding mucous membranes, to combat specific infections or pathologies. Usually undertaken with essential oils that have no issues of dermocausticity or toxicity, that are well tolerated by the body, and that have specific antibacterial, antiviral, or antifungal properties.

Maceration: in herbal medicine, similar to infusion. Most often used to describe preparation of products in which plant material is soaked in an oil base without the use of a direct heat source. Some plant material, e.g.: carrot to create helio-carrot, is macerated in olive oil and placed in the sun to enhance the extraction of the plant properties through the warmth of the sun's rays.

Materia medica: the science or study of the nature, properties, and preparation of healing substances. Also books or documents describing the nature and properties of healing substances or medicines.

Monoterpene: a chemical functional group with ten carbon atoms and one double bond. In aromatherapy, monoterpenes are found in many oils and in the highest quantities in oils from the conifer trees and citrus fruits.

Mucolytic: helping to liquefy, dissolve, or resolve mucus in the body

Muka: term used to describe the residual plant matter remaining after steam distillation of essential oils. Muka is usually left to compost for a period and then spread as a fertilizer or weed retardant in organic and biodynamic agriculture.

Oxide: a chemical functional group characterized by an oxygen atom integrated into a terpene ring system. In aromatherapy the oxide 1,8 cineole is the most common and shows up in high proportions in oils such as ti tree, and the eucalyptus family.

Peroxidation: an oxidation process in which oxygen molecules bind to other oxygen molecules

Phytohormones: plant hormone, or hormones derived from plant sources

Phytomedicine: plant medicine or medicine derived from plant sources

Phytotherapy: therapy using plant products, plant-based medicine

Proving: in homeopathic medicine, the term used to describe the exhibition of symptoms that the remedy is supposed to alleviate or clear up

Prophylactic: guarding from or preventing disease

rH2: a measurement of the electrical conductivity of a substance

Rosacea: an inflammatory condition of the skin where redness, roughness, bumps, and pustules appear across the center of the face, affecting primarily the nose and cheeks

Ruh: hydrodistillation of plant material, usually of exotic flowers such as jasmine, performed almost exclusively in India

SAD: Seasonal Affective Disorder. A series of symptoms including depression, asthenia, problems of the endocrine system, loss of energy and vitality, that combined represent SAD. Believed to be the result of insufficient amount of sunlight entering the eye and reaching the pineal gland.

Safrole: also safrol, a phenyl propane found in essential oil of sassafras and having hepatotoxic effects in rats. Studies on human beings indicate that the hepatotoxicity is not created by safrole in the liver of humans.

Sesquiterpene: a chemical functional group characterized by a terpene molecule with fifteen carbon atoms

Succussion: in homeopathic medicine, the repeated rapping of a bottle to potentize the remedy within. It is believed that the vibrations of the rapping process distributes the energetic vibration of the medicine throughout the substance and increases its potency.

Tincture: an active principle or extract of a plant, usually made with alcohol, for use as a medicine

Tisane: an herb tea or infusion, usually used medicinally or for health-giving properties

THMs: Trihalomethanes. Any of various derivatives CHX_3 of methane (e.g. chloroform) that have three halogen atoms per molecule and are formed especially during the chlorination of drinking water

Bibliography

Abraham, Carolyn. "Scientists Test 'Sixth-Sense' Drugs." *Globe and Mail* (Toronto), November 20, 1999, sec. 1, pp. 1, 2, 20, 21.

Abram, David. *The Spell of the Sensuous.* New York: Vintage Books, 1997.

Ackerman, Diane. *A Natural History of the Senses.* New York: Vintage Books, 1990.

Adams, Douglas, and Mark Cawardine. *Last Chance to See.* London: William Heinemann, 1990; Pan Books, 1991.

Ahmed, Faizan. "Doctors without Diplomas." *Toronto Star,* January 9, 2000, sec B, p. 2.

Alexandersson, Olof. *Living Water.* Bath, England: Gateway Books, 1990.

Arnal-Schnebelen, B., M.D. "La secheresse vaginale." *Vous et votre Sante* 47 (May 1997): 14–15.

Ausubel, Kenny. *Seeds of Change: The Living Treasure.* San Francisco: HarperSanFrancisco, 1994.

Azemar, Jacqueline. "Galenic Forms for Aromatherapy II–Solubol: An Excipient of Choice for Essential Oils." *Les Cahiers de l'Aromatherapie* 2 (September 1996): 92–95.

Balz, Rudolph. *The Healing Power of Essential Oils.* Twin Lakes, Wis.: Lotus Light, 1996.

Barnes-Svarney, Patricia. *The New York Public Library Science Desk Reference.* New York: Macmillan, Stonesong Press, 1995.

Batmanghelidj, Fereydoon, M.D. *Your Body's Many Cries for Water.* Falls Church, Va.: Global Health Solutions, 1992.

Baudoux, Dominique. *Formulaire d'Aromathérapie pratique.* Enghien, Belgium: Surface Utile, 1995.

Berkow, Robert, M.D., ed. *The Merck Manual,* 15th ed. Rahway, N.J.: Merck Sharp and Dohme Research Laboratories, 1987.

Blumenthal, Mark, et al. *The Complete German Commission E Monographs.* Austin, Tex.: American Botanical Council, 1998.

Bown, Deni. *Encyclopedia of Herbs and Their Uses.* London: Dorling Kindersley, 1995.

Bragg, Paul C., N.D., and Patricia Bragg, N.D. *Water: The Shocking Truth.* Rev. ed. Santa Barbara, Calif.: Health Science, 1998.

Breggin, Peter. "Ritalin: Robots on Parade." *What Doctors Don't Tell You* 10 (August 1999): 12.

Brennan, Barbara. *Light Emerging.* New York: Bantam Books, 1993.

Brickell, Christopher, ed. *The Royal Horticultural Society Gardeners' Encyclopedia of Plants and Flowers.* London: Dorling Kindersley, 1989.

Briggs, John. *Fractals: Patterns of Chaos.* New York: Touchstone, 1992.

Brinker, Francis. "Variations in Effective Botanical Products." *Herbalgram* 46 (spring 1999): 36–50.

Brown, Chip. *Afterwards, You're a Genius*. New York: Riverhead Books, 1998.

Bruce, Andrew. "Troubled Water Series: The Bottled Water Phenomenon." *Record On-Line* (www.thekitchener-waterloorecord), January 11, 2000.

Buchman, Dian Dincin. *The Complete Book of Water Therapy*. New Canaan, Conn.: Keats Publishing, 1994.

Carey, John, Ellen Licking, and Amy Barrett. "Are Bio-Foods Safe?" *Business Week* 20 (December 1999): 70–76.

Castro, Miranda, and F. S. Hom. *The Complete Homeopathy Handbook*. London: Macmillan, 1990.

Chappell, Peter. *Emotional Healing with Homeopathy*. Rockport, Mass.: Element Books, 1994.

Charles, H. R. H., Prince of Wales. *Highgrove: Portrait of an Estate*. London: Chapmans, 1993.

Chisholm, Patricia. "Healers or Quacks?" *Maclean's* (September 25, 1995): 34–39.

Collin, Guy J., et al. "Extraction and GC-MS Analysis of the Essential Oil of *Comptonia peregrina*." *Proceedings of the Seventieth Canadian Chemical Conference and Exhibition*, June 7–11, 1987.

Collin, Guy, and F. X. Garneau. *4e Colloque: Produits naturels d'origine végétale*. Chicoutimi, Quebec: LASEVE, 1999.

Cowley, Geoffrey, and Karen Springen. "Is There a Sixth Sense?" *Newsweek* (October 13, 1997): 67.

Damian, Peter, and Kate Damian. *Aromatherapy Scent and Psyche*. Rochester, Vt.: Healing Arts Press, 1995.

Davis, Patricia. *Subtle Aromatherapy*. Saffron Walden, England: C. W. Daniel, 1991.

Day, Christopher. *The Homeopathic Treatment of Small Animals*. Saffron Walden, England: C. W. Daniel, 1990.

Dayagi-Mendels, Michal. *Perfumes and Cosmetics in the Ancient World*. Jerusalem: Israel Museum, 1989.

Duwiejua, M., et al. "Anti-inflammatory Activity of *Polygonum bistorta, Guaiacum officinale*, and *Hamamelis virginiana* in Rats." *Journal of Pharmacy Pharmacology* 46 (1994): 286–90.

EDM. "Satellite Snaps Dire Photo of Canuck Wilds." *Now* (March 9–15, 2000): 21.

Enig, Mary G, and Sally Fallon. "The Oiling of America." *Nexus* (December–January 1999): 19–23, 74–75.

Erdelmeier, C. A. J., et al. "Antiviral and Antiphlogistic Activities of *Hamamelis virginiana* Bark." *Planta Medica* 62 (1996): 241–45.

Fargis, Paul, ed. *The New York Public Library Desk Reference*. 3rd ed. New York: Macmillan, Stonesong Press, 1998.

FDA. *Recalls and Field Corrections: Cosmetics—Class II* (FDA Enforcement Report, September 17, 1997).

Franchomme, Pierre, and Daniel Penoel, M.D. *L'Aromathérapie exactemente*. Limoges, France: Editions Jollois, 1996.

Fumento, Michael. "The Senseless War to End All Scents." *National Post*, April 8, 2000, sec. A.

Gach, Michael Reed. *Acupressure's Potent Points*. New York: Bantam Books, 1990.

Gattefosse, Rene-Maurice. *Gattefosse's Aromatherapy*. 1937. Saffron Walden, England: C. W. Daniel, 1993.

Gibbons, Boyd. "The Intimate Sense of Smell." *National Geographic* 170 (September 1986): 324–60.

Gilbert, Avery N., and Charles J. Wysocki. "The Smell Survey Results." *National Geographic* 172 (October 1987): 514–25.

Gittelman, Ann Louise. "Urgent Detox Bulletin." *Health Sciences Institute: Members Alert* 1 (June 1997): 6–8.

Goeb, Philippe, et al. "Gastro-Duodenal Ulcer Disease." *Les Cahiers de l'Aromatherapie* 2 (September 1996): 56–74.

Government of the People's Republic of China. *A Barefoot Doctor's Manual*. New York: Gramercy Publishing, 1985.

Green, Penelope. "Spiritual Cosmetics. No kidding." *New York Times*, January 10, 1999, Arts sec., pp. 1, 5.

Grieve, Maude. *A Modern Herbal*. London: Tiger Books International, 1931, 1994.

Grosjean, Nelly. *Aromatherapy: Essential Oils for Your Health*. Graveson, France: Editions de la Chevêche, 1987.

———. "The 12 Frictions." Course Notes (November 1996).

———. *Veterinary Aromatherapy*. Saffron Walden, England: C. W. Daniel, 1994.

Haberland, Claudia, and Herbert Kolodziej. "Novel Galloylhamameloses from *Hamamelis virginiana*." *Planta Medica* 60 (1994): 464–66.

Hachey, Jean-Marie, et al. "Extraction and GC/MS Analysis of the Essential Oil of *Achillea millefolium* L. Complex." *Journal of Essential Oil Research* 2 (November/December 1990): 317–26.

Hadlington, Simon. "The Bubbly Sound of Innovation." *Financial Times*, June 2, 1999.

Hartisch, Claudia, Herbert Kolodziej, and Fritz von Bruchhausen. "Dual Inhibitory Activities of Tannins from *Hamamelis virginiana* and Related Polyphenols on 5-lipoxygenase and lyso-PAF: acetyl-CoA acetyltransferase." *Planta medica* 63 (1997): 106–10.

Hildegard von Bingen. *Physica*. Translated by Priscilla Throop. Rochester, Vt.: Healing Arts Press, 1998.

Hoffmann, David. *The New Holistic Herbal*. Rockport, Mass.: Element Books, 1983; 1990.

Huson, Paul. *Mastering Herbalism*. London: Abacus, 1977.

Jack, Lee-Ann. "A Mummy Revealed: The Faces of Djed." *Rotunda* (winter 1995–96): 30–37.

Jackson, Susan. "Alternative Medicine: Not So Alternative Anymore?" *Business Week* (June 2, 1997): 150–51.

Jehl, Douglas. "Tampa Bay Looks to the Sea to Quench Its Thirst." *New York Times*, March 12, 2000.

Jellinek, Stephan J. "Aroma-chology: A Status Review." *Perfumer and Flavorist* 19 (September–October 1994): 25–48.

Jin, Hong. "Examples of Herbs That [Are] Used on Acupoints to Treat Common Illnesses (Disorders)." Paper presented at conference, January 2000.

Kahn, Jenifer, "The Green Machine." *Harper's* (April 1999): 70–73.

Kamen, Betty. "Prozac Takes a Back Seat." *Health Sciences Institute: Members Alert* 1 (June 1997): 6–8.

Kastner, U., et al, "Anti-edematous Activity of Sesquiterpene Lactones from Different Taxa of the *Achillea millefolium* Group." *Planta Medica* 59, supplement 7 (December 1993): A669.

Kazmin, Amy. "Herbal Harmony." *Financial Post*, August 15, 1997, sec 1, p. 14.

Kelner, Merrijoy, and Beverly Wellman. "Health Care and Consumer Choice: Medical and Alternative Therapies." *Shared Scope of Practice Working Paper* 45 (1997): 203–12.

Kettenring, Maria M. *Aromaküche: Gesund und Phantasievoll Kochen Mit Ätherischen Ölen.* Sulzburg, Germany: Joy Verlag, 1994.

Kirk-Smith, Michael, "Therapeutic Uses of Olfaction," n.p., n.d.

Kirsch, Vik. "Troubled Water Series: Feline Finnegan Turns Family on to Filtered Water." *Record On-Line* (www.thekitchener-waterloorecord), January 11, 2000.

Knobloch, K., and H. Strobel. "Effective Concentrations of Essential Oil Components to Scavenge Oxygen Radicals and Inhibit Lipoxygenase Turnover Rates." *Planta Medica* 59, supplement 7 (December 1993): A669.

Kohl, James Vaughan, and Robert T. Francoeur. *The Scent of Eros.* New York: Continuum, 1995.

Korting, H. C., et al. "Anti-inflammatory Activity of *Hamamelis* Distillate Applied Topically to the Skin." *European Journal of Clinical Pharmacology* 44 (spring 1993): 315–18.

Krauss, Lawrence M. *The Physics of Star Trek.* New York: Basic Books, 1995.

Krippner, Stanley, and Alberto Villoldo. *The Realms of Healing.* Berkeley, Calif.: Celestial Arts, 1976.

Kusmirek, Jan. "Floral Waters." *Aromatherapy Quarterly* 49 (summer 1996): 6–8.

Lauriault, Jean. *Guide d'identification des arbres du Canada.* LaPrarie, Quebec: Editions Broquet, 1987.

LeGuerer, Annick. *Scent.* New York: Kodansha International, 1992.

Lewis, Walter H., P. F. Elvin-Lewis, and Memory Elvin-Lewis. *Medical Botany.* New York: John Wiley and Sons, 1977.

Livingstone, David. "A Scent of One's Own." *Images* (winter 1996): 59–61.

Lonsdorf, Nancy, M.D., Veronica Butler, M.D., and Melanie Brown. *A Woman's Best Medicine.* New York: Putnam, 1993.

Lust, John., N.D. *The Herb Book.* New York: Bantam Books, 1974.

Mainguy, Jean-Claude. "Aromatherapy in Everyday Medical Practice: *Thymus vulgaris* b.s. linalool." *Les Cahiers de l'Aromatherapie* 2 (September 1996): 89–91.

Mainguy, Jean-Claude, et al. "Familial Chronic Inflammatory Diseases of the Bowel." *Les Cahiers de l'Aromatherapie* 2 (September 1996): 75–88.

Mainguy, Lucie, and Pierre Mainguy. "Aliksir: le travail d'un producteur Quebecois d'huiles essentielles." *Info-Essence* 1 (February 1996): 3–4.

Mallin, Michael A. "Impacts of Industrial Animal Production on Rivers and Estuaries." *American Scientist* 88 (January–February 2000): 26–37.

Malone, Dawnelle. "Killer Spices." *Herbalgram* 46: 16.

Marcial-Vega, Victor, M.D. "Aromatherapy Oils as Oral Remedies." *Alternative Medicine Digest* 16 (1998): 30–34.

Masaki, Hitoshi, et al. "Active Oxygen Scavenging Activity of Plant Extracts." *Biological Pharmacy Review* 18, no.1 (1995): 162–66.

Masaki, Hitoshi, Takamasa Atsumi, and Hiromu Sakurai. "Protective Activity of Hamamelitannin on Cell Damage of Murine Skin Fibroblasts Induced by UV Irradiation." *Journal of Dermatological Science* 10 (1995): 25–34.

McAndrew, Brian. "Troubled Water Series: Troubled Water." *Record On-Line* (www.thekitchener-waterloorecord), January 11, 2000.

McLaughlin, Patricia. "Smelling Like Dirt." *National Post* (Toronto), January 11, 1999, sec. D, pp. 1–2.

Melody. *Love Is in the Earth*. Wheat Ridge, Colo.: Earth Love Publishing, 1995.

Miller, Light, N.D., and Bryan Miller, D.C. *Ayurveda and Aromatherapy*. Twin Lakes, Wis.: Lotus Press, 1995.

Mitich, Larry W. "Yarrow: Herb of Achilles." *Weed Technology* 4 (1990): 451–53.

Mittelstaedt, Martin. "How Bad Is Canada's Water Problem?" *Globe and Mail* (Toronto), January 11, 2000, sec. A, p. 14.

Mojay, Gabriel. *Aromatherapy for Healing the Spirit.*

Rydalmere, NSW, Australia: Hodder and Stoughton, 1996.

Morfitt, Ian. "Epilepsy." *Globe and Mail* (Toronto), March 28, 2000, sec. R, pp. 8–9.

Morrison, Judith H. *The Book of Ayurveda*. New York: Fireside, 1995.

Murray, Michael, N.D., and Joseph Pizzorno, N.D. *Encyclopedia of Natural Medicine*. London: Optima, 1990.

Myers, Norman, ed. *The Gaia Atlas of Planet Management*. London: Pan Books, 1985.

Naiman, Ingrid. *Cancer Salves*. Berkeley, Calif.: North Atlantic Books, 1999.

Neuray, M., et al., "Extractions des huiles essentielles de rameux d'epicea: Etude comparative du contenu des rameux d'hiver et d'ete." *Landbouwtijdschrift revue de l'agriculture* 2 (1990): 199–204.

Nichols, Mark. "The Enforcers." *Maclean's* (September 25, 1995): 40–41.

Omelia, Johanna. "The Science of Smell Explored." *DCI* (February 1996): 48–51.

Pendick, Daniel. "Aromatherapy for Winters That Won't End." *Globe and Mail* (Toronto), April 12, 2000, sec. R, p. 7.

Phatak, S. R., M.D. *Materia Medica of Homeopathic Remedies*. New Delhi: Indian Books and Periodicals Syndicate, 1977.

Pitcairn, Richard H., D.V.M., and Susan Pitcairn. *Dr. Pitcairn's Complete Guide to Natural Health for Dogs and Cats*. Emmaus, Pa.: Rodale Press, 1982.

Pizzorno, Joseph, N.D. *Total Wellness*. Rocklin, Calif.: Prima Publishing, 1998.

Rasoanaivo, Philippe, and Philippe de la Gorce. "Essential Oils of Economic Value in Madagascar: Present State of Knowledge." *Herbalgram* 43 (1998): 31–39, 58–59.

Robbins, Tom. *Jitterbug Perfume*. New York: Bantam Books, 1984.

Robert, S. "Phytotherapie et affection du systeme uro-genital." Text from a conference proceedings provided by Agriculture Canada.

Roob, Alexander. *Alchemy and Mysticism*. Cologne: Taschen, 1997.

Root-Bernstein, Robert, and Michele Root-Bernstein. *Honey, Mud, Maggots, and Other Medical Marvels*. New York: Houghton Mifflin, 1998.

Rudgley, Richard. *Essential Substances*. New York: Kodansha International, 1994.

Schnaubelt, Kurt. *Advanced Aromatherapy*. Rochester Vt.: Healing Arts Press, 1998.

———. *Medical Aromatherapy*. Berkeley, Calif.: Frog Ltd., 1999.

———, ed. *Proceedings: First Wholistic Aromatherapy Conference on Therapeutic Uses of Essential Oils*. San Francisco, Pacific Institute of Aromatherapy, 1995.

———, ed. *Proceedings: Third Aromatherapy Conference on Therapeutic Uses of Essential Oils, October 30–November 1, 1998*. San Francisco: Pacific Institute of Aromatherapy, 1998.

Seddon, Quentin. *A Brief History of Thyme*. London: Coronet Books, 1994.

Sellar, Wanda. *The Directory of Essential Oils*. Saffron Walden, England: C. W. Daniel, 1992.

Spoerke, David G., Jr. *Herbal Medications*. Santa Barbara, Calif.: Woodbridge Press, 1990.

Steele, John J. "The Fragrant Hospital." Aroma '93 Conference, Sussex, England, July 2–4, 1993.

Suzuki, David. *The Sacred Balance*. Vancouver: Greystone Books, 1997.

Svoboda, Robert. *Prakruti: Your Ayurvedic Constitution*. Albuquerque, N.M.: Geocom, 1989.

Talbot, Michael. *The Holographic Universe*. New York: HarperPerennial, 1991.

Thoss, M., et al. "Storage and Photostability of Cyclodextrin Inclusion Compounds of Lemon, Orange, Hop, and Chamomile Oil." *Pharmazie* 49 (1994) H4: 252–57.

Tierra, Michael, N.D. *Planetary Herbology*. Twin Lakes, Wis.: Lotus Press, 1988.

Tisserand, Robert, and Tony Balacs. *Essential Oil Safety*. New York: Churchill Livingstone, 1995.

Tracy, Eileen. "Wonder Drug or Playground Curse." *Manchester Guardian*, October 12, 1999, Education sec., pp. 2–3.

Trainer, Thomas. "A New Prescription." *Report on Business* (supplement to the 1996 chief information officer summit).

Urquhart, Ian. "Troubled Water Series: Brace Yourselves for a Water Fight." *Record On-Line* (www.thekitchener-waterloorecord), January 11, 2000.

Valnet, Jean, M.D. *The Practice of Aromatherapy*. Rochester, Vt.: Healing Arts Press, 1990.

van Rijn, Nicolaas. "Troubled Water Series: What We Have Is All There Is." *Record On-Line* (www.thekitchener-waterloorecord), January 11, 2000.

Waresh, Julie. "The Natural Law." *Palm Beach Post*, June 11, 2000, sec. F, pp. 1, 5.

Warren, Susan. "Production Set for 'Natural Plastic' Made from Plants." *Wall Street Journal,* in the *Globe and Mail* (Toronto), January 11, 2000, sec B, p. 10.

"Wealth of Opportunity Emerges from a Root System." *Financial Times* (London), September 24, 1998, p. 14.

Weiner, Michael, and Kathleen Goss. *The Complete Book of Homeopathy.* New York: Bantam Books, 1982.

Wirth, Dyann F., and Jacqueline Cattani. "Against Malaria." *Technology Review* (August–September 1997): 53–61.

Index